Contents

Companion website: http://www.contentextra.com/hair/home.aspx
Login details:
Username – HairdressingL2
Password – scissors

Foreword by Andrew Barton

Andrew Barton is known as hairdressing royalty. With his own flagship London salon, product range and electrical tools, and a reputation as a makeover guru, he is TV's favourite hairdresser. Andrew started his career in Yorkshire, where he grew up, and has since circumnavigated the globe, flying the British hairdressing flag by presenting hair shows and seminars. Known as Best Of British, and with a string of hair awards including British Hairdresser Of The Year and Ultimate Hairdresser, his career has spiralled to dizzy heights from his humble beginnings in a village salon in Yorkshire.

There is no such thing as a typical day for Andrew, who is passionate about the craft and profession of hairdressing and is Ambassador for The Hairdressing Council. "One day my life involves working with celebrities on a glamorous photo shoot, the next filming for makeover magic for a TV show or styling hair in my salon. I love my work and the opportunities that hairdressing gives me every day." So how did all this come about?

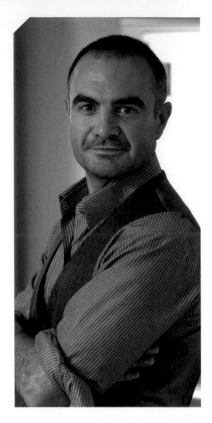

"I started a very traditional hairdressing apprenticeship in my home town in Yorkshire, which was tough and very disciplined, but years later I'm still grateful for it. Along with attending college to study for my hairdressing qualifications, it was the best possible start.

Learning all the key skills to the highest standard has undoubtedly helped me further down the line in my career. Whether working on everyday clients, supermodels, superstars or creating hair for top designers at the catwalk shows, it's so important to have a good foundation of knowledge.

I think I have the best job in the world and I'm amazed by just how much excitement I get from my work every day. Possibly the best advice I can offer anyone is to make sure you work with a great team, never accept an average standard and always push your own creativity through experimentation and trial and error.

Hairdressing is competitive, it's fast and it's ever-changing. Of course, it's about providing a service... but the service of making someone feel great about themselves through their hair is wonderful. I swear the smile a client shows you on her face when you've done her hair is magical and addictive!

Because hairdressing is always changing, there's always something to learn and discover. You'll never be bored and, as British hairdressing and training are widely acknowledged as the best in the world, you're guaranteed to have the best start for the career of your dreams!

Level 2, for me, was all about perfecting the skills I had learned so far and never accepting anything less than the best that I could do. I had started to imagine where my career could take me and the experiences I could have... a world of opportunities were opening up for me, and could be for you too!"

Andrew Barton x

Andrew Barton
Andrew Barton Hair Group

About the authors

Leah Palmer

I started working in a salon as a Saturday girl aged 13. I used to earn £5 for my day's work shampooing, cleaning, tidying, mixing colours and making tea. I was offered an Apprenticeship at the salon but was inspired to go to college full-time by Joan Champion during a school careers visit. I loved my two years at college and was honoured as Student of the Year. I learned a wealth of skills and experience from my tutors, Joan Champion and Mary Pearson, both of whom became wonderful friends and colleagues. I also made some exceptional friends at college, one of whom is my co-author of this book, Nicci Perkins. I left college, started work in a salon and continued my studies one day a week to complete my Advanced Hairdressing. I was then asked to do some teaching at college, which was something I had never even considered. I did some part-time teaching alongside working in the salon and eventually built up my hours at college to full time. In 2005, I was honoured to receive an 'Outstanding lecturer of the year' award. Along the way I have had my children, Brandon, 17, and Phoebe, 14, and continued to work with the help of my husband and my wonderful parents. I have been teaching for 23 years and I am now Director of Faculty for Vocational Studies at Fareham College. I'm privileged to work with an amazingly committed and talented team of hairdressing staff who are continually inspirational. I'm extremely glad I chose to teach hairdressing, as the industry is very exciting and I love making a positive impact on students' lives.

Nicci Perkins

From a very young age, I always had a love of hair, beauty and fashion. It came as no surprise to my parents when I applied for a place on a hairdressing course at Fareham College. I was both amazed and nervous when I was accepted. After two years I completed my full ladies and gents hairdressing qualification and achieved the 'top cutter' of the year. I continued with an Advanced course and secured a job in the industry. After working for three years, I decided I would like to have a go at running my own business and bought a salon, which I owned for 10 years from the very young age of 21! A very good friend – Leah Palmer – encouraged me to go back to college and complete my teacher training and I've never looked back. I have now been teaching for 10 years and enjoy a full and rewarding life alongside my husband Mark, and two children, Jessica aged 6 and Ben aged 4, who support me in my role. Hairdressing has been a challenging and rewarding career; I have particularly enjoyed watching the students' skills evolve daily and working with an inspired and motivated team of people. I have loved every minute.

Acknowledgements

The publisher would like to thank the following for their kind permission to reproduce their photographs:

(Key: b-bottom; c-centre; l-left; r-right; t-top)

Alamy Images: Agencja FREE 307/2, Blue Jean Images 75, Butch Martin 444r, Graham Dunn 307t, Photofusion Picture Library 232b, steve skjold 233/4, View pictures Ltd 83; **Babyliss:** 301bl; **Chris Honeywell:** Chris Honeywell 313, 313/2, 313/3, 313/4, 313/5, 313/6; **Corbis:** iodrakon / Veer 42, TOPAS 243; **cut2white:** 331c, 444l; **globalskinatlas.com:** 147/2; **Glow Images:** 411, 435, 436, 461, 476b, 481, Jerome Corpuz 1, 81t, 105, 119, 133, 157, 271; **Goldwell:** 2, vii, viii, x, xi, xvi, xvii, 27, 170b, 194b, 199, 200, 213, 216b, 250b, 282, 318b, 341, 363, 423, 446b, 482; **Hair by JFK:** ix; **Hair ToolsTM Ltd www.hairtools.co.uk:** 260tc, 261/3, 273/5, 273/6; **Icon Consultancy:** 486/1, 486/2, 486/3; **Getty Images:** AFP / KARIM SAHIB 443cl, Alexey Ivanov 15, 175, Barry King / Film Magic 472, Brad Barket 331, 372, Dave Hogan 284c, 307/3, Eamonn McCormack / WireImages 140tr, Evan Agostini 284t, Federick M. Brown 465, Fotos International 443r, Frazer Harrison 462, GABRIEL BOUYS / AFP 221b, Jason LaVeris / Film Magic 444cr, Jon Kopaloff / Film Magic 140tl, Kevin Mazur / WireImages 233/2, Lambada 297t, Lester Cohen / WireImages 307b, Paul Warner / Getty images 283, Ralf Nau 124, Rob Loud 443cr, Stephen Shugerman 468, Steve Granitz / WireImage 140bl, Stuart Wilson / WireImage 140br, WireImage / Gilbert Garrigue 443l, WireImage / sGranitz 378; **iStockphoto:** Izabela Habur 9r, Joey Nelson 9, Umbar Shakir 9l; **John Carne:** John Carne xiv, xv; **L'Oreal UK:** 177/1, 177/2, 177/3, 177/4, 177/5, 186t, 186cl, 186cr, 186bl, 186br; **Nature's Dream:** 415, 415tl, 415br; **Pearson Education Ltd:** Stuart Cox 19, 21, 28, 30, 34l, 35bl, 36bl, 37tr, 38, 39, 46, 73, 86, 86b, 108, 108c, 122, 123, 134, 149, 152, 183t, 183b, 185/1, 185/2, 185/3, 185/4, 185/5, 185/6, 188l, 188r, 189, 191, 191t, 191b, 204, 207, 207l, 211, 217t, 226/1, 226/2, 226/3, 226/4, 226/5, 226/6, 252t, 288/1, 288/2, 288/3, 288/4, 288/5, 288/6, 289, 289r, 309c, 309bl, 309br, 314/1, 314/2, 314/3, 314/4, 314/5, 314/6, 332/1, 332/2, 332/3, 332/4, 332/5, 332/6, 333, 333/2, 333/3, 333/4, 333/5, 333/6, 351, 351b, 384, 395, 448b, 449/3, 450/1, 450/2, 451/3, 451/4, 451/5, 451/6, 451/7, 451/8, 451/9, 452/1, 452/2, 452/3, 452/4, 452/5, 452/6, 485/1, 485/2, 485/3, 488, Stuart Cox 19, 21, 28, 30, 34l, 35bl, 36bl, 37tr, 38, 39, 46, 73, 108, 108c, 122, 123, 134, 149, 152, 183t, 183b, 185/1, 185/2, 185/3, 185/4, 185/5, 185/6, 188l, 188r, 189, 191, 191t, 191b, 204, 207, 207l, 211, 217t, 226/1, 226/2, 226/3, 226/4, 226/5, 226/6, 252t, 288/1, 288/2, 288/3, 288/4, 288/5, 288/6, 289, 289r, 309c, 309bl, 309br, 314/1, 314/2, 314/3, 314/4, 314/5, 314/6, 332/1, 332/2, 332/3, 332/4, 332/5, 332/6, 333, 333/2, 333/3, 333/4, 333/5, 333/6, 351, 351b, 384, 395, 448b, 449/3, 450/1, 450/2, 451/3, 451/4, 451/5, 451/6, 451/7, 451/8, 451/9, 452/1, 452/2, 452/3, 452/4, 452/5, 452/6, 485/1, 485/2, 485/3, 488; **Pearson Education Ltd:** 382/2, Gareth Boden 64, 64b, 115, 124t, 142t, 142b, 143b, 194t, 208, 209, 247/1, 247/2, 247/3, 248/1, 248/2, 250t, 253b, 282t, 310/1, 310/2, 310/3, 311t, 331b, 345, 349t, 350b, 374t, 444b, 454/1, 454/2, 454/3, 466, 476t, 484, 484/2, 484/3, Image Source 388b, Imagesource 115b, 170t, 488t, Jules Selmes 65, 216t, 400, Mind Studios 471cr, Mindstudio 54/1, 54/2, 54/3, 54/4, 100, 108b, 112, 143t, 143c, 181, 192/1, 192/2, 192/3, 192/4, 192/5, 192/6, 201, 202l, 202r, 205, 205b, 214, 219t, 219b, 220l, 220r, 221, 224/1, 224/2, 224/3, 225/1, 225/2, 225/3, 228/1, 228/2, 228/3, 228/4, 228/5, 230/1, 230/2, 230/3, 230/4, 230/5, 232/1, 232/2, 232/3, 244b, 248/4, 248/5, 252, 253t, 254/1, 254/2, 254/3, 254/4, 254/5, 254/6, 257, 257cl, 257cr, 257r, 258/1, 258/2, 258/3, 259/1, 259/2, 259/3, 259/4, 259/5, 259/6, 260, 260tr, 260l, 260r, 261/1, 261/4, 261/5, 261t, 262, 263l, 263r, 273/3, 275, 277l, 277c, 277r, 280t, 280b, 281l, 281c, 281r, 284b, 286t, 286b, 298, 299t, 299b, 300bl, 301t, 308l, 308r, 309t, 310t, 310c, 311c, 311b, 312/1, 312/2, 312/3,

312/4, 312/5, 312/6, 315/1, 315/2, 315/3, 315/4, 315/5, 315/6, 315/7, 318t, 326, 329, 334/1, 334/2, 334/3, 334/4, 334/5, 334/6, 334t, 346, 349, 350t, 352, 355/1, 355/2, 355/3, 355/4, 356/1, 356/2, 356/3, 356/4, 356/5, 356/6, 357/1, 357tl, 357tr, 357bl, 357br, 358/1, 358/2, 358/3, 360t, 360c, 360cl, 360bl, 371, 371t, 379b, 380/1, 380/2, 380/3, 380/4, 380/5, 381/1, 381/2, 381/3, 381/4, 381/5, 382/1, 382/3, 382/4, 382/5, 383/1, 383/2, 383/3, 383/4, 386, 396, 412c, 412b, 417, 420, 422/1, 422/2, 422/3, 422/4, 422/5, 422/6, 424/1, 424/2, 424/3, 424/4, 426/1, 426/2, 426/3, 426/4, 426/5, 426/6, 427/1, 427/2, 427/3, 427/4, 428, 448t, 449/1, 449/2, 449cr, 449b, 454l, 454c, 454r, 455, 463, 470/1, 470/2, 470/3, 470/4, 470/5, 470/6, 471, 471/1, 471/2, 471/3, 474, 474t, Mindstudio 54/1, 54/2, 54/3, 54/4, 100, 108b, 112, 143t, 143c, 181, 192/1, 192/2, 192/3, 192/4, 192/5, 192/6, 201, 202l, 202r, 205, 205b, 214, 219t, 219b, 220l, 220r, 221, 224/1, 224/2, 224/3, 225/1, 225/2, 225/3, 228/1, 228/2, 228/3, 228/4, 228/5, 230/1, 230/2, 230/3, 230/4, 230/5, 232/1, 232/2, 232/3, 244b, 248/4, 248/5, 252, 253t, 254/1, 254/2, 254/3, 254/4, 254/5, 254/6, 257, 257cl, 257cr, 257r, 258/1, 258/2, 258/3, 259/1, 259/2, 259/3, 259/4, 259/5, 259/6, 260, 260tr, 260l, 260r, 261/1, 261/4, 261/5, 261t, 262, 263l, 263r, 273/3, 275, 277l, 277c, 277r, 280t, 280b, 281l, 281c, 281r, 284b, 286t, 286b, 298, 299t, 299b, 300bl, 301t, 308l, 308r, 309t, 310t, 310c, 311c, 311b, 312/1, 312/2, 312/3, 312/4, 312/5, 312/6, 315/1, 315/2, 315/3, 315/4, 315/5, 315/6, 315/7, 318t, 326, 329, 334/1, 334/2, 334/3, 334/4, 334/5, 334/6, 334t, 346, 349, 350t, 352, 355/1, 355/2, 355/3, 355/4, 356/5, 356/6, 357/1, 357tl, 357tr, 357bl, 357br, 358/1, 358/2, 358/3, 360t, 360c, 360cl, 360bl, 371, 371t, 379b, 380/1, 380/2, 380/3, 380/4, 380/5, 381/1, 381/2, 381/3, 381/4, 381/5, 382/1, 382/3, 382/4, 382/5, 383/1, 383/2, 383/3, 383/4, 386, 396, 412c, 412b, 417, 420, 422/1, 422/2, 422/3, 422/4, 422/5, 422/6, 424/1, 424/2, 424/3, 424/4, 426/1, 426/2, 426/3, 426/4, 426/5, 426/6, 427/1, 427/2, 427/3, 427/4, 428, 448t, 449/1, 449/2, 449cr, 449b, 454l, 454c, 454r, 455, 463, 470/1, 470/2, 470/3, 470/4, 470/5, 470/6, 471, 471/1, 471/2, 471/3, 474, 474t, PhotoDisc / Kevin Peterson 388, 446; **Salons direct:** 190b, 211b, 301cr, 419; **Science Photo Library Ltd:** 147/1, 148/5, 233/3, BIOPHOTO ASSOCIATES 147/5, Dr Chris Hale 148/1, Dr H.C Robinson 146/3, Dr. P. Marazzi 145, 145/2, 145/3, 145/4, 146/2, 148/3, 327, Eye of Science 146/4, John Radcliffe Hospital 148/4, Medical RF.com 229, ST BARTHOLOMEW'S HOSPITAL 146/1, ST. BARTHOLOMEW'S HOSPITAL, LONDON 148/2, 232c, Steve Gschmeissner 146/5; **Shutterstock.com:** Denis Vrublevki 336, dpaint 370, FlexDreams 369, hightowernrw 401, lev dolgachov 402b, lithian 79br, 103br, 118, 132, 156, 172, 198, 241, 269, 295, 322, 340, 367, 391, 408, 434, 458, 479, 490, Luba V Nel 402t, Mars Evis 273/4, masson 363t, Mayer George Vladimirovich 45, 153b, 393, Mayer George Vladimirovich 45, 153b, 393, Mehmet Dilsiz 248/3, 273/2, Noraluca013 233/1, Olga A 247/5, Salim October 334c, Sheftsoff 403, szefei 23, Tassh 403b, Valua Vitaly 272, Zvyagintsev Sergey 247/4, 273; **Simon Lidstone:** 147/3, 232t, 444; **Wahl:** 261, 301br; **www.imagesource.com:** Fstop 423t

Cover images: *Front:* **Barry Jeffery:** Barry Jeffery

All other images © Pearson Education

Picture Research by: Pearson Education Ltd and Susi Paz

For her Key Skills and Functional Skills expertise, thanks are also due to Karen Smith.

Every effort has been made to trace the copyright holders and we apologise in advance for any unintentional omissions. We would be pleased to insert the appropriate acknowledgement in any subsequent edition of this publication.

Introduction

How to use this book and the companion website

This book has been designed with a dual purpose:

1   To lead you through a Hairdressing Level 2 qualification, providing you with background and technical guidance, suggested evidence collection and key skills and functional skills information.

2   To provide you with a range of Level 2 Barbering units, to help you develop your skills further in this area. Many of the skills and techniques you will learn in the hairdressing units can be applied to barbering and some colleges and training providers will give you the opportunity to achieve a Level 2 qualification in barbering as well as hairdressing.

Important information about the hair and skin is provided at the start of the book in 'Facts about hair and skin'. Please read this thoroughly before you do anything else. The information it gives applies to many of the units throughout the book, so if you learn and understand this first, all the other areas should make sense. Remember that you only have to learn the information once and then apply your knowledge to the practical skills unit you are working through. You will also find the information in 'Facts about hair and skin' important when carrying out consultations with clients. It is vital that you can apply what you have learned about the hair and skin structure, hair texture, condition, hair growth and chemical structure of hair when advising clients.

The free website that accompanies this book provides worksheets to accompany many of the tasks in the book, enabling you to generate extra evidence for your portfolio. When you see the website icon in the book, you'll know that there is an associated worksheet on the website for you to access. It also contains a range of video clips, which include demonstrations of the skills described in the book as well as interviews with celebrity hairdresser Andrew Barton.

When you see the video icon, you'll know that there is an associated video clip on the companion website for you to watch.

Some helpful features

To reinforce your learning process and get you thinking, there are several features included throughout the book to help you.

*   *Top tips* **Top tips**

    These offer a guide to good practice and help you anticipate any problems that may arise. They cover health and safety as well as good professional practice.

*   *Tasks* **Task 1**

    These provide activities that apply the theory in a practical situation and can be used to provide portfolio evidence, as well as evidence towards your Key Skills and Functional Skills. Many of the tasks have accompanying worksheets on the website for you to use to record your findings for inclusion in your portfolio of evidence. Check the 'Task mapping' table at the end of each unit (on the 'Getting ready for assessment' page) to see how the task links to the unit and any Key Skills. Functional Skills mapping can be found on the website.

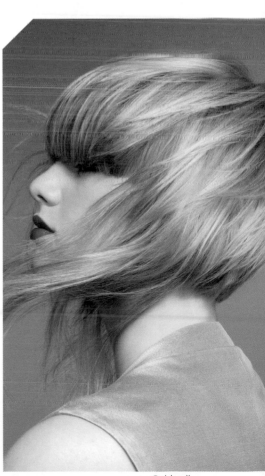

Goldwell

- *Key terms*   `Key terms`

  These highlight terms that are central to your understanding of the topic that you may not have come across before.

- *Fact or fiction?*   `Fact or fiction?`

  These are designed to help you check your knowledge by providing a statement which is either true (fact) or false (fiction). You can check your answer in the back of the book.

- *Salon life*

  This is a full-page feature designed to look like the page of a magazine. It covers a key issue or problem, including an account of a stylist's experience in the salon and expert guidance on the issue or problem covered.

- *Ask the expert*

  These appear in the Salon life feature page, where students have asked for expert advice on particular problems.

- *Personal, learning and thinking skills*   `Personal, learning and thinking skills –`

  If you are taking an Apprenticeship you will also need to demonstrate personal, learning and thinking skills. Opportunities to do this as part of your Level 2 Diploma have been highlighted in the book.

- *Check your knowledge*

  This is a list of multiple choice and/or short answer questions provided at the end of each unit to help you check your knowledge and understanding of that unit. Answers are provided in the back of the book.

- *Getting ready for assessment*

  At the end of each unit you will find helpful information and advice about how that unit is assessed. Also included is a Task mapping table, showing you how each Task provided in that unit links to the Performance Criteria, Range and Knowledge in that unit, as well as any Key Skills and Functional Skills.

A Hairdressing Diploma – Understanding NVQs/SVQs and VRQs

Taking a Level 2 Hairdressing or Barbering course can mean a number of different things. It's important that you understand the type of qualification you are working towards, what will be required of you and the options available to you after you have completed the course.

There are two types of Diploma at Level 2:

- NVQ/SVQ – National Vocational Qualification or Scottish Vocational Qualification
- VRQ – Vocationally-Related Qualification.

Both qualifications are highly successful methods of gaining your Level 2. They do not involve an exam at the end of the course with a pass or fail outcome. There is no one-off, scary day of reckoning! They use continual assessments in each unit, building up to a qualification – another option for those of us who panic at the thought of an exam room! However, you will still need to sit written assessments set by your awarding organisation (for example, City & Guilds, VTCT, Edexcel, SQA).

Goldwell

The qualifications can be taken at different levels – 1, 2 or 3. (Apprenticeships are only offered at Levels 2 and 3.) Your college or training institution will be able to guide you through the requirements of the particular awarding organisation it uses, but the National Occupational Standards do not vary and the information within this book should cover all eventualities of a Diploma at Level 2.

NVQ/SVQ

NVQs/SVQs are generally taken whilst you are also in employment in a salon, or you are undertaking a temporary work placement. By working in a salon you will be gaining plenty of valuable experience. However, it is also important that you take the time to properly learn the skills and gain the knowledge which will serve as the foundation on which you build your career. You may be taught at college or by another learning provider during working hours, or you may be taking the course in the evening. Either way, this will allow you to benefit from the guidance a tutor can provide, complementing what you are learning at your salon or work placement. Your work experience will provide opportunities to collect evidence for assessment, helping you to obtain your qualification. Once you have achieved your Level 2 Diploma qualification you will have the skills and experience necessary to begin working at this level.

VRQ

VRQ qualifications are usually taken as a full-time or part-time course at college. You won't need a job to study a VRQ but work experience in a salon would be highly beneficial. You must have enthusiasm and a keen interest in hairdressing or barbering. The aim of the qualification is to prepare you for taking a work qualification. You will gain the knowledge and practise the skills you will need to work in the industry, but you will need to move on to a work qualification before gaining employment. You may be assessed by carrying out your new skills on your peers, rather than paying clients, or in an environment which simulates the conditions of a salon. This is so that you can progress to a work based qualification with your key skills or functional skills and background knowledge in place, as well as confidence in your own abilities and knowledge.

Both qualifications are based on the same National Occupational Standards (NOS) as set out by HABIA. HABIA is the government-appointed body responsible for standards in hair, beauty, nails, spa therapy, barbering and African-type hair. Awarding organisations such as City & Guilds and VTCT will use these standards to develop the qualification you are taking.

Apprenticeships

Apprenticeships are a popular way of gaining the experience and skills necessary to start work in the hairdressing and barbering industry. An Apprenticeship is made up of a framework of different qualifications which you will need to obtain in order to gain your Apprenticeship.

If you are taking a Level 2 Hairdressing or Barbering Apprenticeship you will be assessed on:

- the knowledge and competence necessary to work in the industry – by taking a Level 2 NVQ Diploma in Hairdressing or Barbering
- Functional Skills, or Key Skills – these are skills in English and mathematics

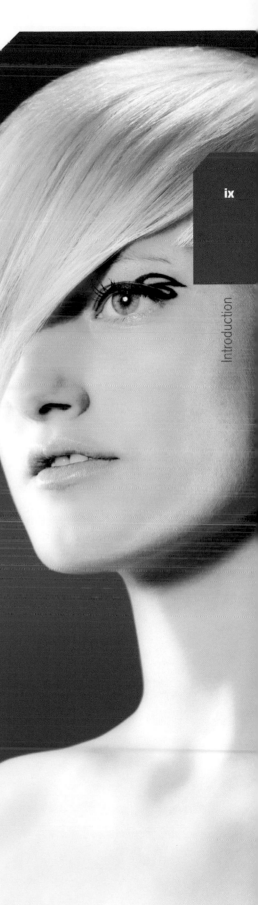

ix

JFK

- Personal, learning and thinking skills — where you will need to demonstrate skills in independent enquiry, creative thinking, reflective learning, team working, self-management and effective participation
- Employee Rights and Responsibilities — important information that you will need to know and apply in your salon.

How to gain your Level 2 Diploma

To gain these qualifications, you will need to show plenty of evidence that you have undertaken each unit. They are practical qualifications, so each student gets a thorough grounding in all the skill areas. This means that when you go into a salon, you will have dealt with most client requests and have lots of confidence to perform the various services.

How do I get my evidence?

Many forms of evidence are acceptable — your tutor will be able to guide you through the best options for your individual, or personal, learning programme. Each of the following types of evidence is valid:

- *Observation* — direct observations by your assessor watching you work.
- *Witness testimony* — a detailed record of the work you have produced, which must be signed by both yourself and a witness.
- *Oral questions* — questions asked directly by your assessor to check your understanding.
- *Written questions* — questions that you must answer in order to check your understanding of the subject area.
- *Assignment* — a piece of written work that must be produced to assess your knowledge of the subject area.
- *Mandatory written test paper* — a written test that must be taken under examination conditions.
- *Online Assessment testing* — questions that are answered online. These are taken under examination conditions.
- *Product evidence* — any evidence that is a product of the assessment, for example a consultation sheet or record card.
- *Simulation* — simulation of an activity may be used only under specific circumstances and for particular units. Simulation cannot be used as evidence for all assessments.
- *Recognition of Prior Learning (RPL)* — this enables you to claim knowledge and skills you have already acquired from previous work or study. Evidence must be produced to prove your competence and knowledge in a particular area. This could be statements from employers and clients, or photos of work you have completed.

You should record your evidence on the evidence sheets provided and these will form your portfolio, which is simply a collection of all your evidence.

Organising your portfolio

It is essential to present your work in a clear format so that it can be assessed easily. For this reason, you should produce an index which lists what is in your portfolio.

An assessor will observe or guide you through the types of evidence listed previously. He or she will have had special training and will hold a specific qualification designed to help you present your evidence in a format suitable for your awarding organisation.

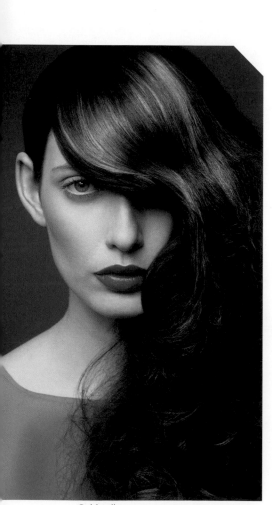

Goldwell

For quality control and fairness across the subject areas, an internal verifier will check the assessor and the portfolio of evidence. This will be performed at your place of training and should take place regularly.

The awarding organisation also has an external verifier who will visit your college or training institution regularly and check that both assessors and internal verifiers are giving the correct information to you, the candidate. Then your portfolio can be accredited with a qualification certificate. This can be achieved one unit at a time or applied for all at once. So, a clear and well-organised portfolio is vital!

What evidence do I need?

Ask your assessor to explain the most suitable method for the work you are doing. Most portfolios contain a mixture of evidence.

If you have external previous experience — Recognition of Prior Learning (RPL) or recent qualifications — this can be counted as evidence. For example, if you work part-time in a shop (not necessarily a salon) and have experience using the till and dealing with customers and complaints, then a witness statement from your employer that is current, valid, signed and dated (such as the one shown below) is acceptable evidence.

Ali's Grocery Store
12 Arcadia Avenue
Little Town
Surrey

12 January 2012

To whom it may concern:

Angela Smith has been working for me for two years and is a trustworthy and honest employee. In the course of her duties she operates the till, deals with cheques, credit cards and cash, and regularly cashes up. Angela has dealt with returned faulty goods, difficult customers and occasional complaints. I find her to be helpful and courteous, and she works well with colleagues. She follows instructions and works well on her own.

Yours faithfully
Ali Shubuala
(Owner)

The evidence shown in the sample letter would cover some of the reception outcomes, as well as some of the communication and interpersonal skills required. It also covers some of the ranges required in your assessment book.

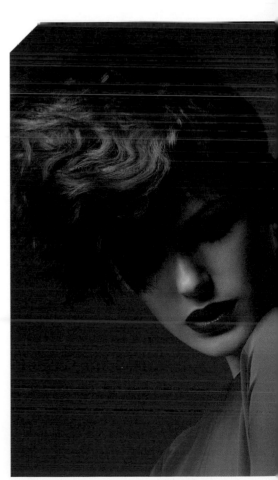

Goldwell

What do I have to achieve?

Now let's take an overall look at what you are going to need to do to gain your Level 2 qualification.

Your college or training institution will register you with its awarding organisation. The awarding organisation will then issue you, the candidate, with your assessment book. Treat it like gold, as this, together with your portfolio, is your source of evidence of your hard work.

The assessment book contains guidance on how to achieve each unit. Each unit is divided into outcomes.

Units that are mandatory and optional

To achieve your Level 2 in Hairdressing, you will need to complete certain mandatory and optional units. The tables below provide you with a quick reference guide to match the qualification you are taking with the units covered in this book.

Level 2 NVQ/SVQ Diploma in Hairdressing

Unit title	Credit value	Chapter
Mandatory – you must achieve each of these units		
Make sure your own actions reduce risks to health and safety	4	G20 page 45
Give clients a positive impression of yourself and your organisation	5	G17 page 105
Advise and consult with clients	4	G7 page 133
Shampoo, condition and treat the hair and scalp	4	GH8 page 175
Change hair colour	11	GH9 page 199
Style and finish hair	6	GH10 page 243
Set and dress hair	6	GH11 page 271
Cut hair using basic techniques	8	GH12 page 297
Optional – you must achieve units adding up to a credit value of 6		
Fulfil salon reception duties	3	G4 page 81
Promote additional services or products to clients	6	G18 page 119
Develop and maintain your effectiveness at work	3	G8 page 157
Plait and twist hair	4	GH13 page 325
Perm and neutralise hair	8	GH14 page 341
Attach hair to enhance a style	3	GH15 page 369

Level 2 NVQ/SVQ Diploma in Barbering

Unit title	Credit value	Chapter
Mandatory — you must achieve each of these units		
Make sure your own actions reduce risks to health and safety	4	G20 page 45
Advise and consult with clients	4	G7 page 133
Shampoo, condition and treat the hair and scalp	4	GH8 page 175
Cut hair using basic barbering techniques	8	GB3 page 435
Cut facial hair to shape using basic techniques	4	GB4 page 461
Dry and finish men's hair	4	GB5 page 481
Optional — Group 1. You must achieve units adding up to a credit value of 9 from this group		
Perm and neutralise hair	8	GH14 page 341
Change men's hair colour	11	GB2 page 411
Optional — Group 2. You must achieve units adding up to a credit value of 9 from this group		
Fulfil salon reception duties	3	G4 page 81
Develop and maintain your effectiveness at work	3	G8 page 157
Give clients a positive impression of yourself and your organisation	5	G17 page 105
Promote additional products or services to clients	6	G18 page 119

Level 2 VRQ Diploma In Womens's Hairdressing

Unit title	Credit value	Chapter
Mandatory — you must achieve each of these units		
Follow health and safety practice in the salon	3	G20 page 45
Working in the hair industry	4	Page 15
Client consultation for hair services	3	G7 page 133
Shampoo and condition the hair and scalp	3	GH8 page 175
Colour and lighten hair	10	GH9 page 199
Cut women's hair	8	GH12 page 297
The art of dressing hair	5	GH10, GH11 pages 243, 271
This unit is mandatory if you are taking your qualification with City & Guilds, or optional if you are taking it with VTCT		
Promote products or services to clients in a salon	3	G18 page 119
Perm and neutralise hair	7	GH14 page 341
Optional — you must achieve units from below adding up to a total credit value of 8 if you are taking this qualification with City & Guilds. If you are with VTCT you can choose from the optional units above and below to add up to a total credit value of 16.		
Create an image based on a theme within the hair and beauty sector	7	Page 393
Display stock to promote sales in a salon	3	G18 page 119
Salon reception duties	3	G4 page 81

Level 2 VRQ Diploma in Barbering

Unit title	Credit value	Chapter
Mandatory — you must achieve each of these units		
Follow health and safety practice in the salon	3	G20 page 45
Working in the hair industry	4	G8 page 157
Client consultation for hair services	3	G7 page 133
Shampoo and condition the hair and scalp	3	GH8 page 175
Cut men's hair	6	GB3 page 435
Cut facial hair	4	GB4 page 461
Styling men's hair	5	GB5 page 481
This unit is mandatory if you are taking this qualification with City & Guilds, or optional if you are taking it with VTCT		
Colour hair	10	GB2 page 411
Promote products and services to clients in a salon	3	G18 page 119
Optional — you must achieve units below adding up to a credit value of 13 if you are taking this qualification with City & Guilds. If you are with VTCT you can choose from the optional units above and below to add up to a total credit value of 27		
Perm and neutralise hair	7	GH14 page 341
Create an image based on a theme within the hair and beauty sector	7	Page 393
Display stock to promote sales in salon	3	G18 page 119
Salon reception duties	3	G4 page 81

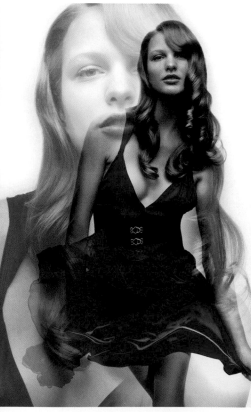

John Carne

Why hairdressing?

A Level 2 qualification is the foundation for a career in hairdressing, an industry that is ever-changing and has no boundaries to success or the avenues that may be followed. Your qualification will give you the basic elements that you need to help you become a qualified hair stylist. However, it is important to make sure that you gain your qualification either through a reputable salon or college/training institution. Once completed, your qualification will open up a world full of opportunities within the fashion and media industries, such as:

- salon stylist/colour technician
- photographic work for magazines
- television work
- fashion shows
- films/theatre work
- salon owner
- hairdressing shows and seminars
- working on cruise ships.

The hairdressing industry has a very flexible employment pattern. As well as working in a salon as a stylist or a technician, many people working in hairdressing are self-employed and enjoy the range of benefits that this brings.

Earning possibilities have improved immensely in recent years. Hairstyles are now classed as a fashion accessory. Clients who buy designer clothes now look to buy designer hairstyles, and will pay the appropriate price for a top stylist to create their image. This has led to improved salaries for the hairdressers.

After completing your Level 2, you will take the role of a junior stylist. Here you will put into practice the basic skills that you have learned and find out what fun the hairdressing industry can be. You will gain excellent customer service skills in monitoring and looking after your clientele as well as creating your own artistic flair and style in hairdressing. When you start work, you will find that you need to develop the skills you began to acquire as you trained.

Hairdressing is a 'people profession' as well as being creative and innovative. It is fun and rewarding, as well as hard work! There are many avenues open to you In terms of careers. Below are four very different career paths that individuals have followed. A profile of each of these people may indicate the range of options available.

A salon manager with a specialist interest in colour

John Carne started his career at the age of 16 years in a small barber shop in Surrey. This was his first experience in hairdressing and it was here that he started reading *Hairdressers Journal*, which opened his eyes to the exciting world of the hairdressing industry. He completed a City & Guilds Apprenticeship and opted for an in-house training scheme at a well-known London salon. All the shampooing, coffee making and floor sweeping was a bit of a shock. Gradually it all fell into place and he realised that all the training was worthwhile. He took full advantage of the opportunities to assist at shows and seminars as well as mastering all the essential skills covered in the basic training.

Before he started his own business in Guildford, John had travelled around the globe for four years, working in Japan, America and Switzerland, performing shows and seminars. He had also been involved in producing photographic work for magazines, which immediately gave him international recognition.

He opened the Guildford salon in 1981 and his first priority was to build a strong team of technicians and stylists. He had always been interested in colour as a specialist aspect of styling. Another interest was in establishing salons with a calm, spacious and comfortable feel. He believes that managing a salon gives a unique opportunity for a stylist to express his or her own personality and interests in a very particular way.

Opening your own salon

Have you ever had dreams of opening your own salon? Lucia describes the path that led her to doing just that.

'I'm Lucia Fabrizio. I left school after my GCSEs when I was 16 years old and went straight to college. I had worked as a Saturday girl in a salon in our town and had loved it even though I had to get up really early every Saturday morning. I enjoyed meeting different clients and came to know some of them well in the year and a half I worked at Cuts 4 U.

I found the work for Level 2 quite hard because there was so much to learn and get right, but all my friends enjoyed the course and we had lots of practical experience. I did find it quite tiring; it can mean standing up all day! It's especially difficult when you don't really feel well or are wearing uncomfortable shoes.

But I passed the course and was offered a job back at my old salon. However, I decided to return to college to join the part-time Level 3 course and also broaden

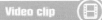
Video clip

Watch video clip 'Best advice' on the website to hear what celebrity stylist Andrew Barton has to say about the best advice he received when starting his career in hairdressing.

xv

Introduction

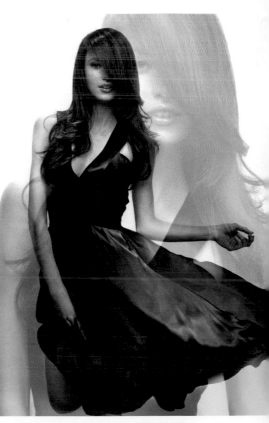
John Carne

my experience. I wanted to concentrate on cutting techniques, but I also aimed to own my own salon one day — the Level 3 course provided opportunities for both. I really enjoyed the course. I was able to expand on my strengths and overcome my weaknesses. By the end, I felt ready to stand on my own two feet!

I spent the next couple of years in the salon developing the skills I had learned, then last week I finally took the step I had been waiting for and opened my own salon.'

Working in television and films

You may find that your forte is to become a session stylist working all over the world doing hair for television and films. Hanna Coles describes her path into this exciting world.

'I'm Hanna Coles and my first introduction to hairdressing was as a Saturday girl in a London salon. I continued my apprenticeship there, built up a clientele and worked as a stylist for five years, particularly enjoying my involvement in the salon shows and session work.

It was this type of work that I decided to pursue, so after a year at sea, hairdressing on cruise liners (a fantastic and fun way to see the world), I set about making my goal a reality. It took time and determination — I made endless calls to people in the media industries, gathered lots of advice and information, assisted established session stylists and show designers, and often worked for free.

It was suggested that I broaden my knowledge, and therefore increase my work potential, by studying wig making and make-up. This I did, and with my new skills was soon working in the wig department of a West End musical, where I discovered the importance of being able to work quickly and intuitively, because theatre is 'live' and anything can happen.

Meanwhile I got a fashion portfolio together by 'testing' with up-and-coming models and photographers, and began to have my work published in the fashion pages of magazines such as *Tatler* and *Arena Homme*. Working in this medium taught me that attention to detail and being aware of forthcoming trends is vital.

Each job presented an opportunity to make new contacts, learn new things and experiment with new ideas. If people like your pace and style of work they use you again, so eventually I found myself being booked for music videos, commercials and television programmes. Then came my first feature film, *A Passion for Life*, shot in beautiful locations in Paris and the south of France.

Now my work is incredibly varied — one day I could be backstage at Fashion Week creating contemporary looks on a model; the next day I could be fitting an actor's wig for a seventeenth-century drama or working with a band on television!

It's definitely fulfilling to see your work come to life 40 feet wide at the cinema, or on a billboard or the cover of a book — it can even be a bit scary! But the most important things for me are the fun I have, the colourful and eclectic people I meet and the extraordinary places this work can take me to.

It is hard work and a very competitive industry; I would not like anyone to believe that it's all glamour and going to wonderful parties. Sometimes I am so tired I can scarcely crawl up the stairs to bed. But if you have the determination and you really want to make it happen, then why not?'

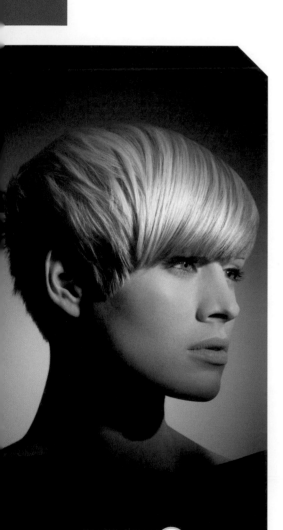

Goldwell

Video clip

Watch video clip 'Staying motivated' on the website to hear what celebrity stylist Andrew Barton has to say about how he stays motivated.

Working as a PA within the hairdressing industry

Amanda West started with John Carne as a Saturday girl and went on to complete her Level 2 through the in-salon training system. Unfortunately, Amanda developed dermatitis (inflammation of the skin). This was provoked by an allergy to hair products, meaning that she could no longer work with hair.

Disappointing though this was, Amanda still wanted to be involved with the hairdressing industry, so she moved on to become a PA (personal assistant). This involves many of the skills needed in hairdressing, for example people management and public relations, so the basic skills learned in her Level 2 were to stand her in good stead when liaising with newspapers and magazines about beauty tips. As in any industry, the people working at the marketing end of a business need to have done their groundwork.

A typical day for Amanda now involves using the following skills:

- customer service in day-to-day personal interaction
- working with beauty editors from fashion magazines if the salon is doing a photo shoot or a show
- organising personnel within the salon
- arranging shows
- talking to model agencies
- liaising with international companies
- writing press/advertising features
- controlling stock to ensure nothing runs out.

xvii

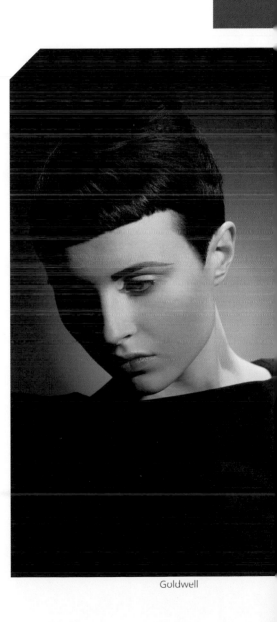

Goldwell

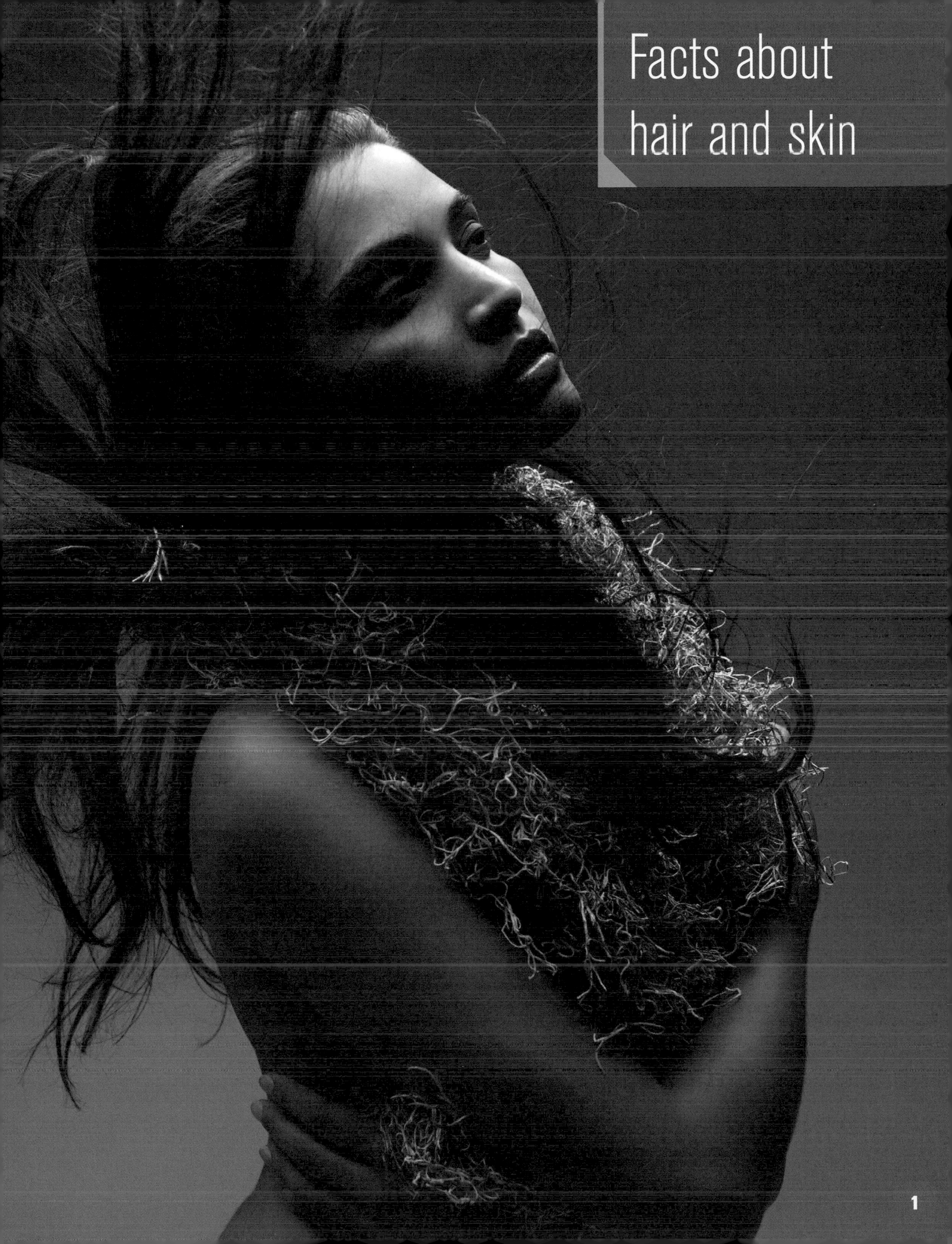

Facts about hair and skin

What you will learn:

- **The structure of hair**
- **The structure of skin**
- **Bones of the face and skull**
- **The growth cycle of hair**
- **The chemical structure of hair**
- **The pH scale**

Introduction

This section contains some exceptionally important facts about hair and skin and it is crucial that you learn them. As you begin to work with hair, you need to know about its structure, how it grows and the effect that we, as hairdressers, can have on it. This will help you understand what effects styling and the use of chemicals will have on the hair. The information contained within this chapter is the foundation to all the units and it is therefore vital that you understand these important facts before moving further on in this book. For example, it is important for you to be aware that chemicals used in hairdressing can badly damage the hair and skin, so you should not use these until you fully understand the structure of hair and skin.

The activities in this section will help you to learn these important facts in a practical way.

Cuticle

The outermost layer of the hair shaft.

Cortex

A major component of the hair shaft, providing strength and elasticity.

Medulla

The central part of the hair shaft.

The structure of hair

A single hair is called a hair shaft. It is made up of:

- the **cuticle**
- the **cortex**
- the **medulla.**

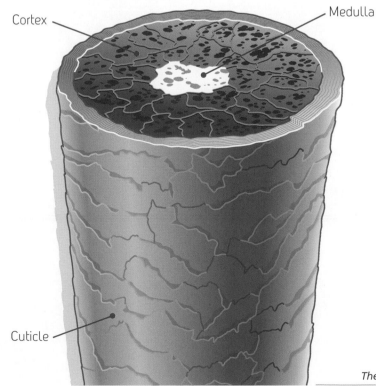

Cortex

Medulla

Cuticle

The hair shaft

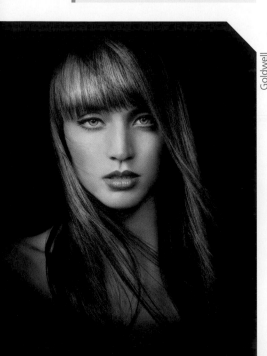

Goldwell

Look at the diagram of a hair shaft below. It has been magnified many times to show this much detail.

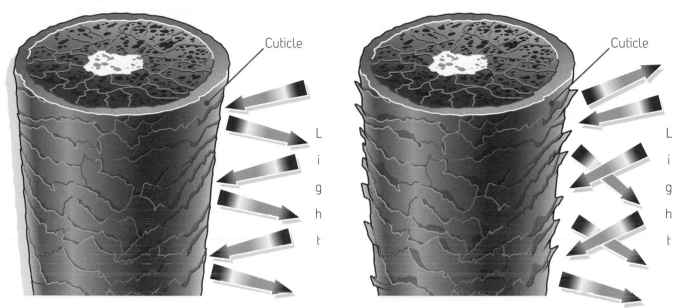

Hair in good condition	Hair in bad condition

Cuticle

Light

Cuticle

Light

Task 1

Porosity test

Take one strand of hair from your head. Hold it firmly by the root between the thumb and forefinger of one hand. With the thumb and forefinger of the other hand, slide from the root to the end of the hair. If the hair feels rough in places that means the cuticle scales are open or raised and the condition of the cuticle is poor. If the hair feels smooth all the way along, the cuticle scales will be closed and flat and the hair will be in good condition and look smooth and shiny. You have just carried out a porosity test to check the condition of the cuticle scales.

Healthy cuticle scales reflect the light to show shiny, healthy hair. Scales in poor condition bounce the light back in all directions, giving the hair a flat and dull appearance

Porosity

The hair's ability to absorb moisture/products.

The cuticle

The cuticle is the outside layer of the hair shaft. Its main function or purpose is to protect everything underneath it. It is very tough and holds the insides of the hair shaft together. The diagram above shows that the cuticle is made up of many layers of overlapping scales. The number of layers varies but there is an average for each of the different types of hair:

- European/Caucasian hair has 4–7 layers of cuticle scales
- African-type hair has 7–11 layers of cuticle scales
- Oriental/Asian hair has more than 11 layers of cuticle scales.

Cuticle scales look like the overlapping scales of a fish or tiles on a roof. The scales are translucent, rather like frosted glass, so the hair's natural colour can be seen through them. The edges of the scales lie away from the scalp.

Elasticity

The condition/strength of the cortex determines the hair's ability to return to its normal shape after being stretched.

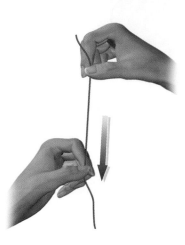

The elasticity test

Although the layers of cuticle scales are tough they can be damaged permanently by the use of strong chemicals such as perms, bleaches and relaxers. However, if the correct service procedures are followed the hair will not be damaged. Excessive heat or overuse of hairdryers and straightening irons will cause heat damage to the cuticle scales and harsh physical services such as over-backcombing or the use of elastic bands can also lift and permanently damage them.

Healthy cuticle scales lie flat and are closed tightly round the hair shaft. The hair will appear lustrous and shiny. Damaged cuticle scales lift away from their closest partner. When this happens the hair's appearance will be dull and the hair will feel rough. In this state any chemicals put on to the hair will be absorbed too quickly through the cuticle and into the next layer of the hair shaft — the cortex region.

Task 2

Elasticity test
Take a single strand of your hair and hold each end tightly between the thumb and forefinger of each hand. Now gently pull. The hair should stretch slightly and then return to its original length. If the hair stretches and does not return to its original length, or if the hair snaps, this means the hair is in poor condition. You have just carried out an elasticity test.

The cortex

The cortex lies underneath the cuticle and is a very important part of the hair shaft. All the changes take place within the cortex when hair is blow-dried, set, permed, coloured, bleached or relaxed.

The cortex is made up of many strands that are twisted together, like knitting wool. These can stretch and then return to their original length. However, only hair in good condition will be able to do this.

In European/Caucasian hair the cortex runs evenly through the hair shaft. Naturally curly African-type hair has two different types of cortex due to the curl. The cortex on the outside of the curve has a less dense structure than the cortex on the inside of the curve, which is compacted and therefore more dense. The flatter shape of the cortex of European/Caucasian hair means that chemicals will process more quickly.

Notice the difference between these two hair shafts

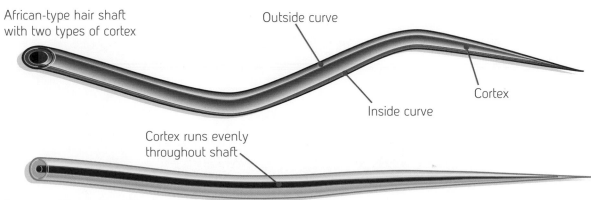

African-type hair shaft with two types of cortex

Outside curve

Cortex

Inside curve

Cortex runs evenly throughout shaft

European/Caucasian hair shaft

The cortex contains all the colour pigments in the hair. These are called **melanin**. Melanin is broken down into two types of colour pigments:

- eumelanin — natural black/brown
- pheomelanin — natural red/yellow.

The medulla

The medulla is found in the centre of the hair shaft. It is not always present (there is no known reason for this), particularly in fine hair, and scientists have found that it does not have any known function.

Task 3

Colour pigments
Look at your own or a colleague's hair. Is the hair colour made up of mainly black/brown pigments or mainly red/yellow pigments?

All natural (not artificially coloured) hair is made up of a combination of lots of different colour pigments. If the hair is blonde it will still have other colour pigments in it as well as yellow pigment. It is the amount or ratio of the different colours that will decide the actual colour of the hair

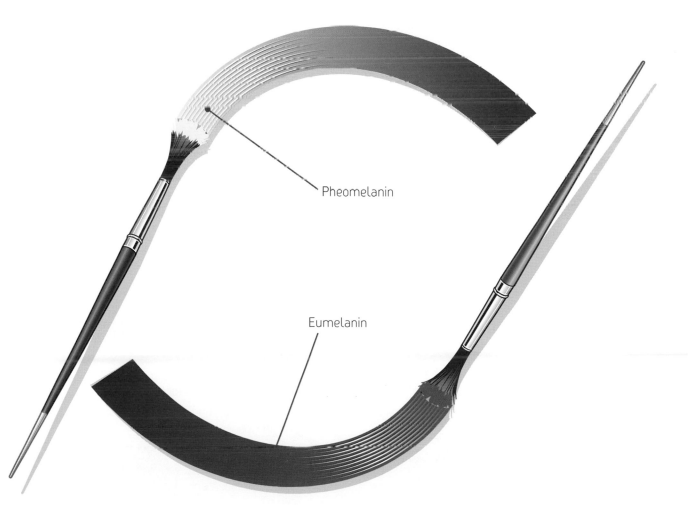

Natural hair colour pigments

Pheomelanin

Eumelanin

Facts about hair and skin

The structure of skin

The skin is made up of different parts, which are described below.

Part of skin	Structure and function
Blood capillary vessels	Consist of arteries, veins and capillaries. Found in the dermis. Carry nutrients and oxygen.
Nerve endings	Found in the dermis. Respond to pain, pressure, heat and touch.
Sweat pore	Opens onto the epidermis. Releases sweat to cool the skin. Also removes waste products.
Hair root	Found in the dermis. Attaches to hair bulb.
Hair follicle	The pocket in which the hair grows.
Hair shaft	The part of the hair above the skin or scalp.
Sebaceous gland	The gland that produces sebum, the hair's natural oil, which is secreted into the follicle where it lubricates the hair and the skin of the scalp.
Epidermis	The outer layer of the skin. It consists of five layers: horny layer, clear layer, granular layer, prickle cell layer, basal layer.
Horny layer	These three layers are dead and are constantly being shed.
Granular layer	
Prickle cell layer	
Clear layer	Three to four rows of dead cells which are flattened. Only found on the palms of the hands and soles of the feet. Found above the granular layer. Protects in areas of friction.
Basal layer	Deepest layer of the epidermis. Continuously producing new cells.
Papillary layer	Joins the epidermis and dermis layers together. Has a rich supply of blood vessels and nerve endings.
Arrector pili muscle	Muscle to erect hair. If you are cold or frightened, this muscle contracts (pulls tight) and the hair stands on end creating 'goose pimples' on the skin.
Subcutaneous layer	Fat layer. Protects muscles, bones and internal organs, provides insulation and a source of energy.
Lymph vessels	Transport lymph fluid through a series of glands to filter toxins and waste.
Nerve fibre	Leads from nerve endings and connects to nervous system.
Sweat gland	The gland that produces sweat to cool the body.
Dermal papilla	Promotes cellular activity with nutrients from the nerves and blood vessels.
Hair bulb	Created as new hair cells form.
Adipose tissue	Fat cells which make up the subcutaneous layer.
Blood vessels	Tiny blood vessels that bring food, oxygen and nutrients to feed the hair and skin.
Dermis (true skin)	The inner layer of the skin. It lies under the epidermis.
Reticular layer	Found beneath the papillary layer. Protects and repairs injured tissue. Contains collagen and elastin.

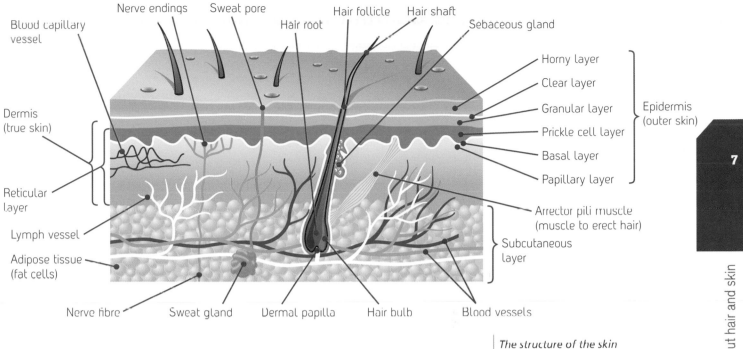

Blood capillary vessel

Nerve endings

Sweat pore

Hair root

Hair follicle

Hair shaft

Sebaceous gland

Horny layer

Clear layer

Granular layer

Prickle cell layer

Basal layer

Papillary layer

Epidermis (outer skin)

Dermis (true skin)

Reticular layer

Lymph vessel

Adipose tissue (fat cells)

Arrector pili muscle (muscle to erect hair)

Subcutaneous layer

Nerve fibre

Sweat gland

Dermal papilla

Hair bulb

Blood vessels

The structure of the skin

Bones of the face and skull

The part of the body that protects the brain and forms the framework for the face is called the skull. It is made up of several different bones fused together. The joins are known as sutures. The skull is attached to the body by the vertebral column, which enables the head to turn and tilt. The weight of the head is supported by the neck, the shoulder girdle bones and muscles.

Bones of the skull

Facial muscles

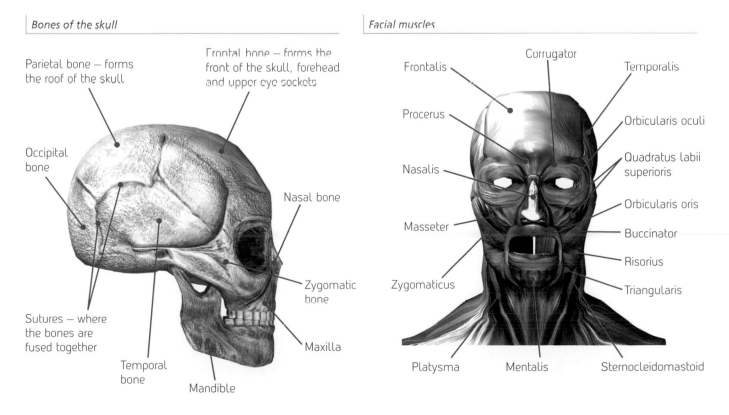

Parietal bone — forms the roof of the skull

Frontal bone — forms the front of the skull, forehead and upper eye sockets

Occipital bone

Nasal bone

Sutures — where the bones are fused together

Zygomatic bone

Temporal bone

Mandible

Maxilla

Frontalis

Corrugator

Temporalis

Procerus

Orbicularis oculi

Nasalis

Quadratus labii superioris

Masseter

Orbicularis oris

Buccinator

Zygomaticus

Risorius

Triangularis

Platysma

Mentalis

Sternocleidomastoid

The growth cycle of hair

On average, hair grows 1.25 cm (½ inch) per month and we lose an average of 80–100 hairs a day. However, a single strand of hair does not grow continuously throughout its life. Hair follicles (where the hair grows from) undergo alternate periods of activity when the hair is growing. The stages in the life cycle of hair are known as:

- anagen
- catagen
- telogen
- anagen.

Anagen

When a hair follicle is active and the hair is growing, this is known as anagen. The period of active growth for scalp hair is from 1.25 years to 7 years. New hairs in early anagen grow faster than old hairs, the average growth being 1.25 cm per month. Between 80 and 90 per cent of scalp hairs are in the anagen state at any one time.

Catagen

Anagen is followed by a short period of change called catagen. During this time, hair follicles undergo a period of change and do not grow. Catagen lasts for about two weeks during which activity (growing) stops and new cells are formed. At any one time only about 1 per cent of follicles are in the catagen state.

Telogen

Finally, the follicle enters a period of rest (dormant like a squirrel in winter hibernation – but still alive) known as telogen. This stage lasts for about three to four months. About 13 per cent of follicles are in the telogen state at any one time.

The growth cycle of hair. Hair cycles undergo alternate periods of activity

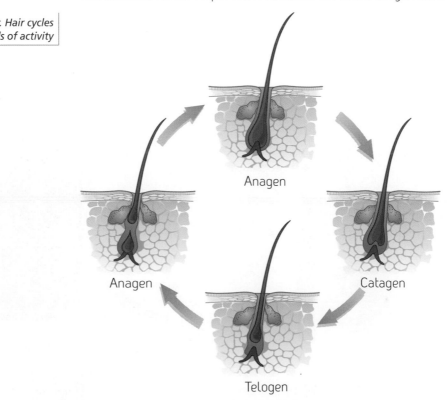

Anagen

Catagen

Telogen

Anagen

Anagen

When the resting phase is complete the follicle begins to lengthen. When the follicle reaches full length a new hair begins to grow. If the old hair is still in the follicle the new hair pushes it out.

Changes in the growth cycle

The growth cycle of hair can change. For example, during pregnancy increased hormone levels can cause the hair's growth cycle to change and may mean that many hairs change into the anagen (active growth) phase that would, under normal circumstances, not be in anagen. When the hormone levels return to normal, after the baby is born, the hairs that would not normally have been in anagen will return to their previous state and stop their active growth.

This explains why some clients lose excessive amounts of hair after their baby is born. You can, therefore, explain the reasons for this unusual amount of hair loss as hair that your client would not 'normally' have had anyway. You should try to ease your client's fears as hair loss can be very worrying.

Types of hair

There are three main types of hair, as shown in the table below. There are many variations on these hair groups.

Hair type	Natural characteristics
Asian/Oriental	• Usually very straight • More than eleven layers of cuticle scales • Coarse and resistant
Caucasian/European	• Usually wavy but can be straight or tightly curled • Four to seven layers of cuticle scales • Can be fine, medium or coarse, depending upon the amount of cuticle layers
African-type hair	• Usually very tightly curled • Seven to eleven layers of cuticle scales • Fragile

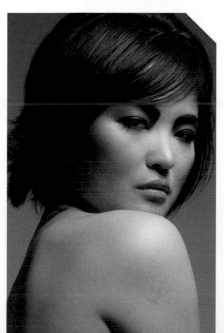
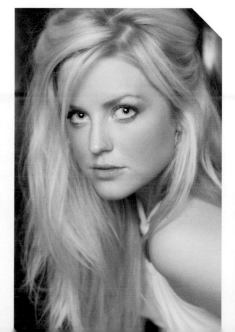
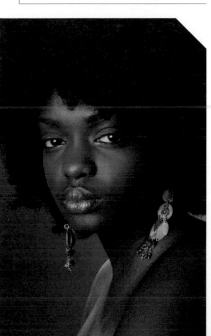

The different textures of hair

There are three kinds of hair on the body.

- Fine vellus hair grows on the body.
- Stronger terminal hair grows on the scalp.
- Lanugo hair is only found on unborn or premature babies but this type of hair usually falls out before the ninth month of pregnancy. You can sometimes see this type of hair on the heads of balding men.

The average person loses 80 to 100 hairs a day.

Factors affecting the growth cycle

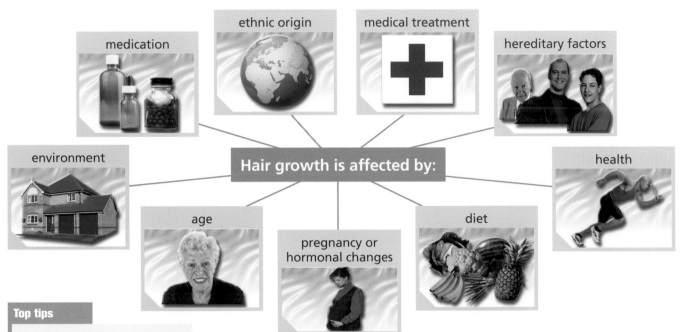

Top tips

A client is worried that more of her hair than usual seems to be falling out. You need to find out the answers to the following questions.

- Is your client taking any medication?
- Has she recently had a baby? The client may lose an excessive amount of hair after the baby is born as hormone levels begin to return to normal.
- Is she suffering from stress or worry? Severe stress has been proven as a reason for hair loss.
- Has she recently had a major shock? Shock can affect hair growth and can, in severe cases, cause all the hair to fall out.
- Has she just had hair extensions removed?

The following factors can affect a person's hair growth cycle:

- *Ethnic origin* – see the table on page 9.
- *Hereditary factors* – your hair growth cycle is programmed into your genes. For example, if everyone in your family has curly hair, you will probably have curly hair too.
- *Medication* – this can affect the hair growth and may have long-term effects.
- *Medical treatment* – this can significantly change many original factors of hair growth. For example, chemotherapy will cause the hair to fall out and regrowth may have a different colour or texture.
- *Environment* – harsh weather, climate and pollution can damage hair.
- *Age* – natural pigment and keratin changes with age.
- *Pregnancy or hormonal changes* – hormones can alter the growth cycle.
- *Diet* – poor diet results in poor hair condition.
- *Health* – the state of your health will be evident in the level of shine and thickness of your hair.

The chemical structure of hair

Hair consists of a hardened protein called **keratin**. Its function is to make the hair elastic and flexible. Keratin is also found in the skin and the finger- and toenails. It is made up of amino acids and peptide bonds. Together they form **polypeptide chains** or links. These chains are found in the cortex of the hair and look like a spiral staircase.

To prevent this spiral from falling down, the polypeptide chains are supported by cross-links of **hydrogen bonds** and **disulphide bonds** acting like scaffolding poles.

Hydrogen bonds are weak and can be easily broken by water. Therefore, the shape of the hair can be changed temporarily by shampooing and then blow-drying or setting.

Disulphide bonds are very strong and only another chemical can break this stronger link. This change will be permanent and takes place when you perm or relax hair.

Keratin

Protein found in hair, nails and skin.

Polypeptide chains

Tiny molecules intertwined creating keratin within the cortex.

Hydrogen bonds

Weak bonds found in the cortex, broken by shampooing and atmospheric moisture. Forms part of keratin.

Disulphide bonds

Two sulphur atoms joined together to make a strong bond which helps form part of keratin.

The structure of keratin

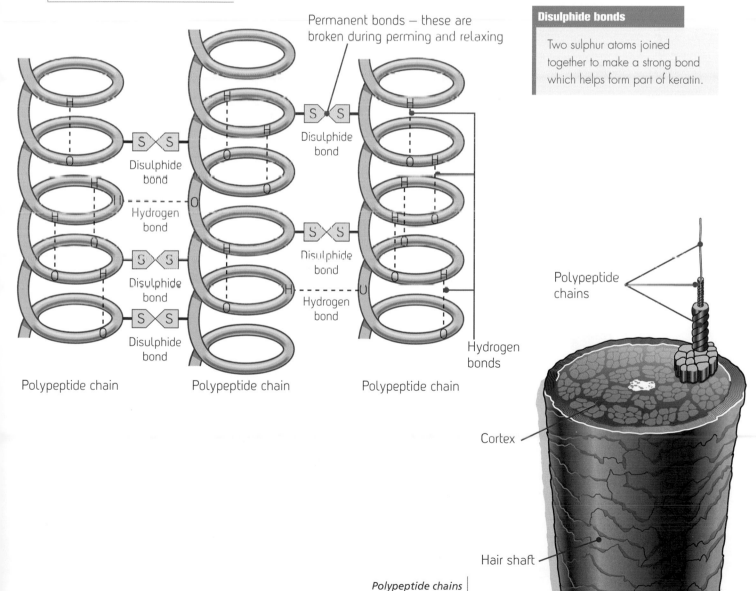

Permanent bonds – these are broken during perming and relaxing

Disulphide bond

Disulphide bond

Hydrogen bond

Disulphide bond

Disulphide bond

Disulphide bond

Hydrogen bond

Hydrogen bonds

Polypeptide chain

Polypeptide chain

Polypeptide chain

Polypeptide chains

Cortex

Hair shaft

Polypeptide chains

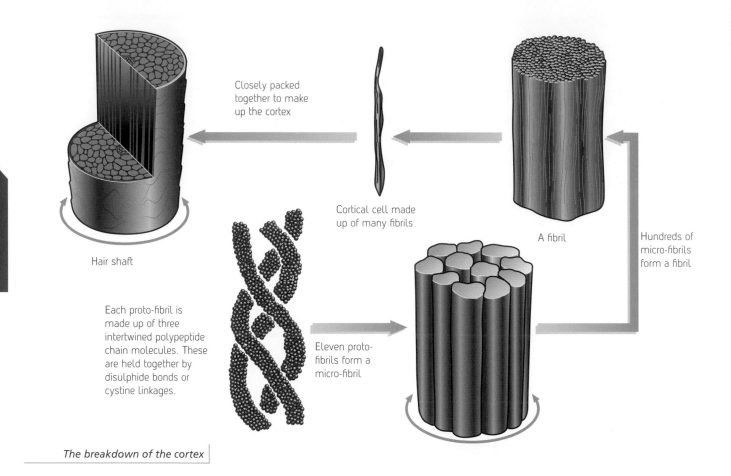

Closely packed together to make up the cortex

Cortical cell made up of many fibrils

A fibril

Hundreds of micro-fibrils form a fibril

Hair shaft

Each proto-fibril is made up of three intertwined polypeptide chain molecules. These are held together by disulphide bonds or cystine linkages.

Eleven proto-fibrils form a micro-fibril

The breakdown of the cortex

Alpha keratin and beta keratin

Hair that has been shampooed and left to dry naturally is described as alpha keratin. This is the natural hair state. If you shampoo and then set or blow-dry hair into a stretched or unnatural state, this is called beta keratin. This shape changes back easily to alpha keratin by either wetting or being in a damp atmosphere, which breaks the hydrogen bonds.

Moving from alpha to beta keratin

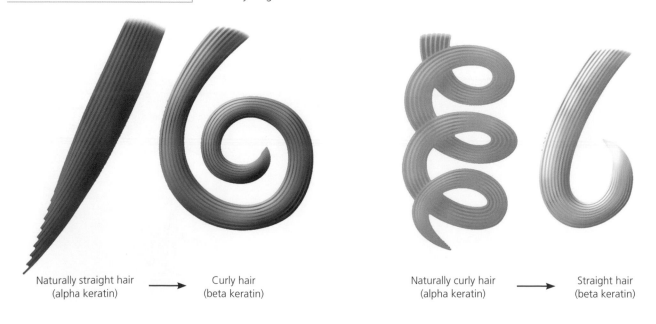

Naturally straight hair (alpha keratin) → Curly hair (beta keratin)

Naturally curly hair (alpha keratin) → Straight hair (beta keratin)

The pH scale

It is very important that you understand the pH scale because it will help you appreciate how different products affect the hair and skin.

The scale measures whether a product is acidic or alkaline, with 1 on the scale being the most acidic and 14 the most alkaline. The more alkaline a product, the more damage it can do to the hair and skin. The halfway point on the scale, 7, is classified as neutral so pH 7.1–14 is alkaline and pH 1–6.9 is acid. Pure water has a pH of 7.

Generally, an acid-based product will close the cuticle scales to make the hair smooth and shiny (for example conditioner). The exception to this rule is an acid perm which needs heat to open the cuticle scales in order to penetrate the cortex, whereas an alkaline perm will automatically open the cuticle scales. Therefore, an acid perm has a gentler, more conditioning action on the hair but will not improve the condition of the hair as a conditioning treatment would.

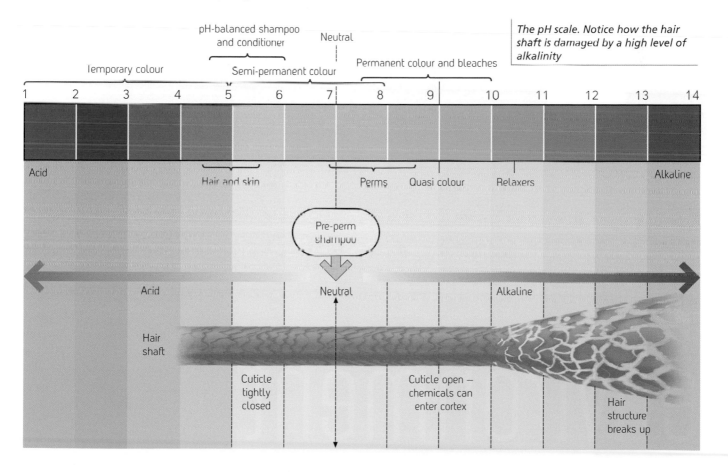

The pH scale. Notice how the hair shaft is damaged by a high level of alkalinity

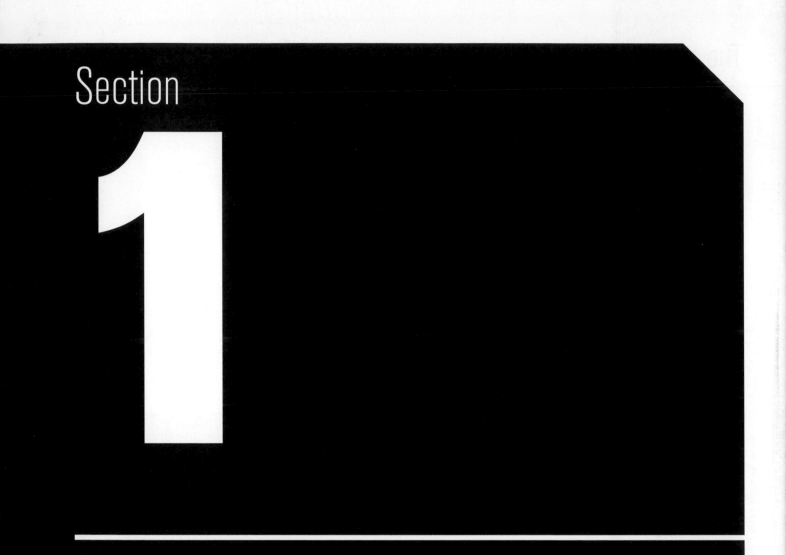

Section

1

The workplace
environment

Working in the
hair industry

What you will learn:

- **How to describe the key characteristics of the hair industry**
- **How to describe working practices in the hair industry**

Introduction

This unit aims to help you understand the scope of opportunities for working in the hairdressing industry. There are over 400 million client visits to hair and beauty businesses each year (HABIA statistics). By understanding the breadth of the hairdressing industry – including its career prospects, development opportunities and the basic employment rights and responsibilities – you will gain the knowledge and skills to allow your full potential to develop. The industry turnover is currently a massive £6.2 billion (HABIA statistics) which demonstrates the size of the industry and shows it is a potentially great career choice as long as you are enthusiastic and prepared to work hard. Throughout this unit you will be required to progress as an independent learner, taking responsibility for your own development while working in the hairdressing industry.

The key characteristics of the hair industry

Sources of information

Accessing sources of information on organisations within the hairdressing industry

It is important for you to have an understanding of the many different types of **organisations** in the hairdressing industry. This will give you a good understanding of the opportunities available to you for your future career. Some of the sources you can access to help you investigate the career options within the industry are available through websites on the internet. This includes the industry's leading body, the Hair and Beauty Industry Authority (HABIA) and hairdressing awarding organisations such as VTCT, City & Guilds and Edexcel.

You can research the industry using magazines and industry publications including trade journals. An example is the *Hairdressers Journal* (also available online at www.hji.co.uk) which contains a huge amouont of information about:

- high-profile salons
- new products advertised by manufacturers and wholesalers
- job vacancies
- how to become part of the industry's **professional** membership organisations
- awards and events.

Participation at **hairdressing exhibitions** and shows (which are held throughout the country) can provide exciting opportunities to witness up-to-date techniques and new products by well-known and celebrity industry professionals. Work experience with local salons, spas and health resorts will also provide you with valuable observation opportunities to make informed decisions about where you would like to work. Attending local open evenings/days at organisations will also provide you with word-of-mouth opportunities to learn more about the potential employment prospects

Organisations

A number of people or groups joined and organised for some purpose.

Characteristics

Any distinguishing features.

Top tip

- The key to good research is to investigate thoroughly. Always use more than one source when researching. For example, don't just rely on the internet – use trade magazines and journals to get a good breadth of information from different sources.
- Another form of research is in person with career guidance from career advisers and job centres.

Professional

Maintaining appropriate standards.

within your area. Simple everyday habits, such as reading newspapers and watching TV, can also inform you of industry trends, including celebrity-**endorsed** products marketed by industry suppliers and manufacturers.

Task 1

Spend some time researching the hair industry and answer the following questions:

1 What types of organisations are there within the hair industry?
2 State the main services offered by the hair industry.
3 Describe the different occupational roles available to you in the hair industry.

A worksheet to help you complete this task is provided on the website.

The main services within the hairdressing industry

It is important for you to understand the main services offered by professionals within the hairdressing industry.

As professionally qualified stylists we are able to offer many services. It is important that this should always start with an initial client consultation service. This is the basis of all the other services we offer and it is important to spend sufficient time on the consultation to allow you to fully discuss and explore all the information required from your client.

Once you have carried out this consultation you can work with your client to decide on the services appropriate to your client's requirements, hair type, texture and condition.

Services you can offer include shampooing and conditioning, scalp massage, Indian head massage, hair cutting, styling, dressing, colouring, perming, relaxing, hair extensions and colour correction. If you are qualified in barbering you can also offer services such as shaving, face massage, specialist **patterns in hair** and cutting facial hair.

Employment in the hairdressing industry

Occupational roles within the hairdressing industry

There are many occupational roles available to you within the hairdressing industry. Hairdressing is an exciting and fast-moving career which can hold a world of opportunities for professionals who develop a passion for hairdressing. Most professionals start at the bottom as a shampooist, salon junior or trainee apprentice and work their way up the career ladder once qualified by becoming a junior stylist. This is known as a 'building block career' — each job role gives you the skills and experience you need to progress to the next role.

Once experience of working with a body of clients is gained there is the opportunity to progress to senior stylist or artistic director status. Other opportunities include:

- becoming a salon manager or salon owner
- work-based or in-house trainer/assessor
- working in salons, spas, health resorts, on cruise ships, abroad or holiday resorts
- passing skills and experience on to others by teaching hairdressing as a lecturer or assessor/instructor
- specialising in services or skills you particularly enjoy such as colour technician, receptionist or barbering.

Hairdressing exhibition

A public show or display of hairdressing products, tools, techniques and hairdressing-related items.

Endorsed

Given approval or support.

Patterns in hair

Specialist work produced by using clippers or a razor to cut shapes and patterns into short hair.

Top tips

Other opportunities in teaching hairdressing include becoming an internal/external verifier, or course team leader.

17

Working in the hair industry

Hairdressing product companies like to employ qualified professionals to market and educate salon stylists due to their knowledge and technical experience. Therefore there are also opportunities to become company representatives for major retailers such as Wella, L'Oréal, Schwarzkopf, Goldwell, Tigi etc.

Career patterns within the hair industry

Most hairdressing salons and product manufacturers offer employment opportunities over a variety of working patterns such as full-time, part-time and seasonal work. Some stylists decide they would like to work for themselves and become self-employed independent or freelance stylists.

Employment characteristics of working in the hair industry

As a stylist you will require many different skills to become a successful professional. Some of the skills you will need are shown below.

Communication skills

The skills required to communicate effectively with others.

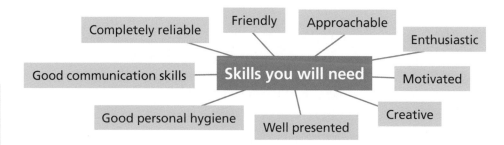

You will need to consistently employ good customer service skills and excellent client care. Ultimately, you need to enjoy working with others as the hairdressing industry is based on working with lots of different people including clients, colleagues, bosses, educators, company representatives and industry professionals. You will need to be able to build effective relationships with all these different people in order to have a successful career in the industry.

Education and training opportunities within the hairdressing industry

It is important for you to understand the education and training opportunities within the hairdressing industry. As much of the industry is client-focused you will acquire many transferable client care and communication skills which are the foundation or basis of many other employment opportunities and can be used in a variety of other sectors and industries. There is lots of flexibility in the hairdressing industry and you will have opportunities to transfer to other sectors of the industry. This means you will always have lots of different career paths open to you.

These include working for:

- hairdressing product manufacturers such as Wella, L'Oréal, Schwarzkopf, Goldwell, Tigi etc.
- hairdressing wholesalers
- beauty therapy salons

- spa industries
- hairdressing awarding organisations
- technical writing for the hair industry or relating essential knowledge and understanding of the hairdressing industry into hairdressing manuals or textbooks as an author.

There is even the possibility of using technical transferable skills such as cutting and clipper work by becoming an animal groomer.

There are different types of qualifications that you can take in the hairdressing industry. VRQs (Vocationally-Related Qualifications) are likely to be taken in a college, while NVQs (National Vocational Qualifications) and Apprenticeships are usually taken in the workplace.

Training opportunities

You are never too old to learn and there are endless opportunities for further training within the industry. This is partly because of the fast-paced changes in technology, techniques and products. If you are always striving to improve your knowledge and practical skills you will be more successful within your career.

For successful career progression you need to ensure you are always motivated and enthusiastic. To keep your motivation levels high it is helpful to have realistically set **targets** to work towards. These are set by your line manager, usually during appraisal. Individual targets can be set to achieve a variety of training opportunities which will stretch and challenge you. It is helpful to have a specific deadline to complete training activities as this makes both outcomes and achievements easier to measure.

Training opportunities can include:

- entering competitions
- Continuing Professional Development courses
- long or short courses
- specialist awards, certificates or Diplomas, VRQ, NVQ, certificate of attendance/ competence
- in-house training.

All evidence of participation in training activities, such as qualifications certificates or certificates of attendance, should be kept in your portfolio of evidence or your Record of Achievement. The more proactive you are about training opportunities the more likely you are to be successful when interviewed by a prospective employer. Employers will wish to employ a member of staff who is willing to update and advance their employability skills. A proactive approach to training and development may also make it easier for you to make a career change to a different sector of the industry and may even lead to you being headhunted by a potential employer who will recognise your value as an asset to their salon.

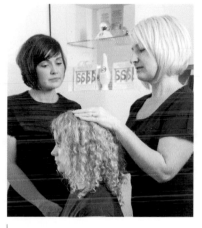

Observing the work of others will help you to learn

Targets

Goals that are aimed at, for example learning a new skill.

Working practices in the hair industry

Following good working practices within the salon

It is vitally important to have the necessary understanding of safe and hygienic working practices. To do this you will need to be familiar with some of the key pieces of legislation affecting the industry. More information on the following key pieces of legislation can be found on pages 52–62 of G20: Make sure your own actions reduce risks to health and safety. This section will briefly summarise the impacts this legislation will have on your working practices.

- **Health and Safety at Work Act** – clean up spillages, report slippery surfaces, report/remove obstacles, provide good all-round access to trolleys and equipment, clean, sterilise/disinfect tools, equipment and work surfaces
- **COSHH** – replace the lids of product containers, provide ventilation for vapour and dust, avoid exposure to chemicals and use them correctly
- **Electricity at Work Act** – visual check of equipment, ensure no trailing wires, carry out regular PAT testing
- **RIDDOR** – employer must keep an accident book, and report accidents or diseases (e.g. HIV, Hepatitis B)
- **Personal Protective Equipment at Work Act** – avoid latex, use powdered gloves taking precautions to avoid dermatitis.

In addition to these key pieces of legislation, your salon should also have policies on the following:

- **Storage Handling Use and Disposal (SHUD)** – sharps box, check end date/packaging of products, store away from heat, damp and direct sunlight, dispose of contaminated waste in a closed-top bin, follow relevant manufacturer's instructions.
- **Manual Handling** – focus on moving stock correctly, lift safely, working at heights, ensure posture and deportment (balance weight, preserve back, prevent slouching) are both correct
- **Liability Insurance** – covers employers, the public and provides professional indemnity
- Smoking
- Eating and drinking
- Drugs in the salon
- Personal hygiene.

Your salon must follow local byelaws (set by the council) and codes of conduct, have a clear risk assessment policy and manage health and safety at work.

Task 2

Understanding the reasons behind the rules and regulations of the salon will help you to remember to observe them. Think about why health and safety guidance is necessary.

A worksheet is provided on the website to help you complete this task.

Importance of personal presentation and reflecting a professional image within the hair industry

Due to the nature of the work you will carry out as a professional it is essential for you to understand the importance of personal presentation within the hairdressing industry. It is very important that you present a professional image to reflect the highly fashion-conscious industry hairdressing is. Your image will help to shape the client's first impressions of you, and will affect how they are likely to think about you and your work. How would you feel if your first impression of a salon was to be greeted by a stylist who looked as though they had not made any effort with their own hair for their day at work?

Your personal presentation promotes both you as a person and also the salon where you are working. It can help to increase business opportunities, the salon's income and your own commission, making you a 'walking advert' for the salon. Looking professional also positively promotes your personal enthusiasm and motivation for the job. Feeling good about the way you look also boosts your self-esteem and will increase your client's trust and confidence in your ability as a professional. This in turn will increase your clientele.

It is also important that you are friendly to clients and present yourself as approachable and cooperative, helping clients to resolve any problems. Clear communication, being easy to talk to while keeping a professional attitude in consultations will promote a trusting and loyal relationship with clients.

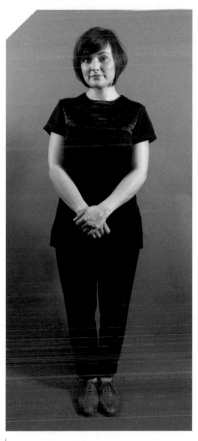

Promoting a professional image

Working in the hair industry

Developing and promoting your own professional image within the hair industry

However, it isn't just about looking and feeling good. There are other ways of promoting a professional image which often take you out of your comfort zone! This can include activities such as taking part in a competition or exhibition work and organising or volunteering your skills at hair or fashion shows or charity events. Even activities that involve sharing good practice within the team at the salon like demonstrating or cascading skills and techniques to other members of your team can help you to develop personally through building your confidence.

Self-development is all about recognising your strengths and weaknesses and working hard to improve on areas that require development. This can be addressed by the appraisal process or work reviews which could include constructive feedback from your line manager or the salon owner/trainer. Other forms of measuring developmental progress include the completion of individual learning/development plans which contain targets, and developmental actions such as attending practical seminars, training sessions or courses to improve your weaker areas or to address agreed developmental targets.

Fact or fiction?

Is this statement fact or fiction?

Self-development is important for you only, not your employer.

To check your answer see page 491.

Fact or fiction?

Is this statement fact or fiction?

Your employer can decide the minimum amount they pay you per hour.

To check your answer see page 491.

Employment rights and responsibilities

It is important for you to understand what is required of you in your job role and what your working day responsibilities are. If you are not aware of your responsibilities it is unlikely you will achieve what your boss expects of you. To ensure you understand what is expected of you by your employer you must be aware of what is contained within your contract of employment and job description.

There are lots of rules and regulations that employers have to adhere to. The chapter Employment awareness in the hair and beauty sector (see page 27) gives a full explanation of these requirements.

Safe working environment

Please refer to pages 45–75 of G20 to ensure you are aware of your responsibilities to work safely ensuring you meet salon and legal requirements. Some of the legislation that affects those working in the hair industry includes:

- Health and Safety at Work Act
- Manual Handling Operations Regulations 1992
- COSHH 1992
- Electricity at Work Act 1989
- RIDDOR 1995
- Data Protection Act 1998
- Consumer Protection Act 1987
- Cosmetic Products (Safety) Regulations 1996
- Trade Descriptions Act 1968
- Sale of Goods Act 1979
- Supply of Goods Act 1994
- Employers' Liability (Compulsory Insurance) 1969
- Equal Opportunities Act
- Discrimination Acts
- Working Time Regulations
- National Minimum Wage
- Employment Rights Act
- Employment Act

Salon life

Getting out of my comfort zone

Nanami's story

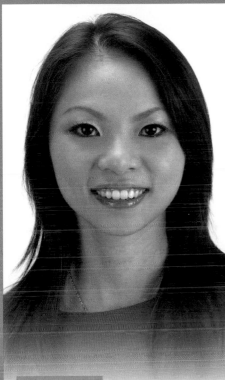

When my boss sent me to London for a training session I was really pleased that he felt I was worth investing in and this gave me a real feel-good factor. However, when he told me he wanted me to teach the rest of the salon team what I had learned I was petrified!

All my colleagues have been hairdressing for ages and knew so much more than me. As the training evening approached when I was going to show all the others the techniques I had learned, I felt sick with nerves. My boss told me not to worry so much and said there is an old saying 'You are never too old to learn.'

At the training evening, although I was really nervous and my hands were shaking, the rest of the team made me feel really comfortable. As I got into the session I even started to enjoy teaching the new techniques I had learned. It just goes to show that even though my colleagues were much more experienced than me, they were interested in what I had to say and they all said they learned something new, enjoyed the session and that I did well.

I feel I have more confidence now and would do it again if asked as I actually enjoyed getting out of my comfort zone – even though I wouldn't have chosen to!

Working in the hair industry

Top tips

- If you feel nervous when you have to speak in front of an audience, take a few deep breaths and imagine that you are just chatting to your friends. Adding humour to your presentation will help you to feel relaxed.
- Before your presentation, imagine that the audience will really enjoy listening to you and will give you positive feedback. Focusing on a positive outcome will make you more likely to succeed.

Ask the expert

Q *How should I prepare for a presentation at a training evening?*

A Write clear notes on what you want to say. Organise the information into brief bullet points and write them on small note cards to take into the presentation room with you. This should help you to feel confident that you will not forget what you had planned to say, but also stop you from staring down at a piece of paper. Practise with a friend several times before the training evening, particularly focusing on keeping eye contact and remembering to smile. The more familiar you are with your material, the more relaxed you will be.

24

Check your knowledge

The following questions will help you to check your understanding of this unit. The answers can be found on page 491.

1 What sorts of things would you see at a hairdressing exhibition?

_____

_____

_____

_____

2 What are Wella, L'Oréal, Schwarzkopf, Goldwell and Tigi types of?

_____

3 State the variety of working patterns in the hairdressing industry.

_____

_____

4 What does CPD stand for?

_____

5 What does COSHH stand for?

_____

6 Why is it important for you to understand what is required of you in your job role and what your working day responsibilities are?

_____

_____

_____

_____

7 Where should all your job responsibilities be recorded?

_____

8 During which processes should your strengths and weaknesses be reviewed?

_____

9 What regulation states how long you can work before you must have a break?

_____

10 What regulation states the least amount employers can pay their staff?

_____

Getting ready for assessment

You will be assessed using a combination of assessment methods, as described below. Remember that within each of the services you carry out with a client, you will cover different units. For example, when carrying out a shampooing and conditioning or treating service (GH8), you will also have to be aware of health and safety (G20) and advise and consult with clients (G7). If you are not sure what you have covered in your service, always ask your assessor or supervisor for advice.

	NVQ	VRQ
Credit value	N/A	4
Guided Learning Hours	N/A	35

	VRQ
Practical demonstrations, to be observed by assessor	VTCT – This unit will be internally assessed. You will be guided by your tutor and assessor on how to achieve the unit's outcomes. You must demonstrate competent performance of all practical outcomes on at least three separate occasions. All outcomes and assessment criteria must be achieved (no specified range for this unit). Evidence should be gathered in the workplace or a realistic working environment. Simulation should be avoided where possible. C&G – Evidence should be gathered in a realistic working environment. Simulation is not allowed for any performance evidence in this unit.
Service timings	There are no maximum service times for this unit.
Additional evidence	VTCT – Knowledge and understanding will be assessed by internally assessed workplace performance using a variety of methods including oral questioning and portfolio of evidence. There are no mandatory written questions required for this unit. C&G – You must demonstrate that you have met the required standard for all the outcomes. Knowledge and understanding will be assessed by oral questioning.

Task mapping

When you have completed the tasks in this unit, check the table below to see which Performance Criteria (purple), Range (red), Knowledge (green) and Key Skills (blue) you have covered within Unit G4 to use as additional evidence within your portfolio. Information about which Functional Skills you have covered is available on the website.

Task and page reference	Mapping to Performance Criteria, Range, Knowledge and Key Skills
1 (page 17)	Performance Criteria: 1a Range: N/A Knowledge: 1b, 1c, 1d Key Skills: N/A
2 (page 20)	Performance Criteria: N/A Range: N/A Knowledge: 2a, 2b, 2c Key Skills: N/A

Employment awareness in the hair and beauty sector

What you will learn:

- **How to explore hair and beauty organisations**
- **How to explore the hair and beauty sector**
- **Employment rights and responsibilities in the hair and beauty sector**

Legislation

Laws.

Introduction

This unit aims to prepare you for a career in the hair and beauty sector. It will give you an understanding of your employment rights and responsibilities in the organisation where you work and in the hair and beauty sector. By understanding the breadth of employment rights and responsibilities you will have the knowledge and skills to allow your full potential to develop.

Throughout this unit you will be required to progress as an independent learner, taking responsibility for your own development whilst working in the hairdressing industry. By achieving the outcomes in this unit you will gain knowledge of:

- the hair and beauty sector
- the many organisations within it
- the huge range of potential career and employment opportunities available to you
- the **legislation** relating to our industry.

Exploring hair and beauty organisations

In this section you will learn about:

- the structure of your organisation and the lines of reporting
- the key aims and objectives of your organisation
- your contribution to your organisation's aims and objectives
- the opportunities for entry, professional development and progression within your organisation.

The structure of your organisation and the lines of reporting

Hierarchy

A system or structure in which the members of an organisation are ranked from the person who holds the highest position of authority to the person who has the lowest.

It is important that you understand the **hierarchy** of your salon to enable you to approach the correct member of the team with any specific queries. Your employer has the ultimate responsibility for you and the rest of their employees. With that responsibility come strict rules and regulations which they must follow. However, not all salon owners are qualified in the hair and beauty sector so they may devolve the day-to-day running of their salon to a manager. Larger companies may have an organisational chart to show the different levels of management and their responsibility for different parts of the organisation.

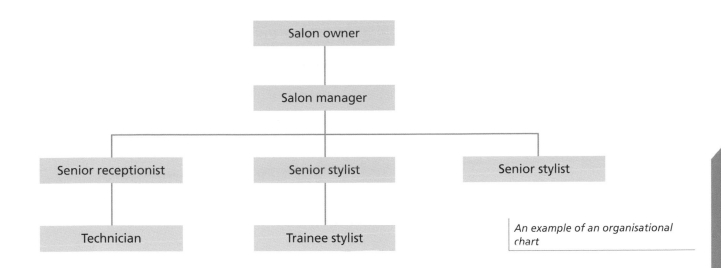

An example of an organisational chart

Staffing and organisation

Task 1

Create an organisational chart which shows the hierarchy within your salon. Write down the correct members of staff that you would go to with any queries to show your knowledge of lines of reporting. Keep this in your portfolio of evidence

The key aims and objectives of your organisation

Key aims

All organisations have a key **aim** which is more easily described as the most important purpose or intention of the organisation. For some it will be to attract more clients to ensure the business makes as much profit as possible. For others it will be to become the first choice of salon in the local area. For new salon owners it may be to improve their local reputation. Some larger organisations will have a mission statement or core values.

Targets

Having specific **targets** helps a business measure its success or define the areas the business needs to improve. Your salon's targets could include increasing the amount of clients who come to the salon over a specific period of time or for a specific service (especially if it is a new service which the salon has just launched). The target for your salon could simply be to ensure all clients receive excellent and consistent customer service which will result in customer satisfaction and a good reputation. Other targets could include increasing retail sales, financial growth or reducing staff turnover.

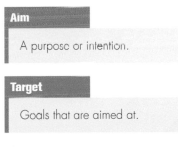

Aim

A purpose or intention.

Target

Goals that are aimed at.

Job description

Written statement that describes all the duties and responsibilities which together make up a particular job.

Appraisal

A process where your progress is reviewed by your manager. An opportunity to celebrate your strengths (your best personal and professional skills and attributes) and identify areas for improvement.

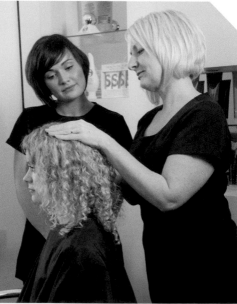

Mentoring aids improvement

Your contribution to your organisation's aims and objectives

It is vital for you to understand the part you are expected to play to help your salon meet its aims and objectives. If you do not know what is expected of you, how can you ever achieve this?

Job objectives

When salons are recruiting for new staff they can advertise internally and/or externally. Whichever type of advert is used, the job role is officially described within a **job description**. The job description should state everything that is expected of the person taking up this job role, including:

- duties
- responsibilities
- most important contributions and outcomes needed from the job role
- required qualifications
- lines of reporting, e.g. specified line manager.

Once you know exactly what is expected of you in your job role you can then set yourself personal targets. These should be a mixture of personal goals and your salon's organisational aims. For example, if your salon has started to offer a new service, your personal target could be to complete the training necessary to offer this new service. This will link with your salon's objectives to offer this new service to as many clients as possible.

Task 2

Write down the objectives of your job role.

What is your long-term goal?

Performance evaluation and development

Your manager will help you evaluate your performance at work by giving you regular work-related reviews or **appraisals**.

An appraisal involves a discussion of your performance to help your development as an individual and as an employee. It will also benefit your employer.

It is important to react in a positive way to any feedback or review. Nobody likes criticism, but it is important to listen carefully to what is being said. Try to view this as constructive criticism which will make you a better stylist if you embrace these comments; listen to how you can improve and develop by acting upon them.

Appraisal will lead to you setting personal goals and targets in negotiation with your manager. This can include staff development opportunities, work experience, job shadowing and mentoring opportunities.

For more information on appraisal see G8 Develop and maintain your effectiveness at work, page 157.

Assisting the evaluation and development of your own work

Before your appraisal you should spend some time evaluating your current duties. You can identify what is going well and whether any additional support is needed from your employer to help improve your work performance. You can then discuss this with your manager during your appraisal which will help to develop your personal action plan for the future.

The opportunities for entry, professional development and progression within your organisation

Continuing Professional Development

The hairdressing industry is extremely fast-moving and exciting due to continual developments in new products, techniques and equipment. Therefore, it is important to keep up to date with current trends and technological developments within our industry so you can continue to offer expert guidance and up-to-date services to your clients.

The personal benefits of keeping up to date include maintaining the currency of your skills and knowledge, improved career progression and opportunities, meeting professional requirements and improving your skills base, which enhances your personal development portfolio. Benefits to your salon include enhanced employee performance, improved standards and services offered by the salon and, as a result, improved customer satisfaction and profits.

Induction

Before you first start work at a salon you should attend an induction session. This will give you all the information you will need when you are working for the company. This should include a tour of the salon where you are introduced to the other members of the team who will be your new colleagues.

During this session you will also be informed about many areas of the new job including the terms of the employment you have accepted. These will include sickness and absence rules and procedures, health and safety guidance, salon amenities, welfare, first aid information, administration and the IT facilities available to you.

Some employers also assign a mentor to new members of staff. He or she will be an experienced member of the team with whom you can discuss any queries or problems.

Training and development

All good salons offer their employees ongoing training to facilitate personal progression and build salon business.

Product companies such as Wella, L'Oréal and Schwarzkopf offer training opportunities. These will either be internal training at the salon or external training at a larger venue, such as a college, to promote training and the correct use of their new products and techniques.

Apprentices should also be given information about their college/training day and their salon's in-house training session/evening as this is a requirement of the Apprenticeship programme.

Continuing Professional Development (CPD)

Ongoing personal training which allows you to keep up to date with techniques and new trends within the hairdressing industry.

31

Employment awareness in the hair and beauty sector

Task 3

What training and development do you receive in your salon and when does this take place? A worksheet for this task is provided on the website for you to complete and add to your portfolio.

Career opportunities and progression

Most salons have a hierarchical structure in place so it is possible to apply for internal promotion opportunities when they occur.

If you aspire to promotion it is important to prove that you are worthy of a higher position where newer members of the team will look up to you. Your employer will look favourably on you for internal promotion if you have shown an interest in a more senior position. You could do this by asking to shadow senior colleagues to help you understand what is involved in their job roles.

To be successful for any type of promotion opportunity you will need to prove you have gained the qualifications and experience required before you can enter the application process.

Fact or fiction?

Is this statement fact or fiction?

To be successful working in the hairdressing industry you need to enjoy working with others.

To check your answer see page 491.

Task 4

What career progression is available in your salon?

- What are the key factors that help people progress?
- What career pathways are available to you?
- If you decided to change your career, what skills have you got that would be transferable?

A worksheet for this task is provided on the website for you to complete and add to your portfolio.

Exploring the hair and beauty sector

In this section you will learn about:

- the diverse nature of the hair and beauty sector
- the key features of the industry in which you work
- employment and career opportunities in the industry in which you work.

The diverse nature of the hair and beauty sector

It is important for you to have an understanding of the many and varied types of organisations within the hairdressing industry. This will help you to recognise the opportunities available to you for future career options.

Some of the sources which will help you to investigate career options can be found on the internet, including the website of our industry's Sector Skills Body, the Hair and Beauty Industry Authority (**HABIA**). You could also visit the websites of the hairdressing awarding organisations such as VTCT, City & Guilds and Edexcel.

Read magazines and industry publications, including trade journals such as the *Hairdressers Journal International* which hosts a huge source of information on high-profile salons, advertisements for new products, wholesalers, training opportunities, job vacancies and how to become part of our industry's professional membership organisations.

The internet is also a good source of information on your local further education colleges, independent training schools and local training providers.

HABIA

Hair and Beauty Industry Authority – the standards-setting body for hairdressing, beauty, barbering, African-type hair, nails and spa qualifications.

Fact or fiction?

Is this statement fact or fiction?

The Hairdressers Journal International *is a trade magazine containing a huge amount of industry information.*

To check your answer see page 491.

Size and scope

HABIA has produced the following industry statistics. This information presents a snapshot of the hair, beauty, nails and spa sector in the UK. It is the most current and up-to-date information available (November 2008).

Industry statistics

All the information and statistics shown in the table below are credited to HABIA.

Industry size and turnover:	Statistic
Annual turnover	£5.25 billion (2006 – not including spas)
Total employment	245,795 (2007) = 0.87% of the total UK workforce
Hair salons	35,704
African-Caribbean hair salons	302
Barbering salons	2,967
Nail bars/technicians	1,512
Beauty salons/consultants	13,107
Beauty therapists (mobile)	947
Spas	400
Gender of employees	female 90%, male 10%

Contribution to society

Clients can enter the salon feeling negative about the way they look but, after having an expert professional service or treatment, they can leave the salon feeling like a new person. This is why the hair and beauty industry is often referred to as the 'feel-good factor' industry. The most rewarding aspect of working in the hair and beauty industry is the ability to make clients feel fabulous.

As fashion has a huge influence within the hair and beauty industry, and many clients also want to look younger, it has led to many people spending some of their disposable income in salons. Therefore the hair and beauty industries are continuing to make a positive contribution to the UK economy.

Roles of HABIA

The key objectives for Sector Skills Bodies are to:

- reduce skills gaps
- improve productivity and performance in businesses
- increase the skills and productivity of the workforce
- improve the quality of learning through Apprenticeships, higher education and National Occupational Standards
- represent industry on skills and business issues to government and its agencies
- act as a first point of contact on industry issues for the media and other organisations.

Fact or fiction?

Is this statement fact or fiction?

HABIA is the hairdressing industry's awarding organisation.

To check your answer see page 491.

Awarding organisation

An organisation that issues an educational award, following formal assessment, including organisations that certify professional competence.

The main industries that make up the hair and beauty sector

The hair and beauty sector is made up of several industries including hairdressing, barbering, African-type hairdressing and barbering, nail services, beauty therapy and spa therapy.

The key features of the hair and beauty industry

The composition of your industry

The hair and beauty industry is made up of many different organisations including public, private and voluntary organisations; representative, regulatory and professional bodies; trade unions; and user and consumer groups.

The size of the hair and beauty industry in terms of employment

Please refer to the table on page 33 for information and statistics.

Principles, values or codes of practice

Within our industry we are heavily influenced by culture, media and religious beliefs and therefore we may need to adapt our services to ensure we meet individual needs.

Codes of practice provide us with industry-endorsed guidance to encourage good practice.

Key organisations and their roles

As listed above, there are many key organisations, each with vital roles within the hair and beauty industry. They provide services and consumer support and protection.

Vital to the professionalism of our industry is high-quality, standardised education and training. This is robustly monitored by awarding organisations who award qualifications when the set standards have been achieved.

It is also important to have the necessary government bodies, responsible for research, setting industry standards, law enforcement and inspection.

Task 5

Research key organisations that link with the hairdressing and beauty industry. Complete a mind map of these organisations showing how they link to the hairdressing and beauty industry.

State their roles within the hair and beauty industry.

Issues of public concern

The standard of the services you provide is not only vital to continue to generate salon income but also to meet health, safety and hygiene standards.

It is important to provide clients with quality services which are carried out with the highest professionalism possible, using professional-quality products.

The environment in which services and treatments are provided must be safe and have a pleasant atmosphere with enough privacy to maintain client dignity.

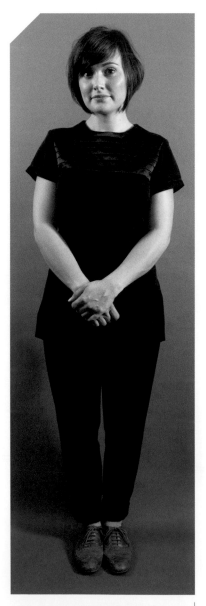

Presenting a professional image

Employment and career opportunities in the industry in which you work

Sources of information

Refer to page 41 for good sources of information when researching the different organisations with the hairdressing industry.

You should also carry out your research in person and seek career guidance from careers advisers and job centres.

Visit industry exhibitions and shows to witness up-to-date techniques and demonstrations of new products by celebrity and well-known industry professionals.

Apply for work experience with local salons, spas and health resorts. This will give you valuable opportunities to make informed decisions about where you would like to work.

Attend local open evenings or days at organisations within the industry. This will provide you with word-of mouth opportunities to learn more about the potential employment prospects within your area

Simple everyday habits such as reading newspapers and watching TV will also keep you up to date with industry trends including celebrity-endorsed products marketed by industry suppliers and manufacturers.

Main job roles and career pathways

The occupational roles within the hairdressing industry are many and varied.

Most professionals start at the bottom as a shampooist, salon junior or trainee apprentice and work their way up the career ladder once they are qualified by becoming a junior stylist. Once you have gained experience of working with clients, there is the opportunity to progress to senior stylist or artistic director status.

However, there are many alternative career paths to this typical route. See pages 17–19 for some ideas.

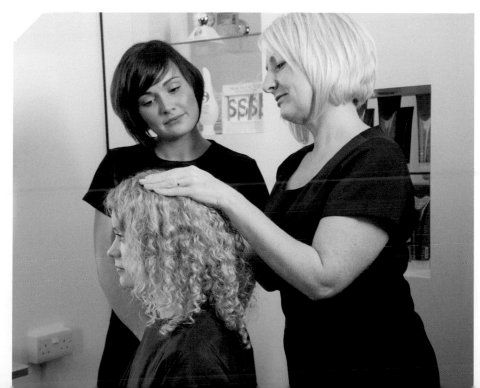

A salon junior learns from the artistic director

Progression and transferring between sectors

As much of our industry is client-focused, you will acquire many transferable client care and communication skills. These are the foundation or basis of many other employment opportunities and can be used in a variety of other sectors and industries.

Other transferable skills and qualities acquired while working in the hairdressing industry include organisational skills, leadership skills, honesty, motivation and team-working skills. These interpersonal skills and personal qualities are transferable across many industries.

Employment rights and responsibilities in the hair and beauty sector

In this section you will learn about:

- your employment rights and responsibilities under the law
- documents relevant to your employment in the hair and beauty sector
- key employment procedures at work and information sources.

Your rights and responsibilities under the law

It is important for you to understand what is required of you in your job role and what your working day responsibilities are. If you are not aware of your responsibilities it is likely you will not fulfil what your boss expects of you.

Contracts of employment

To ensure you understand what is expected of you by your employer you must be aware of what is contained within your **contract of employment** and job description.

Your employment contract doesn't have to be in writing. However, you are entitled to a written statement of your main employment terms within two months of starting work.

It should contain:

- your name and your employer's name
- your job title or a brief job description
- the date when your employment began
- your pay rate and when you will be paid
- your hours of work
- your holiday entitlement
- where you will be working (if you are based in more than one place it should say this along with your employer's address)
- details of sick pay arrangements
- information about notice periods
- information about disciplinary and grievance procedures
- any collective agreements that affect your employment terms or conditions
- details of pensions and pension schemes
- how long your employment is expected to continue (if you are not a permanent employee) or the date your employment will end (if you are a fixed-term worker).

Top tips

Know your rights as an employee. If you are not sure whether you are being treated fairly by your employer, check out your rights on the following government website: www.direct.gov.uk.

Contract of employment

An agreement between an employer and an employee which sets out their employment rights, responsibilities and duties. These are called the 'terms' of the contract.

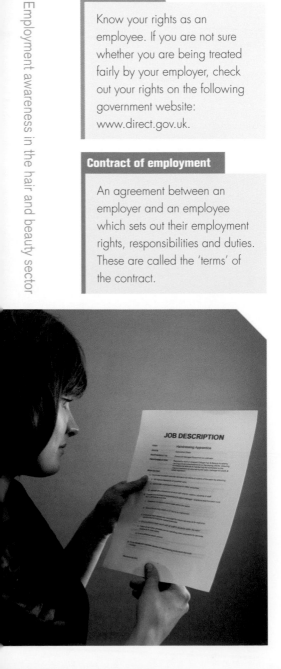

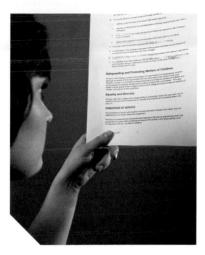

Make sure you read and check the conditions of your contract of employment thoroughly before signing it. Once you and your employer have signed this it becomes a legally binding contract.

Equality and diversity legislation

The Equality Act is the most significant piece of equality legislation to be introduced for many years. It is there to strengthen protection, advance equally and simplify the law. Ninety per cent of the Act came into force on 1 October 2010. The rest of it includes Public Sector Equality Duty (PSED) which came into effect in April 2011. The Equality Act brings together, and significantly adds to and strengthens, a number of previous existing pieces of legislation, including race and disability legislation. One of the key changes is that it extends protection to encompass:

- age
- disability
- gender reassignment
- marriage and civil partnership
- pregnancy and maternity
- race
- religion or belief
- gender
- sexual orientation.

The Act also makes explicit the concept of 'dual discrimination', where someone may be discriminated against or treated unfairly on the basis of a combination of two or more of the protected characteristics. For example, someone might feel they are being discriminated against because they are over 50 and female.

The main provisions which are of interest to local government are contained within the PSED, which came into effect in April 2011. Key aspects of the PSED are:

- a general duty to: (i) eliminate discrimination, harassment and victimisation; (ii) advance equality of opportunity; and (iii) foster good relations
- specific duties to: publish data; assess impact; set equality objectives; report progress at least annually
- new transparency on data to drive culture change
- duty applies to listed public bodies and those discharging public functions (in respect of those functions), for example, third-sector bodies when discharging public functions
- clarification that procurement and commissioning can be used to drive equality.

Working hours

Adult workers cannot be forced to work more than 48 hours a week on average – this is normally averaged over 17 weeks. You can work more than 48 hours in one week, as long as the average over 17 weeks is less than 48 hours per week.

Your working week is not covered by the working time limits if you have a job:

- where you can choose freely how long you will work (e.g. a managing executive)
- in the armed forces, emergency services and police
- as a domestic servant in private houses (in some circumstances)
- as a sea transport worker, a mobile worker on inland waterways or a lake transport worker on board sea-going fishing vessels.

Holiday entitlement

There is a minimum right to paid holiday, but your employer may offer more than this. The main things you should know about holiday rights are that:

- you are entitled to a minimum of 5.6 weeks of paid annual leave — 28 days for someone working five days a week
- part-time workers are entitled to the same level of holiday pro rata (so 5.6 times your usual working week, e.g. 22.4 days for someone working four days a week)
- you start building up holiday allowance as soon as you start work
- your employer can control when you take your holiday
- you get paid your normal pay for your holiday
- when you finish a job, you get paid for any holiday you have not taken
- bank and public holidays can be included in your entitlement
- you continue to be entitled to your holiday leave throughout your ordinary and additional maternity leave and paternity and adoption leave.

Sickness absence and sickness pay

If you are absent from work you should try to speak to your manager within an hour of your normal start time. You should let your manager know about your illness and when you are likely to return to work. If you have been off work sick for seven days or less your employer can ask you to confirm that you've been ill. You can do this by filling in a form yourself when you return to work. This is called self-certification.

Many employers have their own self-certification forms. If your employer doesn't have their own form, they may use an Employee's Statement of Sickness form instead.

If you have been off work sick for more than seven days you will need to get a Statement of Fitness to Work (fit note) from your GP or the doctor who treated you in hospital.

The fit note allows your doctor to provide you with more information on how your condition affects your ability to work. It may suggest ways in which you can return to work, for example, changes to your working hours or different duties for a temporary period of time. This will help your employer to understand how they might be able to help you return to work sooner. You and your employer will be able to talk about how this will benefit your return to work.

Data protection

Refer to page 59 of G20 for information on data protection legislation.

Fact or fiction?

Is this statement fact or fiction?

RIDDOR stands for Reporting of Injuries, Diseases and Dangerous Occurrences Regulations.

To check your answer see page 491.

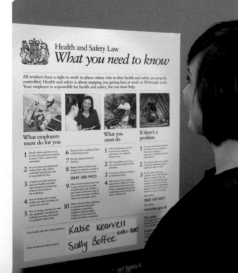

Rights and responsibilities of the employer

Refer to page 49 of G20 for information on your employer's rights and responsibilities.

Legal health and safety requirements

Refer to page 52 of G20 for information on health and safety legislation or visit the following web link:
www.direct.gov.uk/en/Employment/HealthAndSafetyAtWork/index.htm.

Implications

If you do not follow health and safety legal requirements for your job role there could be serious consequences.

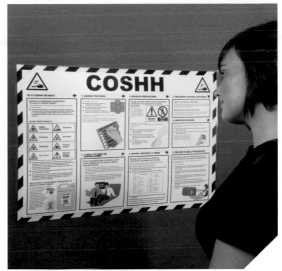

The documents relevant to your employment in the hair and beauty sector

The main terms and conditions of a contract of employment

The terms and conditions of your employment are stated in your contract of employment and this is what you must legally adhere to. That is why it is important to agree these terms with your employer before you sign any legally binding documents.

Job description

The purpose of your job description is to clarify individual roles and responsibilities within your organisation. The contents of your job description should state your job title, your accountability, summarise your job role, location of work, your duties, hours of work and your salary and benefits.

Personnel records

Personnel records contain your personal details, next of kin details, references, application details, payroll information, training records and appraisal forms. They will also include information of your salary/wages, holiday and sickness records and any CRB checks.

Task 6

Find out what type of personnel records your employer keeps for you. Ask how they are updated.

Top tips

If you decide to become a freelance stylist you must get the correct public liability insurance policy to cover any claims that might be made against you.

Fact or fiction?

Is this statement fact or fiction?

COSHH stands for Control of Substances Hazardous to Hands.

To check your answer see page 491.

Employment awareness in the hair and beauty sector

Employment awareness in the hair and beauty sector

Fact or fiction?

Is this statement fact or fiction?

Employers must pay their staff at or above the levels of the National Minimum Wage.

To check your answer see page 491.

A sample payslip

Pay slips/statement of earnings

There are legal requirements relating to the records that employers must keep of their employees' pay. They must record the employee's name, tax code, National Insurance (NI) contributions, gross pay, net pay, PAYE, P60, P45, tax code, pension scheme contributions, pay reference and payment dates.

Pay Statement

Employee Name	Pay date	Tax code
A. N. Other	31/02/2012	522L

Payments		Deductions		Total	
Basic pay	£1041.50	Tax	£149.50	Gross Pay	£1041.50
		National Insurance	£ 76.25	Deductions	£ 297.75
		Pension	£ 66.00		
Total pay	£1041.50	Total deductions	£291.75	NET pay	£ 749.75

Key employment procedures at work and information sources

Taking time off

When you enter into a contract of employment you are entitled to a specific amount of annual leave. You will need to negotiate when you take your holidays/leave with your employer to ensure it fits in with the business – you and your colleagues cannot all take leave at the same time or the business will not survive. Some employers allow time off in lieu (TOIL) when you have worked extra hours – they will allow you to take back the extra time you have worked at their discretion. There are other forms of entitlement to leave/holiday depending on your circumstances including maternity/ paternity/adoption leave, time off for dependants, jury service and public duties.

Grievance procedures

Grievances are concerns, problems or complaints that employees raise with their employer. There is no legally binding process that you and your employer must follow when raising or handling a grievance at work. However, there are some principles you and your employer should observe.

Discrimination or bullying procedures

Bullying at work is when someone tries to intimidate another worker, often in front of colleagues. It is usually, though not always, done to someone in a less senior position. It is similar to harassment, which is where someone's behaviour is offensive. For example, making sexual comments, or abusing someone's race, religion or sexual orientation.

You cannot make a legal claim directly about bullying, but complaints can be made under laws covering discrimination and harassment.

41

> ## Task 7
>
> You shouldn't have to put up with bullying at work. Find out more about what bullying is and what you can do to stop it if you think it is happening to you. Write this down and keep it in your portfolio of evidence.

Disciplinary procedures

Employers use disciplinary procedures to tell employees that their performance or conduct is not up to the expected standard and to encourage improvement.

A disciplinary procedure is a way that your employer can tell you something is wrong. It allows them to explain clearly what improvement is needed and should give you an opportunity to explain your side of the situation. It can lead to disciplinary action, including dismissal in more serious cases.

Before taking formal disciplinary action or dismissing you, your employer may try to raise the matter with you informally. This is often a good way of resolving a problem quickly. Sometimes the problem may be the result of a misunderstanding, and you may be able to provide evidence to clarify the issue.

Your employer can decide to go directly to their formal disciplinary or dismissal procedures.

Sources of information and advice

There are many avenues to explore to find information and advice about work-related issues. You should approach your supervisor, line manager or senior manager with any queries if you cannot find the answers in your staff handbook.

If you work for a large company you may have a Human Resources department which will guide you in company policy and procedures. If you work for a small organisation you may need to contact external agencies to get the information you require.

The Citizens Advice Bureau and ACAS (Advisory, Conciliation and Arbitration Service) are helpful organisations. You can also visit useful websites such as Directgov.

Salon life

Practice makes perfect!

Evie's story

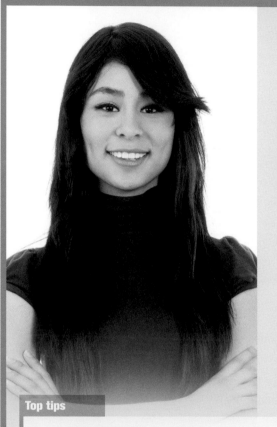

After I completed my apprenticeship I started work as a salon junior in a popular city centre salon. I love my job as I have now got the opportunity to put into practice the skills I learned whilst working towards my apprenticeship. I knew that I would improve my hairdressing skills by working closely with stylists and by starting to work on paying clients. I was surprised that our salon manager, Suzie, also wanted us to take part in special training days. When we started to use a different brand of colour she asked us to spend half a day learning about the product and practising how to use it. A representative from the company which supplied the colour talked us through the new product and showed us the technique to use for mixing and applying the different tones. We then had to practise ourselves, to show we understood exactly what to do when we started using the new product. At first I didn't mix the tones correctly so, rather than the vibrant pink it was meant to be, it looked like brown sludge! However, the rep talked me through how to do it a second time and the colour looked correct. I realised that Suzie knows that spending time on training us to use new products and techniques is really important if we are to do our job well. It means that the salon can offer new products and techniques in the confidence that their staff will carry them out to the client's satisfaction.

Top tips

By taking part in training you will not only show your manager how enthusiastic you are to learn, but you can also add the training to your CV. This will help when you want to move into a more senior role.

Listen carefully to all the instructions you are given as part of your training and ask plenty of questions! This is an opportunity to practise what you will be doing before you start using a new product or techniques on a client.

Ask the expert

Q *How often will I take part in training at my salon?*

A It depends how often your salon launches new products, techniques or buys new equipment. Whenever they do this it is important that you feel comfortable about using these on clients. If you have not had special training, always ask to be shown first and to have to the opportunity to practise.

Check your knowledge

1 What does HABIA stand for?

_____

2 What is HABIA's function?

_____

3 State five personal qualities that your employer will expect you to have.

_____

4 If you decide to become a freelance stylist what must you ensure you have to protect yourself and your clients?

_____

5 What is the National Minimum Wage?

_____

6 State five things you should find in your contract of employment.

_____

_____

7 State five things you should find in your job description.

_____

_____

Getting ready for assessment

The Employment Rights and Responsibilities (ERR) qualification is taken as part of an Apprenticeship. In order to achieve this part of the Apprenticeship framework you will be taking one of the following four qualifications:

- Edexcel Level 2 Award in Work Skills for Effective Learning and Employment
- VTCT Level 2 Award in Employment Awareness in the Hair and Beauty Sector
- City & Guilds Level 2 Award in Employment and Personal Learning at Work
- ITEC Level 2 Award in Employment Awareness in the Hair and Beauty Sector.

	Edexcel	City & Guilds	ITEC	VTCT
Credit value	4	4	6	6
Guided Learning Hours	35–40	35–40	35	35

There are no maximum service times for this unit. Evidence should be gathered in the workplace or a realistic working environment. All outcomes and assessment criteria must be achieved (there is no specified range for this unit). You will be guided by your tutor and assessor on how to achieve the unit's outcomes. Knowledge and understanding will be assessed by internally assessed workplace performance using a variety of methods including oral questioning and portfolio of evidence.

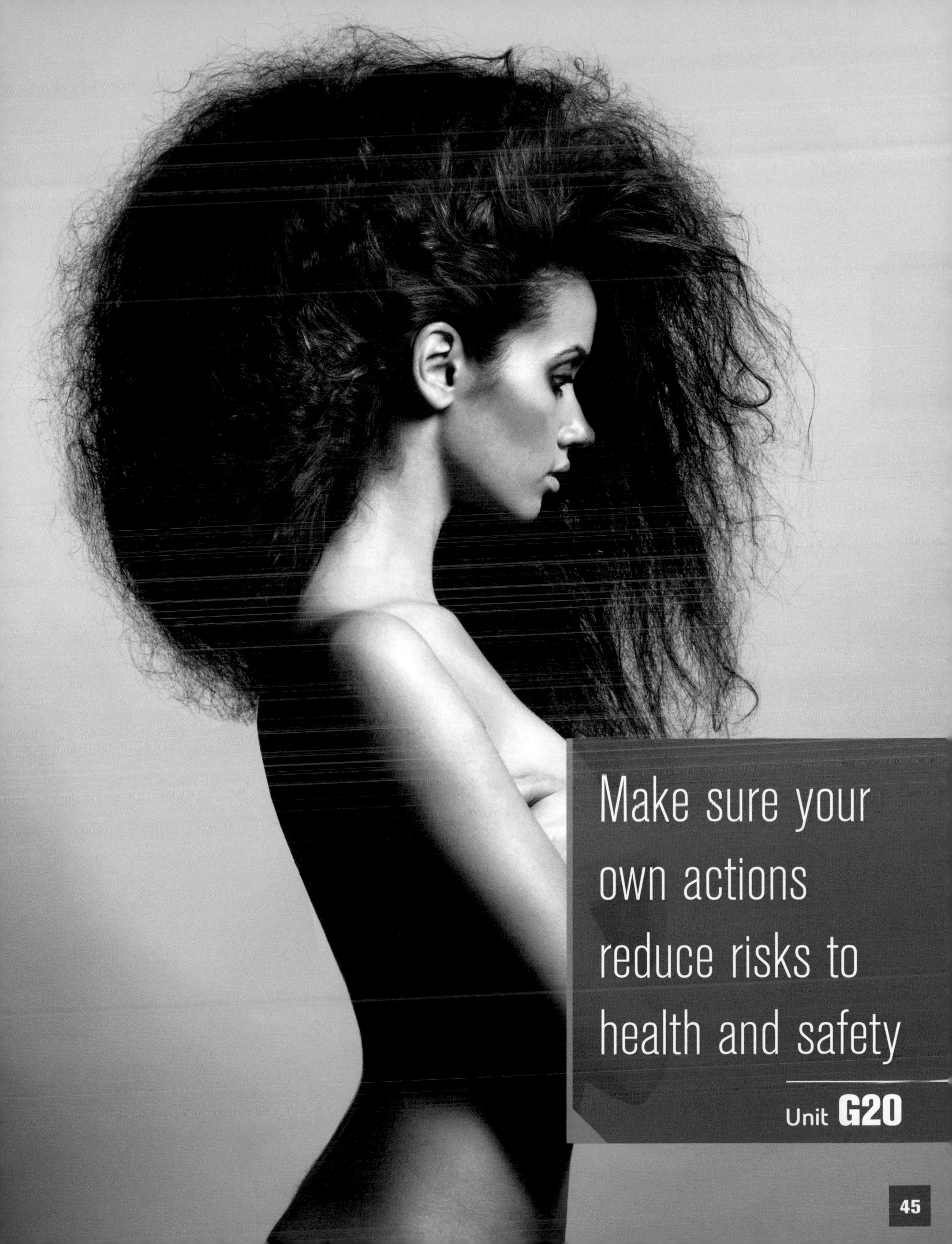

Make sure your own actions reduce risks to health and safety

Unit **G20**

45

Unit
G20

Make sure your own actions reduce risks to health and safety

What you will learn:

- **How to identify the hazards and evaluate the risks in your workplace**
- **How to reduce the risks to health and safety in your workplace**

Introduction

This unit is very important for your working day and focuses on the well-being of the stylist, clients, colleagues and all other visitors to the salon. It is about how you can help to make your workplace a safe, secure environment for everyone.

You must consider the health and safety of the client every time you carry out a service. Whether in the workplace or a college/training institution, you have a responsibility to follow health and safety legislation. To help you, the most important aspects of health and safety laws are explained in this unit. If you ignore health and safety procedures when carrying out an assessment or service, at best the assessment will not be deemed competent; at worst your actions could result in injury or damage, for which you may be legally responsible.

The health and safety laws, regulations and considerations covered in this unit apply to every other unit, so you will be constantly referring back to this information. Health and safety guidance which relates to specific procedures, for example colouring or perming, are covered within the relevant units.

Hazard

Something with the potential to cause harm.

Risk

The likelihood of a hazard actually causing harm.

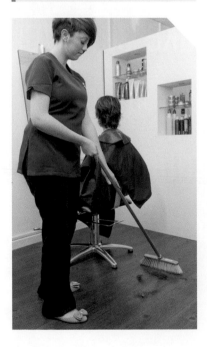

How to identify the hazards and evaluate the risks in your workplace

In this section you will learn about your responsibilities in relation to potential **hazards** in the salon and how you should deal with them. In some cases you will be able to deal with a hazard yourself, but in others you may need to ask the advice of a more qualified member of staff. In these instances you need to know who to approach. You will also need to know your responsibilities for implementing the health and safety policies used in your salon — if you do not know what they are, how can you make sure you follow them?

Almost anything can be a hazard, but it may or may not become a **risk**. For example, a trailing lead from a hairdryer is a hazard. If it is trailing across the path of a client, it has a risk of someone tripping over it; if it is safely out of the path of the client, the risk is much less.

Hairdressing products, such as hydrogen peroxide, stored in the salon are hazards and because they are toxic and flammable may present a risk. However, if they are kept in a properly designed secure storage area and handled by trained stylists, the risk is much less than if they are left out in a busy workshop for anyone to use — or misuse.

Removal of hair cuttings will minimise the risk of slipping for stylists and clients

Reporting and dealing with hazards

As part of personal responsibility, the stylist needs to be able to recognise whether a hazard should be dealt with immediately or if help is needed, and whether it needs to be reported to a supervisor, lecturer, technician or manager.

It is important to be able to identify hazards before they become risks and decide what **controls** should be in place. If they become risks, it is essential to know how to deal with them.

Control

The means by which risks identified are eliminated or reduced to acceptable levels.

47

Unit

G20

Make sure your own actions reduce risks to health and safety

Hazard	How to avoid risk	When referral may be necessary
Machinery or equipment (when using or maintaining)	Make sure machinery and equipment are in good working order. Electrical equipment should be tested for safety every six months and all staff must be adequately trained to use it.	If equipment is faulty, you must make sure all staff are aware of it (each salon will have its own procedure for reporting faulty equipment or machinery). Refer to a manager if the machinery or equipment is vital to the smooth running of the salon, as he or she will need to authorise its repair or the purchase of a replacement.
A spillage	Take care when mixing, pouring and filling.	If spillage material is **corrosive** or an irritant.
Slippery floors resulting from staff not following salon rules for tidying the salon	Make others aware by blocking the area with a chair to prevent an accident. Sweep up powder spills and mop up spills of liquids; refer to **COSHH** sheets for correct method.	If acid, grease or polish are spilt.
Waste materials	Make sure all staff follow COSHH sheets and manufacturers' instructions when disposing of chemical products, **sharps** and infected waste (for example, cut hair infested with head lice).	If staff are not following specific guidelines; when the skin is pierced by used sharps; when infected waste is left.

Identifying risks

Risk assessment sheets

Hairdressing products also require a risk assessment sheet. Usually, most salons keep these sheets together in a folder for easy access.

Risk assessment sheets contain the following information:

- chemical composition (ingredients) of the product
- personal protective equipment (PPE) needed when using the product
- storage instructions
- handling instructions
- the hazard under COSHH
- what the product is used for
- special safety measures to follow
- disposal instructions.

Dealing with hazards and risks in the salon

Corrosive

A substance that will destroy or damage another substance when it comes into contact with it.

COSHH

Control of Substances Hazardous to Health (COSHH) Regulations 2003. These deal with how to handle, store and dispose of chemicals and products (see page 56).

Sharps

The term used in hairdressing to describe the blades used in safety razors.

Unit

G20

Make sure your own actions reduce risks to health and safety

Task 1

To help you to understand how to identify a hazard or risk and what controls need to be considered, complete the following blank risk assessment sheet within your salon or training establishment.

A worksheet for this task is provided on the website for you to complete and add to your portfolio.

CONTROL OF SUBSTANCES HAZARDOUS TO HEALTH ASSESSMENT OF RISK

Expt. Title/No Substance Process		Year	
		Course	

Substance(s) used

Hazard(s) Please tick:

Irritant		Corrosive		Harmful		Very toxic	
Oxidising		Explosive		Flammable			

Where used please tick:

Laboratory	Preparation Room	Chemical Store	Workshop	Other (specify)

By whom please tick:

Lecturer	Technician	Student	Other (specify)	

Document(s) outlining working method(s) e.g. Safety & Science Lecturers Guide etc.

Expected Hazardous By-Product(s)

	Tick	
		Irritant
		Corrosive
		Harmful
		(Very) Toxic
		Oxidising
		Explosive
		Flammable

Likely route(s) of entry:

Inhalation	Mouth	Skin contact	Eyes

Specific safety measures to be taken:

Goggles	Fume cupboard	Apron/coat	Eye-wash bottle	Good ventilation	Safety screen	Wash hands	Gloves	Respirator	Dust mask

Specified procedures for dealing with:

First Aid ST or PH	Emergency Spillage SP	Fire	

Assessor _____ Date of Assessment _____

Head of Department _____ Date of Authorisation _____

Responsibilities – who does what?

It is very important to know who to approach with a salon problem or potential
health and safety issue. All salons will have members of staff with different skills.
Some staff will be trained in first aid while others may faint at the sight of blood! As
a salon trainee, you need to know who to call if your client requires a first aider, how
to fill out the accident report book — and where to find the first aider and the accident
report book!

Task 2

How would you deal with these situations? Who would you report them to?

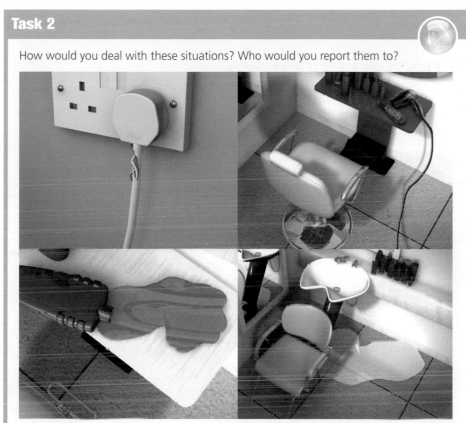

A worksheet for this task is provided on the website for you to complete and add to
your portfolio

Task 3

Find out the following information for the salon in which you work.

Name of first aider	Contact number for first aid help	Location of first aid kit	Location of accident report book	Location of risk assessment sheets

A worksheet for this task is provided on the website for you to complete and add to your portfolio.

Make sure your own actions reduce risks to health and safety

Make sure your own actions reduce risks to health and safety

Policies in your workplace

Every salon should have a set of rules and procedures for everyone to follow. These should be common knowledge for the safety and protection of all within the salon. By law, a salon has to:

- display health and safety rules and regulations on the wall in a prominent position
- display the fire evacuation procedures.

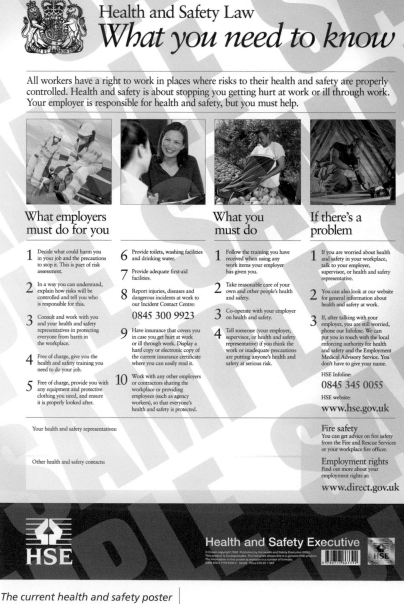

The current health and safety poster

The health and safety poster illustrated here provides bullet point guidance on the legal responsibilities of both employers and workers and what workers can do if there is a health and safety problem. The Health and Safety Executive (HSE) provides a website, (www.hse.gov.uk) where guidance and information can be found on a wide range of issues, including RIDDOR, first aid, and health and safety responsibilities. Traumatic events can be reported to the HSE by calling their infoline (0845 345 0055).

Salons will also have their own individual policies in place and it is your responsibility to follow them, so make sure you know what your salon's policies are. All salons will require employees to follow basic rules, like reading and following manufacturers' instructions. If this rule is not followed, services could go wrong, resulting in loss of clients and damage to the salon's good reputation. The salon owner is legally obliged to put into place the rules covering the health and safety of all employees and clients, and to ensure that safe practice is followed by all staff. The employee must follow these rules.

Salon policies may include:

- *Smoking* – all salons are completely non-smoking zones and clients would need to be informed of this by members of staff. You must be fully aware of the rules and enforce them if a client decides to light a cigarette.
- *Eating and drinking areas* – the preparation of food and drinks should not be in the same area as the mixing and preparation of products. This would cause an environmental health and safety issue, as many chemical products in hairdressing are **caustic** and if accidentally mixed with food or drinks would cause internal medical problems.
- *Drug policies* – remember, only fully qualified, medically trained personnel are allowed to administer drugs or medicines.
- *Salon security* – all staff will be responsible for ensuring that windows and doors are locked at the end of the day, and that money is removed from the till and stored in an overnight safe or banked.

Caustic

A substance that burns or corrodes tissue.

Task 4

Find out and write down four of your workplace policies. One of the policies should include salon security.

A worksheet for this task is provided on the website for you to complete and add to your portfolio.

Professionally, the salon will have certain standards to maintain for insurance cover to be valid. Ensuring effective health and safety in the workplace involves:

- regular training, with staff meetings to update on safety issues – this may be once a week or fortnightly; all staff will be encouraged to contribute and all staff will be expected to attend training when a new piece of electrical equipment is introduced to the salon
- giving future employees a clear outline at their initial interview as to what is expected of them (you will be made aware of the salon's fire evacuation procedures, where the accident book and first aid kit are kept, who to report to in case of an emergency, the procedures for reporting faulty equipment or hazards, where to find manufacturers' data sheets, and general health and safety within the salon)
- maintaining records of injuries or first aid treatment given (you will be given guidance on how to complete an accident report book)
- monitoring and evaluating health and safety arrangements regularly, including regular risk assessment updates and training
- providing a written health and safety booklet – this should be read and understood
- consulting the experts and being knowledgeable – ignorance is not an excuse; you should know and ask the relevant member of staff for help and guidance.

Make sure your own actions reduce risks to health and safety

How to reduce the risks to health and safety in your workplace

This section covers health and safety risks and outlines how to reduce the risks that you may come into contact with in the salon. You need to know how to carry out tasks safely following instructions and workplace requirements. You must also have a good understanding of the health and safety policies within your salon that affect your working day. This includes following manufacturers' and suppliers' instructions when using products, materials and equipment. You also have to prove that your personal presentation and conduct ensures the health and safety of yourself, your clients and colleagues.

Legal requirements (health and safety legislation)

This covers all the Acts of Parliament that relate to a business as set down by the UK government. These Acts of Parliament are being updated continually to fit into modern society, so you will find that Acts have dates after their title stating when they were updated, for example the Trade Descriptions Act 1968 (amended 1987). This means that these Acts are the law of the land and to break them or to ignore them is an offence and you will be punished. The consequences may be payment of a fine, closure of the business or imprisonment.

As well as following British law, you have to follow European law. Local government bye-laws are those decided by the Local Authority and can differ from region to region; for example, London has different local bye-laws from Birmingham.

To be fully competent in employment, it is essential that you have a sound knowledge of consumer protection and health and safety legislation. Do not worry too much about trying to remember the dates attached to the laws; concentrate more on the Acts themselves and how they protect both the stylist and the consumer — that is, the client.

Health and Safety at Work Act 1974 (HASAWA)

This requires all employers to provide systems of work that are, as is reasonably practicable, safe and without risk to health. The employer's duty is to provide:

- premises — a safe place to work
- systems and equipment
- storage and transport of substances and material
- access to the workplace exits
- good practices in the workplace
- first aid facilities and emergency plans.

The employer also has a responsibility to other persons not in employment including contractors and self-employed people.

Employer's responsibilities	Shared responsibilities	Employees' responsibilities
Planning safety and security.	Ensuring safety of the working environment.	Correct use of the systems and procedures.
Providing information about safety and security.	Cooperating to follow the law.	Reporting flaws or gaps within the system or procedure when in use.
Updating systems and procedures, in workplaces with five or more employees.		Taking reasonable care of themselves and other people affected by their work.
Ensuring the safety of themselves, other employees and visitors to the premises.		

Health and safety responsibilities

53

Unit
G20

Make sure your own actions reduce risks to health and safety

The employee has a responsibility to:

- take care during time at work to avoid personal injury
- assist the employer in meeting requirements under the Health and Safety at Work Act
- not misuse or change anything that has been provided for safety.

The Act allows various regulations to be made which control the workplace. The Act also covers self-employed persons who work alone, away from the employer's premises.

In 1992, EU directives updated legislation on health and safety management and widened the existing Acts. These came into being in 1993. There are six main areas:

- provision and use of work equipment
- manual handling operations
- workplace health, safety and welfare
- personal protective equipment at work
- health and safety (display screen equipment)
- management of health and safety at work.

Some of the EU directives are the protection of non-smokers from tobacco smoke, the provision of rest facilities for pregnant women and nursing mothers, and anti-discrimination measures.

Manual Handling Operations Regulations 1992

The Health and Safety Executive (HSE) has drawn attention to skeletal and muscular disorders caused by manual handling and lifting, repetitive strain disorders and unsuitable posture causing low back pain. The regulations require that certain measures be taken to avoid these types of injuries occurring.

Think of all the situations that may apply in the salon. For example:

- stock unpacking and storage — lifting heavy objects
- moving chairs or cutting stools used in the salon.

In each of these types of situations, you need to take action to safeguard your health.

You must also protect the health of your clients. For example, if a client is not sitting correctly in a chair, you should instruct them to ensure that their lower back is in contact with the back of the chair and their feet are flat on the floor or on a foot rest.

Top tips

For more information, go online to www.direct.gov.uk.

Make sure your own actions reduce risks to health and safety

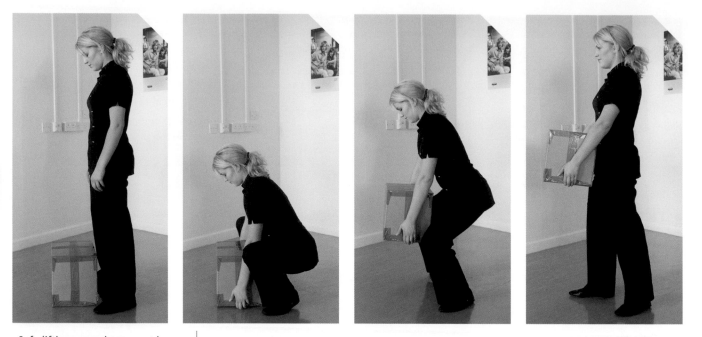

Safe lifting procedures must be observed

Top tips

Follow the golden rule: always lift with the back straight and the knees bent. If in doubt – do not lift at all!

Heat stress

The HSE draws attention to heat stress at work. The best working temperature in hairdressing salons is between 15.5 and 20°C. Humidity (the amount of moisture in the air) should be within the range of 30–70 per cent, although this will vary if your salon has a sauna or steam area. These should be in a well-ventilated area away from the main workrooms, while still being accessible to clients. There should also be sufficient air exchange and air movement, which must be increased in special circumstances, such as chemical mixing and usage.

There are different types of ventilation that may be used within the salon.

- *Mechanical ventilation* – extractor fans, which can be adjusted to various speeds.
- *Natural ventilation* – open windows are fine, but be careful of a draught on the client.
- *Air-conditioned ventilation* – passing air over filters and coolers brings about the desired condition, but of course, this is the most expensive method!

A build-up of fumes, or strong smells from chemical preparations such as perm lotions, bleaches and tints, may cause both physical and psychological problems, which affect not only clients but staff, too!

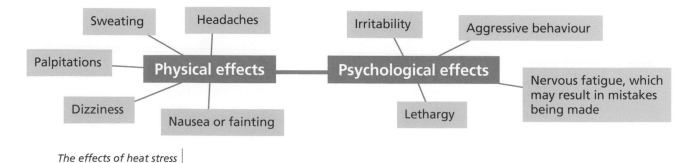

The effects of heat stress

Protective clothing and equipment

This covers both equipment and protective clothing provisions to ensure safety for all those in the workplace. The regulations also state that workplace personnel must have appropriate training in equipment use. Protective clothing ensures cleanliness, freshness and professionalism. For certain services, it may be advisable to wear extra disposable coverings. The client's clothing must also be protected.

Personal Protective Equipment at Work Regulations 1992

You are required to use and wear the appropriate protective equipment or clothing during chemical services. Protective gloves and aprons are the normal requirements for your protection and your employer should provide these for you.

Work-related contact dermatitis

The symptoms can be any of the following:

- itching
- dryness
- redness
- soreness.

In extreme cases, if the skin is excessively dry, the skin will crack, bleed and blister. Hairdressers are more susceptible to developing dermatitis because of the length of time their hands are in contact with water.

Once you have developed dermatitis the symptoms can recur at any time, so prevention is better than cure. Follow these easy steps to protect your hands and skin:

- When using chemicals make sure you wear disposable non-latex gloves.
- When shampooing, ensure you dry your hands thoroughly – especially underneath rings.
- Use a good barrier cream or moisturiser frequently during the day.
- For more advice and guidance, visit www.hse.gov.uk/skin/.

Protection against infectious diseases

Caution: It is important to protect against diseases which are carried in the blood or tissue fluids. Protective gloves should be worn whenever there is a possibility of blood or tissue fluid being passed from one person to another, i.e. through an open cut or broken skin.

Two specific diseases to mention are:

- *AIDS* – Acquired Immune Deficiency Syndrome (AIDS) is a disease caused by the Human Immuno-deficiency Virus (HIV). The virus is transmitted through body tissue. Most people are aware of AIDS because of media coverage. The virus attacks the natural immune system, and therefore carries a strong risk of secondary infection, such as pneumonia, which could be life-threatening. As there is no known cure, prevention through protection is vital.
- *Hepatitis variants (A, B and C)* – this is an inflammation of the liver. It is caused by a very aggressive virus that is also transmitted through blood and tissue fluids. The virus can survive outside the body and can make a person very ill indeed; it can even be fatal. The most serious form of this disease is hepatitis B; fortunately

55

Unit

G20

Make sure your own actions reduce risks to health and safety

you can be immunised against it by a GP. If a person can prove that he or she needs this protection for employment purposes, there is no cost involved. Most training establishments will recommend immunisation against hepatitis.

Task 5

You need to know the personal protective clothing used by both the stylist and the client for all the services you carry out in the salon.

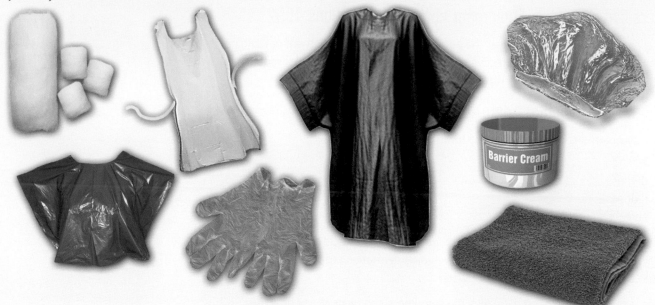

A worksheet for this task is provided on the website for you to complete and add to your portfolio. It asks you to match different items of personal protective clothing to the services for which they are used.

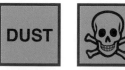
DUST
Dust

Toxic

Irritant

Corrosive

Flammable

Oxidising agent

Dangerous for the environment

Symbols showing types of hazardous substances

Control of Substances Hazardous to Health (COSHH) Regulations 2003

Your responsibilities under the COSHH Regulations are to follow instructions given in:

• manufacturers' data sheets – read the instructions before using a product
• COSHH assessment sheets – which state where to store chemicals.

You also need to follow salon requirements, use the correct PPE (personal protective equipment) and notify a supervisor or manager if a problem arises.

COSHH requires employers to control exposure to hazardous substances in the workplace. Most of the products used in the salon are perfectly safe, but some products could become hazardous under certain conditions or if used inappropriately. All salons should be aware of how to use and store these products.

Employers are responsible for assessing the risks from hazardous substances and must decide upon an action to reduce those risks. Proper training should be given and employees should always follow safety guidelines and take the precautions identified by the employer.

Look at the symbols showing types of hazardous substances (left). COSHH requires that they are found on packaging and containers in beauty and hairdressing salons.

Examples of potential hazards are given below.

- Highly flammable substances, such as hairspray or alcohol steriliser, are hazardous because their fumes will ignite if exposed to a naked flame.
- Explosive materials, such as hairspray, air freshener or other pressurised cans, will explode with force if placed in heat, such as an open fire, direct sunlight or even on top of a hot radiator.
- Chemicals can cause severe reactions and skin damage. Vomiting, respiratory problems or burning could be the result if chemicals are misused.

Information from manufacturers

All manufacturers of hair services and products must, by law, supply manufacturers' data sheets to comply with the Control of Substances Hazardous to Health (COSHH) Regulations 2003 (amended in 2005). These sheets provide you with everything you need to know about the product you are using – the ingredients, the handling and storage of the product, and any disposal considerations.

The sheets will also tell you the first aid measures to follow if the product comes into contact with the eyes or skin, or is swallowed. What would you do if you accidentally got some of the styling products that you were using in the client's eye? Ideally, you should call a first aider, but if one is not available immediately, then you need to take action. By following the first aid measures stated on the manufacturer's data sheet, you will be able to deal with the problem until a first aider is available.

COSHH precautions

Employers must, by law, identify, list and assess in writing any substance in the workplace. This applies not only to products used in the salon but also to products that are used in cleaning, for example bleach or polish. These substances must be given a hazard rating, or risk assessment, even if this is rated zero (no risk).

Finally, you should read all the COSHH sheets used in the salon and be safe: abide by what they say, never ignore manufacturers' instructions, and attend regular staff training for product use – you never know when you might need it!

Electricity at Work Regulations 1989

The Electricity at Work Regulations are concerned with general safety of the use of electricity. They cover the use and maintenance of electrical equipment in the salon. All electrical equipment must be regularly checked for electrical safety. In a busy salon this may be every six months. The check must be carried out by a 'competent person' – preferably a qualified electrician, and is called Portable Appliance Testing (PAT). All checks must be recorded in a book kept for this purpose only.

The safety record book should state the dates, the nature of the repair and who carried it out. It should also contain a list of tests carried out on the equipment under inspection, the results of those tests, and be signed by the competent person who carried them out. The manufacturer may supply its own technical staff to attend to safety checks, as they will be trained in areas of expertise.

If the equipment is found to be faulty, damaged or broken it must be withdrawn from service and repaired. This is essential for insurance purposes for **public liability** and in case of legal action being taken for an accident or negligence. More and more people are demanding court action for **negligence** – do not be liable! Use these regulations to keep you, your colleagues and your clients both out of danger and out of court!

57

Make sure your own actions reduce risks to health and safety

Top tips

Remember these COSHH tips:

- Manufacturers have to supply COSHH data sheets for all their products
- Invest in all the leaflets and latest information regarding COSHH from your local Health and Safety Executive office. *Keep up to date and keep safe.*

Public liability

Part of the law that focuses on civil wrongs; an injured party can sue based upon negligence and/or damages.

Negligence

Lack of proper care and attention.

Fact or fiction?

Is this statement fact or fiction?

Around 1,000 electric shock accidents at work are reported to the HSE each year.

To check your answer see page 492.

Task 6

Using the information in this section, answer the following questions.

1 How do the Electricity at Work Regulations affect the use of electrical equipment in the salon?
2 If electrical apparatus is found to be faulty, what action must be taken?
3 What is the purpose of an electrical safety record book?

A worksheet for this task is provided on the website for you to complete and add to your portfolio.

Reporting of Injuries, Diseases and Dangerous Occurrences Regulations 1995 (RIDDOR)

These regulations cover the recording and reporting of any serious accidents and conditions to the local environmental health officer, whose remit covers hairdressing salons. This officer will investigate the accident and makes sure the salon prevents it from happening again in the future. The officer can also assess the risk factors in each instance.

An accident or death at work must be reported without delay. Even if the accident does not require a hospital visit, but the person is absent from work for more than three days, it should be reported.

If an employee reports a work-related disease, a report must be sent. Work-related diseases include occupational dermatitis, asthma caused through work, and hepatitis. Accidents as a result of violence or an attack by another person must be reported.

A dangerous occurrence in which no one was actually injured must also be reported, for example, if the ceiling of the salon collapses overnight.

If you are a mobile hairdresser in someone's home and you have an accident yourself or injure the client, you must report it.

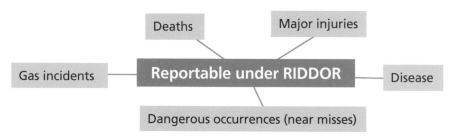

Employer's Liability (Compulsory Insurance) Act 1969

Employers and self-employed persons must by law hold employer's liability insurance. This will reimburse them against any legal liability to pay compensation to employees for bodily injury, illness or disease caused during the course of their employment.

Employers must insure for at least £5 million but check with your own insurance company. The amount depends upon individual risks and liabilities. Also check the recommendations of your professional association.

It is worth remembering the following points:

- A legal claim made against your salon could result in very large financial losses and possibly the sale of the owner's business or even private home.
- Public prosecution results in a heavy fine for those not having this essential insurance cover.
- Damage to the salon could be so great that the business may never recover.
- Some cases take up to ten years to come to court and with inflation the claim against you could be very much more than your original cover if you only go for the minimum requirements.

Insurance

Professional indemnity insurance

Every single professional hairdresser should have **indemnity** insurance protection, regardless of how few or how many services they carry out.

The best deal for all insurance policies is usually found via your professional body. They will be able to offer the best rates as they negotiate on behalf of members and get a considerable discount.

As an employee you need to check with your employer whether you are covered on the business insurance or need to organise your own cover. A salon owner or employer should include this liability in the public liability policy, so that all employees are protected against claims made by clients.

Public liability Insurance

This is not compulsory but it is certainly advisable. It will protect the employer should a member of the public be injured on the premises. This could be something as simple as a roof tile hitting the client on her way into the salon. If this results in the client being unable to work for a long period of time, the client can seek legal advice and the salon owner could be sued for compensation.

Data Protection Act 1998

Businesses that use computers or paper-based filing systems to hold personal details about their staff and clients may be required to register with the Data Protection Registrar.

The Data Protection Registrar will place your business on a public register of data users and issue you with a code of practice. There are eight principles of the Data Protection Act which you must comply with, stating that information should be:

- kept in a secure location
- accurate and up to date
- not kept for longer than necessary
- processed fairly and lawfully
- relevant to your needs
- not transferred to another country without adequate protection in place
- processed within the individual's rights
- released upon request to the individual that the information concerns.

Contact: The Information Commissioner's Office, Wycliffe House, Water Lane, Wilmslow, Cheshire SK9 5AF (tel. 08456 30 60 60; www.ico.gov.uk).

Indemnity

Compensation paid for a loss.

Fact or fiction?

Is this statement fact or fiction?

All employees must take responsibility for their deeds and actions, and are liable if they do not. Insurance cover will be null and void if it is proven that legislation or establishment rules have been broken and an accident or damage has occurred.

To check your answer see page 492.

Top tips

Professional indemnity insurance protects against injury from damage caused by services and covers personal injury. Indemnity insurance could save you a lot of money.

59

Unit
G20

Make sure your own actions reduce risks to health and safety

The information held by an organisation on computer about any one of us can be revealed if requested within 40 days, for a fee not greater than £10. It is possible to gain compensation through a civil court action if you feel there has been any infringement of your data protection rights.

The Consumer Protection Act 1987

This Act follows European Laws to safeguard the consumer in three main areas. The three parts of this Act fall under both criminal and civil law.

1 *Product liability* – a faulty product is one that does not reach the standard of safety you are generally entitled to expect. A customer can claim compensation if the faulty product causes death or personal injury.

2 *General safety requirements* – it is a criminal offence to sell unsafe goods; products must meet a general safety requirement. Traders are strictly liable if they break the general requirements and can be fined or imprisoned. Retailers supplying consumer goods can argue that they took reasonable steps to avoid committing the offence – that is, instructions or warnings were given; specific circumstances were taken into account.

3 *Misleading prices* – it is a criminal offence for a trader to give consumers a misleading indication about the price of goods, services or facilities. Always have an up-to-date price list on display and products with the correct price (including VAT) attached to them. Any special offers must be clearly displayed and worded.

Before 1987 an injured person had to prove a manufacturer's negligence before suing for damages. This Act removes the need to prove negligence. This could be a client getting injured as a result of incorrectly using a product that was bought from your salon. She should have had clear information and advice on how to use the product correctly so that an injury didn't occur.

An injured person can take action against any one of these groups of people

In the salon this means that only reputable products should be used and sold and care should be taken in handling, maintaining and storing products so that they remain in top condition. It is important that all staff are aware of handling, maintaining and storing when selling products and when using products in a service.

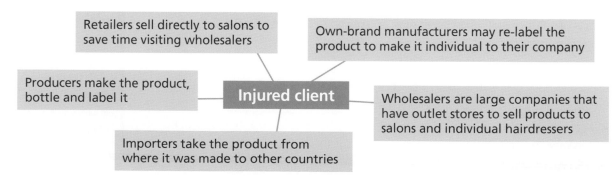

Retailers sell directly to salons to save time visiting wholesalers

Own-brand manufacturers may re-label the product to make it individual to their company

Producers make the product, bottle and label it

Injured client

Wholesalers are large companies that have outlet stores to sell products to salons and individual hairdressers

Importers take the product from where it was made to other countries

Cosmetic Products (Safety) Regulations 1996

These regulations are part of consumer protection. The EU has laid down strict regulations about the composition of products, labelling of ingredients, how the product is described and how it is marketed. American cosmetic companies have had to list all ingredients on their labels for years and Europe is now following suit. This is ideal for the easy identification of products that clients/customers may be allergic to, such as lanolin.

Trade Descriptions Act 1968 (and 1987)

This Act is concerned with the false description of goods and it is important to realise the relevance of this Act.

It is illegal to mislead the general public. This also applies to verbal descriptions given by a third party and repeated. So, if a manufacturer's false description is repeated, you are still liable to prosecution.

The law states that the retailer must not supply information that is in any way misleading, or falsely describe or make false statements about either a product or a service on offer. The retailer must not:

* make false contrasts between present and previous prices
* offer products at half price unless they have already been offered at the actual price for at least 28 days prior to the sale.

Sale of Goods Act 1979, Sale and Supply of Goods Act 1994

This Act has several others under its umbrella of protection:

* The Supply of Goods and Services Act 1982
* The Unfair Contract Terms Act 1977
* The Supply of Goods (Implied Terms) Act 1973.

The Sale of Goods Act recognises the contract of a sale between the retailer and the consumer when purchasing a product. This applies when the salon sells a product to a client, but it can apply to us all as consumers when we purchase any goods. (This Act is a good one to quote when returning something to a shop!)

The Act states that the retailer:

* has a responsibility to sell goods of the very best quality that are not defective in any way
* must refund the money for the purchase if it is found to be defective (some retailers will only offer an exchange of goods if there is no receipt)
* must then make a complaint to the supplier.

There are three main points to the Act:

1 Goods must be merchantable: reasonably fit for normal purpose and not faulty; for example, a hairbrush should not fall apart the first time you use it.
2 Goods must be fit for any purpose made known, either expressly or by implication; for example, a hairdryer should heat up sufficiently to be able to dry the hair.
3 Goods must be as described; for example, a natural bristle hairbrush must not be made of plastic bristles.

The Supply of Goods and Services Act 1982

This Act also deals with rights for the consumer and the trader's obligations towards the consumer. It has two branches: goods and services. Both of these Acts covered consumer rights before the Sale of Goods Act 1979, when definitions became tighter and the law was better defined regarding consumer rights.

Goods

The Act allows the consumer to claim back some or all of the money paid for goods. When we buy something in good faith we expect it to be of merchantable quality, fit for

Top tips

Be careful of using statements like 'our price'. Comparison of prices can be misleading and could even be illegal – you need to be sure that the product is identical in every way. You should also check that products are labelled with their country of origin.

61

Unit
G20

Make sure your own actions reduce risks to health and safety

Unit
G20

Make sure your own actions reduce risks to health and safety

the purpose for which it was sold and as described in the advertising. This applies to all goods, regardless of whether they are on hire, in part exchange or as part of a service.

Services

The Act states that the person or trader providing a service (such as a hairdresser) must charge a reasonable price, provide the service within a reasonable time and give the service with reasonable care and skill. This means no two-hour haircuts, no charging over-the-top prices and no slap-dash services!

Your customer can complain and contact the Trading Standards Office if they feel they have a case against you. Be careful!

The Unfair Contract Terms Act 1977

This Act was prior to the Sale of Goods Act 1979 and defined the term 'of merchantable quality' for the first time.

Water safety

It is essential that clients' safety is a priority during their time in the salon. When shampooing and conditioning, you are using water and possibly electrical equipment (such as a steamer), both of which can cause serious accidents if health and safety rules are not followed.

Workplace environment

The following are standard health and safety rules for the salon environment.

- The salon must always be kept clean and tidy.
- Any spillage of water or product on the floor is a hazard and should be wiped up immediately.
- Your work area should be kept clean and tidy throughout the service and any waste should be removed immediately after shampooing and conditioning.
- Always make client comfort an important issue and position your client carefully at the basin before you begin shampooing.
- You should position yourself to ensure good posture while working to avoid discomfort and the risk of injury.
- Any shampooing or conditioning product entering the eye should be flushed immediately with clean water and first aid attention sought.
- A client suffering from an **infection** or **infestation** must not be treated in the salon, as the problem is likely to cause a **cross-infection** to other clients, colleagues and yourself.

Health and safety rules

These will encompass all aspects of the Health and Safety at Work Act, plus COSHH and the Electricity at Work Act. You should be in no doubt about:

- your responsibility
- salon procedures
- service safety
- equipment safety
- protection against cross-infection.

Infection

The successful invasion and growth of micro-organisms to a degree that causes the symptoms of a disease.

Infestation

A term applied to parasites which live in or on another living creature in large numbers.

Cross-infection

The transfer of a disease or infection from one person to another.

Aspect of working practice	Health and safety procedures
Client safety	• Positioning of the client • Minimise the risk of a hazard happening within the salon • Correct use of equipment • Correct use of products • Correct evacuation procedures
Storage procedures	• Electrical equipment • Chemicals • Valuables • Stock • Money
Stock regulations	• COSHH regulations are followed • First aid procedures in place • Stock rotation • Spillage management • Correct storage and containers

Your employer or head of the training establishment should have all these standard procedures in place. If you are not instructed within your first few weeks of beginning your new post, then ask!

Health, hygiene and sterilisation

Sterilising

There are various methods for **sterilisation** of tools and equipment – see the chart below. Some are more effective than others and not all equipment can be sterilised in the same way. Your tools should be sterilised after every client so that you minimise the risk of cross infection and infestation.

The table below shows the various sterilisation methods available.

Method	Description
Disinfecting	These methods are only effective if used correctly. Disinfectants must be used at the correct concentrations and tools must be left in disinfectants for the correct length of time (read manufacturer's instructions). Different methods include: • hot water (60°C minimum) – for towels and gowns; the hot cycle of a washing machine can be used • disinfectant solutions, e.g. Barbicide®. Note: Brushes and combs should be washed with hot, soapy water before being immersed in the solution for at least 20 minutes (read manufacturer's instructions).
Sterilising wipes and sprays	Best for metal objects, e.g. scissors, clippers and razor handles (not blades) – remove loose hairs before spraying or wiping.
Ultra-violet (UV) radiation cabinet	This method of sterilisation is suitable for all tools. However, the tools must be turned over to ensure that each side has been exposed to the light for 20–30 minutes. (Note: Tools must be cleaned before placing in the cabinet, and the cabinet must be cleaned on a regular basis.)
Autoclave	Very efficient method of sterilising, especially for metal tools. However, some plastics cannot withstand the heat (check manufacturer's instructions). Autoclaves take about 20 minutes to sterilise tools. Not suitable for wooden-handled brushes.

Salon procedures for health and safety

Fact or fiction?

Is this statement fact or fiction?

Barbicide® is approved by the United States Environmental Protection Agency for use as a hospital disinfectant.

To check your answer see page 492.

Sterilisation

The killing of all organisms such as bacteria, fungi and parasites.

Disinfecting

Immersing equipment in a disinfectant solution such as Barbicide® for a certain length of time.

Sterilisation methods

63

Unit

G20

Make sure your own actions reduce risks to health and safety

Unit

G20

Make sure your own actions reduce risks to health and safety

Cleaning equipment

As well as making sure that all of your equipment is sterilised, you need to make sure that it is clean from hair and products. If you are using your equipment regularly, you will find that hair builds up. You may also find that you get a build-up of product residue in between the teeth of brushes and combs. This needs to be removed before you can sterilise your equipment.

Task 7

Using the information below on sterilising techniques, tick the correct box on the chart to show which sterilising method is most suitable for the following pieces of equipment. This will give you a handy checklist that you can refer back to.

	Barbicide®	Boil wash	Sterilising wipes and sprays	Ultra-violet cabinet	Autoclave
Brushes and combs					
Scissors					
Clippers					
Clipper grades					
Water spray bottles					
Towels and gowns					
Sectioning clips					
Razors					

A worksheet containing this chart can be found on the website for you to record your findings. This can then be used as additional portfolio evidence.

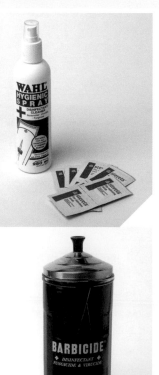

Sterilising solution, wipes and spray

- Brushes should be washed in warm soapy water to remove grease and products then soaked in a disinfectant solution (Barbicide®) for at least 20 minutes. Remember – if the brush has a wooden handle, only immerse the bristles otherwise the wood will swell and crack.
- Combs should be washed in warm soapy water to remove grease and products then soaked in a disinfectant solution (Barbicide®) for at least 20 minutes.
- Scissors should be cleaned regularly to remove hair cuttings and sterilised using medi-wipes or sterilising spray. They are made of surgical steel and can also be placed in an autoclave, immersed in Barbicide® or placed in a UV cabinet.
- Razors and hair shapers should be brushed free of cut hair after use. The replaceable blade must be disposed of in a sharps bin to avoid piercing the skin; this is then collected by the local health authority for incineration. The handle can be sterilised by either wiping with a medi-wipe or sterilising spray. They can also be placed in an autoclave, Barbicide® or a UV cabinet.
- Fixtures and fittings, all chairs, workstations, mirrors, hood dryers, climazones and steamers must be wiped clean daily to remove any hair cuttings, chemical and styling products, and general dust and dirt. If you deal with an infestation, for example headlice or scabies, within the salon you can use sterilising wipes and sprays on the backs of chairs and on work surfaces.
- Floors should be swept at regular intervals throughout the day to avoid slippery surfaces. All spills must be wiped up immediately. Floors should be bleached at the end of each day.

By using effective cleaning and sterilisation methods you can prevent cross-contamination or cross-infection from one client to another.

Disposal of used sharps

Salons should supply a yellow sharps bin for the disposal of blades (sharps). This is a hard plastic bin that cannot be pierced and is collected by the local health authority to be incinerated. If you put a disposable blade from your razor/hair shaper in an ordinary black bin liner, the person emptying the bin may cut themselves.

Disposal of hair cuttings

Normal hair cuttings can be swept up and placed in the salon bin. There is no current legislation on the removal of hair cuttings that might be contaminated with nits, but good practice would be to double-bag the hair to prevent any infestations in the salon environment.

Disposal of chemicals

Most chemicals can be poured down the sink and rinsed away with cold water. If the product packaging is rinsed it can then be disposed of in a recycling bin.

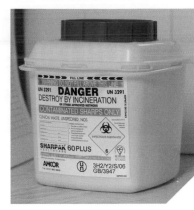

A sharps bin

Salon/workplace policies

Fire policies

Fire Precautions Act 1971

By law, all business premises must undertake a fire risk assessment. If five or more people work together as employees, the assessment must be in writing. Employers must also take into account all other persons on the premises, not just employees. This will include clients and visitors to the salon.

There must also be a fire and evacuation procedure. In every period of one year there must be at least one fire drill, which involves everyone. All staff must be fully informed, instructed and trained in what is expected of them. Some employees will have special duties to perform such as checking rooms.

All employees, trainees and temporary workers must cooperate with their employers so far as is necessary to enable the employers to fulfil the duties placed upon them by law. This means that everyone must cooperate fully in training courses and fire drills, even when everyone knows it is only a practice.

Many fire-training exercises are organised with a fire safety officer from the local fire station. Often fire engines will take part in the exercise to test the firefighters' own attendance time from the station to the premises. Everyone should be made aware of his or her own particular roles for evacuation.

When joining a salon, a new employee should be briefed on all health and safety issues, and especially in fire evacuation procedures. It is standard practice to include the information in a handbook containing all the salon's policies. Look carefully at the following example of a training institution's evacuation procedure.

Make sure your own actions reduce risks to health and safety

BUILDING EVACUATION PROCEDURES IN THE EVENT OF FIRE OR BOMB ALERT

The following procedure has been agreed and must be followed. Any staff member who does not comply is committing an infringement of the college disciplinary code. Whenever a fire occurs, the main consideration is to get everybody out of the building safely. Protection of personal or college property is incidental.

RAISING THE ALARM

Anyone discovering a fire must immediately raise the alarm by operating the nearest fire alarm and report to the controller the fire location.

On hearing the alarm the receptionist will immediately contact the emergency services and then evacuate the building.

In the event of a fire being discovered when the reception is unmanned, the premises officer on duty will contact the emergency services and assume control.

ON HEARING THE ALARM

All those in senior positions proceed to the control point – normally at a main entrance to the building – where one person must take control of the proceedings.

All other staff: close windows, switch off machinery and lights, and close doors on leaving the room.

Assist less able colleagues, leave the building by the nearest marked route and proceed quickly to the appropriate assembly point. Staff must supervise their class.

Staff evacuating the building must check their locality is clear.

ASSEMBLY POINTS

Everyone must remain at assembly points well away from buildings and clear of access roads.

Report to control in person or via two-way radios where allocated.

Everyone must remain at assembly points to await further instructions.

DO NOT re-enter the building until you are told it is safe to do so.

Example of a training institution's evacuation procedure

Emergency fire procedures

Fire drill dependent on the working area

- All electrical equipment to be switched off.
- Shut windows.
- Clients to be led by the stylist to a safe area. Wrap wet hair in a towel and take extra towels for warmth and water sprays in case any chemicals are nearing their full development time.
- If possible, take the client's valuable possessions with her, such as a handbag, but only if it does not put the client or stylist in any danger.
- Be aware of the service being performed before the evacuation – if the client has chemicals on the hair, keep checking the development of the service and dilute the strength of the product using a water spray if necessary. This would need to be at the judgement of the person in charge of the salon – certainly a client having a perm or colour will need constant attention while waiting at the assembly point.

Task 8

When you next hear a building evacuation alarm in your workplace, complete a write-up of the procedure you undertook, ensuring you, your colleagues and clients left the building quickly and safely. Locate the firefighting equipment that is available and state its purpose.

Get this evidence signed and dated by your lecturer or manager to use as evidence in your portfolio.

Sensible fire precautions

- Be informed – know what to do and where to go when the evacuation begins.
- Be sensible and do not panic – this will only make the clients feel panicky too.
- Make sure that the locations of the fire alarm, fire extinguishers and fire exit are familiar.
- Never ignore smoke or the smell of burning – it is far better to have a false alarm than to risk fire.
- Do not misuse or mistreat electrical appliances that are a potential hazard – always treat electrical appliances with respect.
- Do not ignore manufacturers' instructions for the storage and use of highly flammable products, which are very common within the salon.
- Be sensible with naked flames and matches or disposal of cigarette ends – a smouldering tip can burst into flames in minutes.
- Be accountable for clients on the premises – the appointment book should be taken outside as a master check of which clients should be present.
- Do not use a lift for the evacuation – it may be that the fire affects the electrical mechanism and that then becomes another emergency.

Firefighting equipment

Fire extinguishers

Only a person specially trained in the use of a fire extinguisher should attempt to use one. Never put yourself or others at risk – personal safety is more important than saving material items that can be replaced.

68

Unit

G20

Make sure your own actions reduce risks to health and safety

There are different types of portable fire extinguisher for use on different types of fire – using the wrong one can make the situation worse. The latest extinguishers are coloured red with a zone or panel of colour, which indicates the contents of the extinguisher. On older models the colour of the whole fire extinguisher identifies its use.

Extinguisher	Colour	Type of fire	Uses	NOT to be used
Dry powder	Blue marking	Electrical fires	For burning liquid, electrical fires and flammable liquids	On flammable metal fires
Carbon dioxide (CO$_2$)	Black marking		Safe on all voltages. Used on burning liquid and electrical fires and flammable liquids	On flammable metal fires
Vaporising liquid	Green marking		Safe on all voltages. Used on burning liquid and electrical fires and flammable liquids	On flammable metal fires
Water	Red marking	Non-electrical fires	For wood, paper, textiles, fabric and similar materials	On burning liquid, electrical or flammable metal fires
Foam	Cream/yellow marking		On burning liquid fires (e.g. petrol, diesel)	On electrical or flammable metal fires

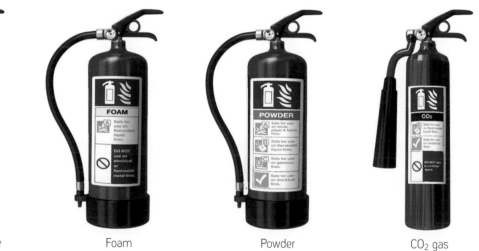

Water with additive   Foam   Powder   CO$_2$ gas

Different types of fire extinguishers

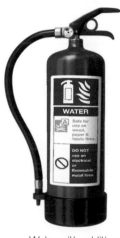

Top tips

If you cannot control a fire, leave the room, close the door, proceed to a safe place, then phone the emergency services. Even small fires spread very quickly, producing smoke and fumes, which can kill in minutes. If there is any doubt, do not tackle the fire, no matter how small.

Hundreds of people die and thousands of people are injured in fires each year, many caused by lack of concentration or carelessness. It is better to prevent a fire starting in the first place, for example by using chemicals safely and maintaining electrical appliances.

Fire blankets

Fire blankets are made of fire-resistant material. They are particularly useful for wrapping around a person whose clothing is on fire. A fire blanket must be used calmly and with a firm grip. If the blanket is flapped about, it may fan the fire and cause it to flare up, rather than put it out. When putting a blanket on a victim, protect your own hands with the edge of the cloth. Remember to place the blanket, never throw it, into the desired position.

Sand

A bucket of sand can be used to soak up liquids, such as chemicals, which are the source of a fire. However, never risk injury. If in doubt, leave the area and phone the emergency services.

First aid

People at work can suffer injuries or fall ill. It does not matter whether the injury or illness is caused by the work they do. It is important that they receive immediate attention and that in serious cases an ambulance is called. First aid can save lives and prevent minor injuries becoming major ones.

The Health and Safety (First Aid) Regulations 1981 set out the essential aspects of first aid that employers have to be responsible for.

As a trainee or student, you must have some basic knowledge of first aid. Unless you hold an up-to-date first aid certificate, you should not treat injuries; but you should know when and how to summon a competent first aider and call for an ambulance if necessary.

Top tips

First aid in the workplace is the initial management of any injury or illness suffered at work. It does not include giving tablets or medicines to treat illness.

Common first aid problems in the salon

Problem	First aid necessary
Chemicals entering the eye, e.g. perm lotion or neutraliser	Immediately flush the eye with cool, clean water, then summon a first aider.
Scissor cut to skin	Give the client a pad to stem the flow of blood. Do not touch the wound, surrounding area or blood without gloves on. If the cut is deep or does not stop bleeding, call for first aid assistance or phone the emergency services for an ambulance.
Client or colleague falls and is knocked out	Put them in the **recovery position** and call for medical assistance from a first aider or summon an ambulance.
Client or colleague faints	Put them in the recovery position and call for medical assistance from a first aider or summon an ambulance.

It is essential that sufficient first aid personnel and facilities are available:

- to give immediate assistance to casualties with both common injuries and illnesses and those likely to arise from specific hazards at work
- to summon an ambulance or other professional help.

Recovery position

First aid technique recommended for assisting people who are unconscious or nearly unconscious but still breathing.

The number of first aiders and facilities available will depend upon the size of the workforce, the type of workplace hazards and risks, and the history of accidents in the workplace. There are two legal aspects of first aid that you need to consider:

- *Trainees* – students undertaking work experience on certain training schemes are given the same status as employees and therefore are the responsibility of the employer.
- *The public* – when dealing with the public the Health and Safety (First Aid) Regulations do not require employers to provide first aid for anyone other than their own employees. Employers should make extra provision for the public. Educational institutions need also to include the general public in their assessment of first aid requirements.

First aid kits

The minimum level of first aid equipment is a suitably stocked and properly identified first aid container. An old biscuit tin just will not do! First aid containers should be easily accessible and placed, where possible, near to hand-washing facilities.

The container should protect the items inside from dust and damp and should only be stocked with useful items. Tablets and medication should not be kept in it. There is no compulsory list of what a first aid container should include but some suggestions are shown overleaf.

Make sure your own actions reduce risks to health and safety

Make sure your own actions reduce risks to health and safety

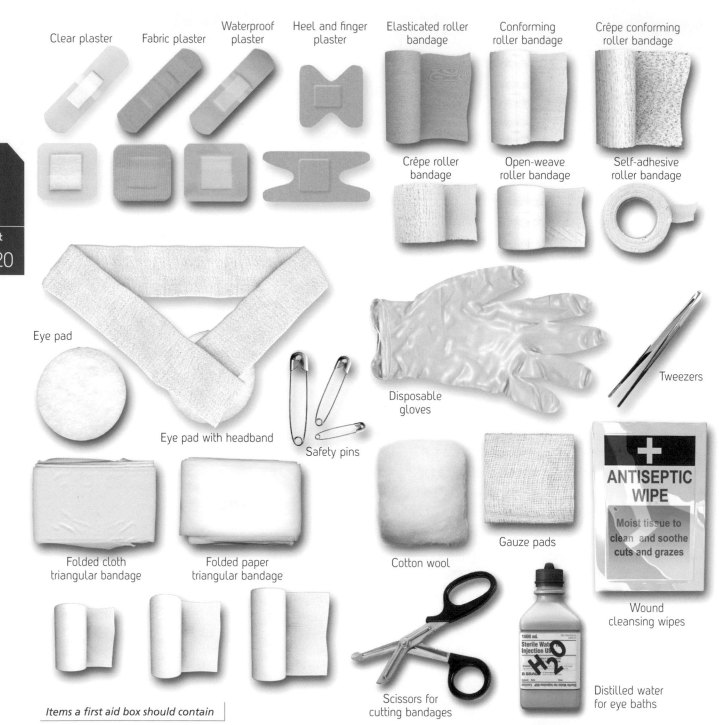

Clear plaster

Fabric plaster

Waterproof plaster

Heel and finger plaster

Elasticated roller bandage

Conforming roller bandage

Crêpe conforming roller bandage

Crêpe roller bandage

Open-weave roller bandage

Self-adhesive roller bandage

Eye pad

Eye pad with headband

Safety pins

Disposable gloves

Tweezers

ANTISEPTIC WIPE

Moist tissue to clean and soothe cuts and grazes

Folded cloth triangular bandage

Folded paper triangular bandage

Cotton wool

Gauze pads

Wound cleansing wipes

Items a first aid box should contain

Scissors for cutting bandages

1000 mL Sterile Water Injection USP

H₂O

Distilled water for eye baths

The number of first aid containers a salon or establishment has will depend upon the size of the establishment and the total number of employees in that area.

Task 9

1　Who is responsible for checking the first aid box in your salon?
2　How often is it checked?
3　What should you do if you have used something from the box?

Make a note of this information for your portfolio of evidence.

First aid training

First aid certificates are only valid for the length of time the Health and Safety Executive (HSE) specifies, which is currently three years. Employers need to arrange refresher training with re-testing of competence before certificates expire. If a certificate expires, the individual will have to undertake a full course of training to be reinstated as a qualified first aider. Specialist training can also be undertaken if the workplace needs it.

Rectifying health and safety risks

Recording incidents

It is good practice for employers to provide first aiders with a book in which to record incidents that require their attendance. If there are several first aid persons in one establishment, then a central book will be acceptable.

If you have to deal with an incident, you should record the following information:

- date, time and place of incident
- name and job of injured/sick person, and contact details
- details of the injury/illness and what first aid was given
- details of the action taken immediately afterwards (for example, did the person go home or to hospital; was she taken in an ambulance?)
- name and signature of the first aider or person dealing with the incident.

This record book is not the same as the statutory accident book, although the two might be combined. The information kept can help the employer identify accident trends or patterns and improve on safety risks. It can also be used to judge first aid needs. It may also prove useful for insurance and investigative purposes.

Salon accident/incident report

This form should be filled in by the first aider/staff member responsible for dealing with the accident/incident. It should be completed as soon as possible after the accident/incident.

Task 10

Complete the accident report form on the website within your training establishment and use for evidence within your portfolio.

71

Unit

G20

Make sure your own actions reduce risks to health and safety

Unit

G20

Make sure your own actions reduce risks to health and safety

THE HAIR STUDIO

ACCIDENT REPORT FORM

SECTION 1 PERSONAL DETAILS

Full name of first aider/staff member: _____

Position held in salon: _____

Date: _____

Accident (injury) ☐ Incident (illness) ☐

Time and date of accident/incident: _____

Full name of injured/ill person: _____

Staff member ☐ Client ☐ Other ☐

Address: _____

Tel. no: _____

SECTION 2 ACCIDENT/INCIDENT DETAILS

Describe what happened. In the case of an accident, state clearly what the injured person
was doing. _____

_____

Name and address/tel. no. of witness(es), if any: _____

_____

Action taken

Ambulance called ☐   Taken to hospital ☐   Sent to hospital ☐   First aid given ☐

Taken home ☐   Sent home ☐   Returned to work ☐

SECTION 3 PREVENTATIVE ACTION

Preventative action implemented ☐

Describe action taken: _____

_____

Date implemented: _____

Signature of first aider/staff member: _____

Signature of salon manager/owner: _____

Date: _____

An accident report form

Accident procedures

Accidents happen, even to the most careful
of people. In the event of an accident in the
salon, stay calm and follow the salon's accident
procedures.

You should be aware of all possible risks in all
aspects of salon life, including:

- preparation of area
- unpacking stock
- clearing up of area
- dealing with stock, equipment and products
- putting stock away/taking stock out of storage.

Top tips

You should continually review the salon for hazards
that might cause an accident. For example, if the
same accident occurs more than once, then you
must ask why.

Health and safety suggestions

The salon should provide lockable storage, filing cabinets or similar so that
staff personal belongings can be locked away. Handbags and purses are always
vulnerable to the opportunist thief, who may come in unnoticed off the street and
leave with someone's valuables. If your salon does not provide somewhere secure
for your belongings, you could suggest this at your next staff meeting.

Staff should be discouraged from bringing large amounts of cash into work and from
wearing expensive jewellery if it has to be removed during services and is therefore
vulnerable to loss or theft.

Carry out banking of money from the till at different times of the day and do not
keep too much money in the till at any one time. Removing large amounts of takings
from the salon into a bank or night deposit safe should be done daily. Avoid taking
the same route to the bank at the same time of day. Someone may be watching!

Be aware of suspicious packages left unattended – inform a supervisor and, if
necessary, call the emergency services. The salon should have a list of telephone
numbers by the phone in case of emergency, such as the local police station or
security guardroom – this will save time when it really counts.

Do not allow yourself to be unprotected – do not leave outside doors open when working in the salon, do not leave the till drawer open, do not be naive enough to think that it could not happen to you! If unsure, seek professional advice from the local police station or crime prevention officer for personal safety hints for staff and clients.

As a professional stylist, do not allow yourself to become a victim – follow your professional guidelines.

Personal presentation

Hairdressing is part of the fashion industry and the image you portray should reflect this. However, your personal appearance should always combine safety with professionalism. For example, high-heeled shoes are not only uncomfortable after a day's standing but also not particularly stable to walk in. Similarly, open-toed sandals will not protect the toes from damage, spillage or impact injury. Shoes should be smart but essentially comfortable.

- Do not wear dangling jewellery which may be a hazard.
- Avoid stooping and slouching; this will prevent back problems occurring.
- Hairdressers often have arms and shoulders raised when cutting, perm winding and setting. This awkward and unnatural posture often leads to hairdressers becoming round-shouldered and in old age can lead to a hunched back. It is important to learn to stand with good posture while working to prevent this from occurring.
- Evenly distribute body weight by standing with feet slightly apart – this will prevent accidents and body damage.
- Always wear the correct protective clothing to shield a uniform.
- Always wear gloves when using chemicals or if there is a possibility of coming into contact with body fluids.
- If a salon provides a uniform as part of a corporate image, wear it with pride!
- Your hair should not interfere with any service you carry out; this avoids the possibility of cross-infection.
- A high standard of cleanliness will ensure no cross-infection can occur
- Wash your hands between dealing with clients.
- Keep your nails tidy.
- Cover cuts or open wounds.
- Do not attend work if you have an infectious disease.
- Do not spread germs by coming into the salon with a cold or flu.

Personal conduct

Good conduct cuts down any risks.

- Do not run or rush around the salon.
- Use equipment properly.
- Follow manufacturers' instructions at all times.
- Ensure the salon and equipment are cleaned thoroughly.
- Always leave equipment ready for use by the next person.
- Do not block fire exits for any reason.
- Behave sensibly.
- Use proper lifting procedures.

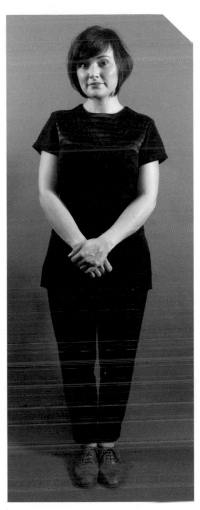

Good personal presentation gives a positive image to the salon

Make sure your own actions reduce risks to health and safety

Top tips

When stock is delivered to the salon it is usually left at reception for staff to check that the order is correct and then it is taken to the storage area for unpacking. Often the stock is delivered in large, heavy boxes and therefore great care must be taken by all salon employees who lift the boxes. This means bending your knees before taking the weight of the box, and keeping your back straight to avoid straining back muscles and more serious long-term back problems. See page 54 for correct lifting and handling procedures.

Make sure your own actions reduce risks to health and safety

- Take responsibility for yourself, machinery and problems such as spillage that may occur – do not expect someone else to clean up after you!
- Always treat your clients with the utmost respect.

Task 11

For each of the points above, write a short statement to explain *why* you should follow the good conduct rules and recommendations.

A worksheet for this task is provided on the website for you to complete and add to your portfolio.

Salon security and reducing workplace risks

There are many areas to keep secure in a business. Possible risk areas include:

- the premises
- stock and products
- equipment
- money
- display materials
- personal safety
- clients' belongings.

The premises

For insurance and mortgage applications the salon owner must have adequate security measures in place for the salon, and it is worth consulting the local police for guidance. A crime prevention officer will come and survey the premises and give advice regarding the most vulnerable areas and the most common forms of entry by a burglar.

External security

- Deadlock all doors and windows.
- Double-glazed windows are expensive but are more difficult to break into – the older the window and frame, the easier the entry.
- Fit a burglar alarm, if possible, or even fit a dummy box on the wall, which may deter a burglar.
- Closed-circuit television (CCTV) may be available if the premises are in a well-known shopping area.
- If the premises have metal shop-front shutters, use them, as they are probably the most effective deterrent to a burglar.

Internal security

- Internal doors can be locked to prevent an intruder moving from room to room.
- Fire doors and emergency exits should be locked at night and re-opened by the first person in at the start of business every morning.
- Stock and money should be locked away or deposited in the bank so that nothing is visible to entice a burglar.
- Lock expensive equipment away in the stock cupboard.
- Very large businesses employ security firms to patrol their premises at night, but, along with alarmed infra-red beams, these are not affordable for the average

small salon owner. If, however, the salon is situated within a shopping centre or business park, night patrols may be included in the lease or purchase agreement or offered for a set fee per year. Costs would need to be considered, but it may save money in the long term.

- The local police station can be contacted and police patrols will regularly check the building as part of their normal evening beat.

Stock and products

This includes both items on display and those in use in the salon. The smaller items may prove most irresistible to the thief as they are small enough for a pocket and are very accessible. Unfortunately, this form of theft costs many businesses a great deal of money, as stock can be expensive to replace and can be a big chunk of the capital outlay of a salon.

Another very sad fact is that the average 'thief' may be rather closer to home than is comfortable. Staff may 'borrow' an item of stock for home use and think that this behaviour is acceptable. There may be some clients who like the look of a re-sale product on display and 'forget' to pay for it!

The following precautions are needed to prevent the salon's stock and products from being stolen:

- Have one person (usually a senior stylist or senior receptionist) in control of the stock, and limit keys and access to stock
- Do a regular stock check – daily for loss of stock and weekly for stock ordering and rotation.
- Use empty containers for displays, or ask the suppliers if they provide dummy stock (this will also save the product deteriorating while on display).
- Keep displays in locked glass cabinets that can be seen but not touched.
- Try to keep handbags (belonging to both staff and clients) away from the stock area, usually reception, to stop products 'dropping' into open bags.
- Have one member of staff responsible for topping up the service products from wholesale-sized containers.
- Hold regular staff training on security and let the staff know what the losses are and how it may affect them – some companies offer bonus schemes both for reaching targets of sales and minimising pilfering. Heavy losses may affect potential salary increases.

Top tips

A light left on in reception may deter a thief – no burglar wants to be seen.

Task 12

Complete the stock check form in your training establishment and use as evidence for your reception unit as well.

A worksheet for this task is provided on the website for you to complete and add to your portfolio.

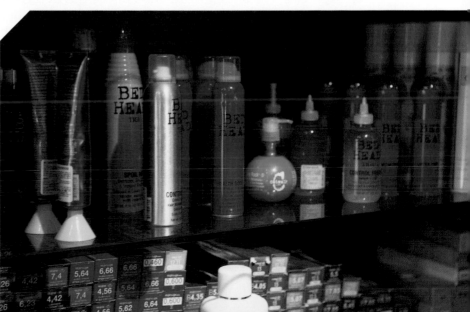

Check your knowledge

The following questions will help you to check your understanding of this unit. The answers can be found on pages 492–3.

1 What does the abbreviation HASAWA stand for?

_____

2 A hazard is:
a) something that makes your job difficult to do
b) something with the potential to cause harm
c) not having the correct equipment to carry out a service
d) a form of consultation.

3 A salon policy is:
a) having rules and regulations for staff to follow to ensure safe practice
b) a timetable stating lunch breaks for staff
c) a risk assessment form
d) a stock check form.

4 What is the purpose of the Manual Handlings Operations Regulations 1992?
a) To state the correct personal protective equipment to be used during a service
b) To ensure all electrical equipment is safe to use
c) To make sure that the correct lifting, pulling, pushing, etc. postures are used
d) To make sure the salon has the correct insurance cover in place for staff

5 What are your responsibilities under the Health and Safety at Work Act?

_____

6 What does RIDDOR stand for?
a) Risks In Day to Day Outdoor Recreation
b) Reporting of Industrial Diseases and Dangerous Occurrences
c) Reporting of Injuries, Diseases and Dangerous Occurrences
d) Replenishing of Injuries, Diseases and Dangerous Occurrences

7 Under the Electricity at Work Regulations 1989 all equipment should be checked every:
a) six months
b) three months
c) five months
d) year.

8 The purpose of sterilising tools and equipment is to:
a) make them look and smell nice
b) kill all living parasites
c) kill all organisms including bacteria, fungi and parasites
d) get the hair out of your tools and equipment.

9 How many people have to be employed at a workplace before a fire risk assessment has to be in writing?
   a) 12
   b) 5
   c) 20
   d) 2

10 What type of fire extinguisher can be used on electrical fires?
   a) Dry powder, foam and water
   b) Dry powder, carbon dioxide and water
   c) Dry powder, vaporising liquid and carbon dioxide
   d) Dry powder, foam and carbon dioxide

11 What is meant by the term 'workplace policies'?
   a) A list of rules set by government to make sure that the workplace pays tax
   b) A set of rules that the salon expects staff to follow to ensure safe working practices
   c) A list of rules set by a collaboration of local salons, applying to all salons within a specified geographical area
   d) A document which states how much of a product should be used on each client

12 What is meant by the term 'code of practice'?
   a) A document stating the behaviour, professional appearance etc. that is expected in the salon
   b) A document stating how many times a stylist must practise a new style before working on a paying client
   c) A bye-law set by the local authority that salons must adhere to
   d) Legislation set by government to determine the maximum number of clients that any salon can serve

13 What are the responsibilities of the employer under the Health and Safety at Work Act?
   a) To report flaws or gaps in systems and procedures, and to pay employee wages
   b) Plan safety and security, provide information, update systems and ensure the safety of individuals and visitors
   c) Not to misuse or change anything that has been provided for safety, and make sure that clients wear safety goggles and yellow helmets
   d) Assist the employee in meeting requirements under the Health and Safety at Work Act, and provide safety manuals for all employees

14 Which of these is the responsibility of the employee under the Health and Safety at Work Act?
   a) To plan safety and security
   b) To provide information about safety and security
   c) To update systems and procedures
   d) To report flaws or gaps within the system or procedure when in use

Make sure your own actions reduce risks to health and safety

15 What is the main purpose of health and safety legislation?
  a) To make sure the stylist does their job correctly
  b) To fine salons if health and safety measures are not followed
  c) To help the salon to manage employees correctly
  d) To ensure employers provide safe systems of work

16 What is a PAT test?
  a) A product allergy test
  b) A porosity and tautness test
  c) A portable appliance test
  d) A personal attention test

17 Which colours of fire extinguishers could be used on an electrical fire?
  a) Red, yellow or green
  b) Blue, red or green
  c) Black, green or blue
  d) Green, yellow or red

Getting ready for assessment

You will be assessed using a combination of assessment methods, as described below. Within every service you carry out with a client, you will address health and safety concerns. You should therefore have plenty of opportunities to collect evidence for your portfolio. If you are not sure what you have covered in your service, always ask your assessor or supervisor for advice.

	NVQ	VRQ
Credit value	4	3
Guided Learning Hours	38	22

	NVQ	VRQ
Practical demonstrations, to be observed by assessor	In this unit you will be expected to gather relevant information during practical performances to support your work. Evidence can include direct observation in the workplace, but there are also many other possible methods for compiling evidence.	Direct observation can make up some of the evidence for this unit. You should avoid simulation where possible.
Service timings	There are no mandatory service timings for this unit.	There are no mandatory service timings for this unit.
Additional evidence	Assessment methods can include: • witness testimony by colleagues or line managers • documentary and other product-based evidence • a personal report endorsed by colleagues • questions • discussions • professional discussion.	You will be assessed by oral questioning and you should compile a portfolio of evidence. There is a mandatory written paper for this unit.

Task mapping

When you have completed the tasks in this unit, check the table below to see which Performance Criteria (purple), Range (red), Knowledge (green) and Key Skills (blue) you have covered within G20 to use as additional evidence within your portfolio. Information about which Functional Skills you have covered is available on the website.

Task and page reference	Mapping to Performance Criteria, Range, Knowledge and Key Skills
1 (page 48)	Performance Criteria: 2, 3, 4, 5, 6, 7, 10, 12, VRQ 1h Range: N/A Knowledge: 1, 2, 3, 4, 5, 6, 7, 8, 9, 10, 11, 12, 13, 17, VRQ m Key Skills: C1.2, C1.3, C2.3
2 (page 49)	Performance Criteria: 6, 7, 10, 13, VRQ 1b, 1h Range: N/A Knowledge: 7, 10, 11, VRQ l, n Key Skills: C1.2

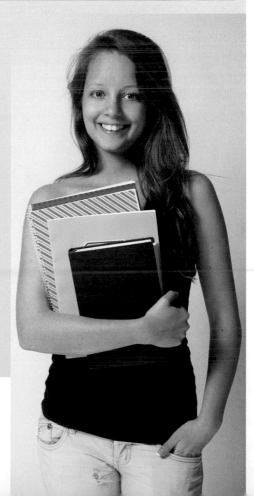

Make sure your own actions reduce risks to health and safety

3 (page 49)	Performance Criteria: 6, VRQ 2a, 2b, 2c Range: N/A Knowledge: 2, 3, 10, 11 Key Skills: C1.2
4 (page 51)	Performance Criteria: 1, 12, 14, 15, VRQ 1d Range: N/A Knowledge: 2, 4, VRQ j Key Skills: C1.2, C1.3, C2.3
5 (page 56)	Performance Criteria: 2, 5, 9, 12 14, VRQ 1a, 1f Range: N/A Knowledge: 8, 9, 12, 14, VRQ p Key Skills: C1.2
6 (page 58)	Performance Criteria: 6, 7, 8, 12, VRQ 1a, 1b, 1h Range: N/A Knowledge: 2, 3, 4, 5, 6, 7, 10, VRQ n, o Key Skills: C1.2, C1.3, C2.3
7 (page 64)	Performance Criteria: 3, 8, 9, 12, VRQ 1e Range: N/A Knowledge: 2, 4, 5, 8, 9, 12, 14, VRQ s, t Key Skills: C1.2
8 (page 67)	Performance Criteria: 1, 14, VRQ 2a, 2b Range: N/A Knowledge: 2, 3, 8, 9, 12, 16, VRQ e, i Key Skills: C1.2, C1.3, C2.3
9 (page 70)	Performance Criteria: 6, 8, VRQ N/A Range: N/A Knowledge: 10, 11, VRQ N/A Key Skills: C1.2
10 (page 71)	Performance Criteria: 5, 8, VRQ 2a, 2b Range: N/A Knowledge: 2, 3, 4, 10, VRQ e Key Skills: C1.2, C1.3
11 (page 44)	Performance Criteria: 5, 8, 9, 11, 12, 14, VRQ 1a, 1c, 1h Range: N/A Knowledge: 2, 3, 4, 8, 9, 12, 14, 15, 16, VRQ q Key Skills: C1.2, C1.3, C2.3
12 (page 46)	Performance Criteria: N/A, VRQ N/A Range: N/A Knowledge: N/A, VRQ N/A Key Skills: C1.3, C2.3

Fulfil salon reception duties

Unit G4

Fulfil salon reception duties

What you will learn:

- **How to maintain the reception area**
- **How to attend to clients and enquiries**
- **How to make appointments for salon services**
- **How to handle payments from clients**

Introduction

This unit covers all aspects of a receptionist's duties. Every salon needs a welcoming reception area, overseen by a confident and effective receptionist. Being part of your salon's team means you will need to employ all sorts of different roles within your working day. When your role is on your salon's reception area it is vitally important that you know what your responsibilities are and have the communication skills to deal confidently and professionally with clients. This is because the reception area (which is often called the 'front of house') is the first impression the client will have of the salon — and first impressions are usually lasting ones. You will need to find out your salon's guidelines for dealing with both general enquiries and specific problems that may occur. You will also have to learn how long each stylist needs for each of the services offered and how to use the appointment system correctly so that the salon is run cost-effectively while maintaining client satisfaction.

Video clip

Watch video clip 'Making the right impression' on the website to hear what celebrity stylist Andrew Barton has to say about the key factors in making the right first impression.

The qualities of a good receptionist

Before starting this unit, you need to look at two essential parts of the salon's working environment:

- the receptionist's role
- the atmosphere of the salon.

The receptionist's role

To be a successful receptionist, you will need to know everything that the job role demands. You should be aware of the limitations of your authority and know when to ask the manager or salon owner for help.

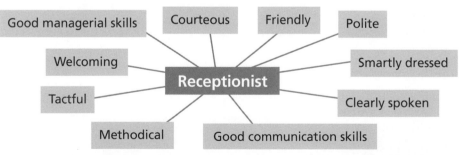

Some receptionists are employed for their managerial and office skills and they may not be qualified stylists. However, to be able to book in a client and talk about services, all receptionists should have some knowledge about the services shown on the salon price list, products used in the salon and the retail product range.

Knowledge of the services will not only allow you to talk with confidence about each service but will also enable you to book appointments correctly, schedule the working day into a logical sequence and advise clients. All this can only be achieved through good training, which should be seen as an investment for the future and necessary to promote healthy and sustainable growth of the business. If the receptionist is not a hairdresser, he or she should have experienced all the services (where possible) as a client to enable him or her to understand fully what is involved and to be able to talk about the services confidently.

A further role of the receptionist is to carry out skin tests on clients wishing to book for colouring processes (see page 207).

Task 1

The receptionist should be able to talk knowledgeably about services and retail products available in the salon.

Using the worksheet provided on the website, complete the diagram to show what the receptionist should know about each service.

The importance of the receptionist

- As the receptionist, you will be the first person the client sees or hears on the telephone. You are therefore the ambassador for the salon.
- The receptionist represents the entire business, and first impressions do count!
- The atmosphere of the salon   good or bad – is set by the receptionist.
- The receptionist can make or break the success and growth of the business. How well you do your job will determine how smoothly the salon will run.
- The receptionist is the lynchpin of the salon, holding everyone (both clients and staff) together.
- The reception area is the central pivot that the business revolves around and its success will largely depend upon the skills of the person in charge of it.

Personal, learning and thinking skills – Creative thinking

In your role as a receptionist you are required to complete tasks to ensure the smooth running of the salon and portray a professional image. You are the first person that clients will come into contact with, so it is important that you maintain high standards. Sometimes it is important to look at your surroundings with fresh eyes, as if you are a client seeing the environment for the first time. With a critical eye, look at your surroundings and use some creative thinking to see if there are improvements that can be made. Inform your manager of your findings to show you are thinking creatively about improvements for your salon.

The atmosphere of the salon

The reception area should be as welcoming and friendly as possible and should be a positive reflection of the rest of the salon. The area should be very clean, warm and tidy, and clients should be able to wait in comfort. It should be inviting and encourage the clients to want to stay.

Part of a receptionist's job is to ensure that the reception area is clean and tidy at all times, as this is the clients' first impression as they walk through the door. Promotional display stands need to be well stocked to allow clients to see what products are available for them to buy in order to maintain services carried out in the salon. Making sure that you have all the correct stationery to carry out your job efficiently and knowing the salon's policies on client care are key to offering a professional service.

83

Unit
G4

Fulfil salon reception duties

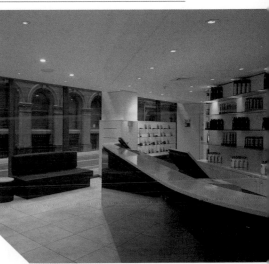

The reception area should be welcoming

How to maintain the reception area

Keeping the reception area clean and tidy

From your own experiences you may have come across businesses that do not appear to be professionally run. This may be for a number of reasons, but may have been as a result of a bad impression when first entering a shop.

Look at the reception area in your salon and see how many positive points you can identify about how your reception area is kept clean and tidy.

Task 2

Receptionist job role

Try to complete all of the following tasks.

- Magazines are up to date and stacked neatly.
- All finished coffee cups are removed and washed up.
- Clients' coats are taken from them upon arrival and hung up.
- If there are cushions in the seating area, these are neatly arranged.
- Tables are kept dust free.
- The floor area is vacuumed or swept regularly.
- Reception area is kept free of obstructions.

A worksheet for this task is provided on the website for you to complete and add to your portfolio.

Even when the salon is really busy it is unacceptable to have the following:

- dirty cups left from previous clients
- magazines scattered over dusty tables
- clients' coats left on seating areas
- hair on the floor all around the salon.

When maintaining the reception area, think how and when you can carry out the jobs required of you in order to keep the area clean and tidy. Should you be vacuuming around clients' feet? Should you wait until you have enough cups to make it worthwhile washing up? The answer is NO. Common sense is required on your part so that the jobs you carry out maintain a professional reception without making clients feel uncomfortable or in the way.

Cleaning the floor and dusting can be carried out last thing at night or first thing in the morning before clients arrive. Cups and saucers can be picked up in a regular hourly round-up to ensure you do not run out. Magazines can be tidied when cups are collected from reception. Coats can be taken from clients when you know that they are having a service.

Top tips

First impressions count! It is a well-known fact that people make a judgement about you within the first 30 seconds to two minutes of meeting you. We form our opinion about someone on the following basis:

- 55 per cent appearance, facial expression and body language
- 38 per cent tone of voice
- 7 per cent what you say.

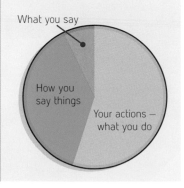

What you say

How you say things

Your actions – what you do

Keeping stationery stock up to date

You will need certain stationery items when you are working on reception. These will probably include:

- a memo pad for taking messages
- appointment cards
- loyalty cards
- price lists
- retail product price list
- a cashing-up summary sheet.

When you are taking a message for a colleague, either over the phone or from a client in person, you will need to take all of the relevant details. Which item of stationery will you need from the list above?

If you ran out of the correct forms on reception and the message was written down on a scrap piece of paper, the chances are that the message would be lost. It is important to make sure that you have all of the relevant forms and stationery so that reception can function professionally.

Your job may be to ensure that there are enough price lists for clients to be able to take them away with them if required. They may be regular clients and know the prices of their own services, but what if they want to introduce family or friends to the salon?

Many salons have computerised tills which have a variety of functions to benefit the salon. Some computerised tills calculate different stylists' commission on general salon income from client services and retail sales. This information may also be recorded manually.

If you have not notified the person in charge who orders in the stationery that it is running low and requires reordering you will run out. This could potentially lose the salon business, especially if a client has been promised or is expecting a new loyalty card or discount voucher.

These are just some examples of how important it is to make sure that you know what stationery your salon uses.

> **Top tips**
>
> It is important that you use the correct stationery so that the salon's records are kept accurate and up to date.

Task 3

Find out who you report stationery shortages to within your salon and what is the minimum amount of stationery that the salon may keep at any one time.

Product displays

Another important job of the receptionist is to make sure that all product display stands are kept well stocked with the right levels of products at all times.

In order to make the correct retail product recommendations, you will need to make sure you are knowledgeable about what the products do and their suitability for different hair types to maintain the services carried out. If you are selling products to clients you also have to know the rules that affect you. See page 61 for legislation on the Sale of Goods Act.

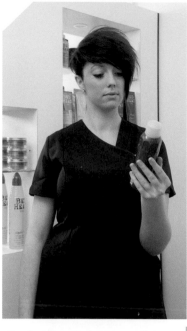

Product knowledge is essential when selling to clients

Task 4

Using a copy of the grid below, make a list of:

- all the products your salon has for sale
- the benefits of each product
- what service the product is suitable as aftercare for
- the cost of the product to the client.

Product type	Benefits of the product	Aftercare for which service	Cost

A worksheet containing this chart can be found on the website for you to record your findings. This can then be used as additional portfolio evidence.

Task 5

Who do you report stock shortages to in your salon and what is the minimum amount of stock you can run to?

Client hospitality and client care

We have all been into a shop at one time or another where the staff have been more interested in having a conversation between themselves than serving us. How has this made you feel? Good hospitality and client care are essential to ensure clients will return time and time again and the salon will grow and sustain its business.

Most salons offer drinks to their clients. At some salons they may be free of charge while at others there may be a small charge. You may find that salons that do not charge for drinks may only offer them to clients who are having chemical processes or a service over a certain period of time.

Would it make sense to offer a hot drink to a client who is only having a dry trim? By the time you boil the kettle and make the drink she may be leaving the salon. However, if the stylist is running a little late and the client has to wait, you may decide that it is appropriate to offer her a drink while waiting. You need to use your common sense when deciding.

Hospitality extends beyond offering a client a cup of tea! Make a list of how else you can make clients feel welcome when they enter your salon. Some of the things you have on your list may include:

- greet every client with a smile, even when you answer the telephone, because this reflects in your voice
- make sure you have positive body language by looking the client in the eye and sitting up straight at reception
- always ask the client how you can help
- offer to take the client's coat and ask her to take a seat
- offer the client a drink or magazine while she is waiting
- find out how long the stylist is going to be and inform the client of this
- if the client has to wait a little longer than usual, check that she is aware of this.

Remember to smile when greeting clients on the telephone too – hospitality and client care are essential to a successful salon

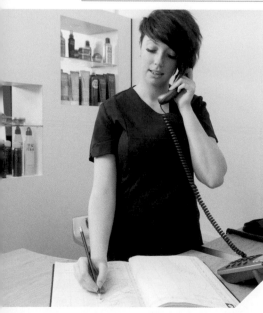

Task 6

What is your salon's code of practice for hospitality and client care?

Find out what beverages your salon has to offer and what it charges, if anything.

How to attend to clients and enquiries

Receiving clients into the salon is rather like welcoming a guest into your home. The hospitality and friendliness should be the same. Whether it is the client's first visit or their fifteenth, the polite and welcoming atmosphere should be the same. This is achieved through verbal and non-verbal communication skills, listening skills and questioning techniques. In this section you will look at good practice in handling a range of clients and enquiries.

Handling enquiries

The approach to clients and all visitors to the salon can be summed up in the word PLEASE, which stands for:

- **P**osture
- **L**isten
- **E**xpression
- **A**ppearance and attitude
- **S**peech
- **E**agerness to help others.

Posture should be good and body language open. Nothing is more off putting to a visitor than someone slouching over a desk. It says, 'Can't be bothered with you,' and sends out entirely the wrong message.

Listen with your ears, 'listen' with your eyes by looking at the client to show you are paying attention, and 'listen' with your body language so that you are saying, 'You are important to the salon and I am taking notice of you.'

Expression should be welcoming, smiling and open, not hostile with a frown or scowl.

Appearance and attitude should reflect total professionalism and indicate the high standing of the salon.

Speech should be clear, without a patronising tone, and jargon free! (Do not use technical terms that the client will not understand.)

Eagerness to help others is an excellent quality — use it whenever you can!

When greeting clients you need to quickly identify the enquiry.

- Is the client in your salon because she has come to make an appointment, or has an appointment?
- Is the client there to pick up a price list?
- Is the client a regular client who has called in to purchase some retail products?
- Is the client actually a representative from a company wishing to see your boss to show a new range of products?
- Has the client come in to complain about a previous service?

Unit

G4

Fulfil salon reception duties

Task 7

How many other reasons can you think of as to why a client would be in your reception area? How many of these reasons can you deal with and which ones need to be referred to a senior member of staff?

A worksheet for this task is provided on the website for you to complete and add to your portfolio.

Balancing the needs of individuals

Customers may have special needs that have to be considered. For example:

- Clients with physical disabilities may require some help negotiating doorways and getting into the salon. Always offer to help, but do not assume the client cannot manage — and never patronise or 'talk down' to the client.
- Clients who are hearing impaired are usually good lip readers, so the receptionist should face the client and speak clearly; this allows the client to see the words forming. Depending upon the severity of the disability, a notepad could be provided to jot down a message. A price list can be a good visual aid to help clarify the client's needs.
- Visitors from overseas may have slight problems being understood, although some cultures have a better command of English if they have been taught it in school. Again, speak clearly, use visual materials to help clarify what is required and seek help if available.
- Older clients may have problems with mobility or hearing, but do not assume this to be the case — do not pre-judge!

Dealing with telephone enquiries

Good telephone communication skills are very useful for business, and it is worthwhile learning how to use the telephone well.

Good telephone manner

There are some key steps to acquiring a good telephone manner, thereby ensuring that the person on the end of the phone is treated courteously, efficiently and accurately. These include the following:

- Always have a pen and paper handy so that you are prepared to take messages.
- Answer the phone promptly, even if you are busy. If you do feel harassed, pause, take a deep breath before lifting the receiver and put a smile in your voice — it is very easy to sound abrupt on the telephone.
- Identify the salon quickly, after making sure you are connected properly and the caller can hear you.
- Be cheery — no matter how pressurised you may feel, it should not be obvious from the tone of your voice. No one wants to be greeted with a miserable-sounding receptionist! Redirect the call quickly if going through to another extension. If the call cannot be put through, ask if the caller wishes to leave a message.

You may answer the telephone to an unhappy or disgruntled client. Below is a list of points to remember.

- Stay polite at all times.
- Take down as much information as you can about the problem.

- Take the client's details and contact number.
- Reassure the client that someone who can deal with the complaint will phone her very shortly.
- Inform a member of staff immediately after the phone call.
- Know the limits of your own authority and when you should seek advice from a more senior colleague.

Dos	Don'ts
✓ *Do* answer with a smile on your face – just as if you can see the caller's face.	✗ *Don't* sigh into the phone – it gives the impression that the caller is a nuisance and that you are doing a huge favour by answering.
✓ *Do* write a message clearly so that it can be read easily and make sure that it includes all information such as the name of the caller.	✗ *Don't* be curt, rude or irritated when you first pick up the phone – you never know who is on the other end and no one deserves rudeness.
✓ *Do* remember that all calls are from existing or prospective clients.	✗ *Don't* lie to the caller – if you do not know something or where someone is, then be honest. If you make something up, you will only get caught out and lose credibility.
✓ *Do* ask to use the phone if you need to make a quick personal call.	✗ *Don't* ever slam down the phone in temper, cut someone off or talk about the caller in a rude manner – the caller will most certainly hear and be offended.
✓ *Do* remember that there might be telephone calls outside of office hours or when everyone is genuinely busy. An answer machine is a simple solution. Revenue may be lost if there is no one to answer that important phone call.	✗ *Don't* use the telephone for long-distance or private calls. Itemised phone bills will show who made a call, for how long and to whom. No employer would mind the odd local call or emergency message, but do not abuse an employer's goodwill.

Dos and don'ts when using the telephone

Task 8

Use the grid on the website to make a list of all the enquiries you answer throughout a working day. How many were telephone enquiries? How many were face-to-face enquiries? Keep a note of these by writing down a brief account of the nature of the enquiry, the client's name and the date and time, and include this as evidence for your portfolio.

Confirming appointments

You should always confirm the details of an appointment with a client to make sure that you have understood each other. By doing this, you are double-checking that all of the information received is accurate and that the client is happy with the date and time of the appointment.

You should remember to do the following:

- Repeat back to the client the details of the appointment by stating clearly the date, time and service she will be receiving. Most salons have an appointment card system.
- If there is a potential problem with the stylist's column in the appointment system, discuss this with the stylist before confirming the appointment.
- Make sure that any confidential information is recorded in the appropriate place and not broadcast to the whole salon!

What is confidential information?

This includes the client's address, telephone number, health status, medication and any other private information you might have access to. You are allowed to give these details to authorised people only, such as the salon owner, manager or employees. No person outside of the salon must have access to your clients' personal details.

Client Record Card

Name:

Address:

Post Code: Telephone:

Date	Service/Product/Perm Colour Condition etc.	Application/Rod size/Timing/Result	Stylist

Client record

Fact or fiction?

Is this statement fact or fiction?

You do not need to keep your client records secure.

To check your answer see page 493.

Many salons have computerised systems which incorporate a computerised appointment system and till. There are many benefits to using this type of technology as once the client details are entered into the system there are programs which can generate mail shots and texts to clients, produce special offers and loyalty vouchers, etc. However, if you are storing client details on a computerised appointment system it should be protected by a password so that only authorised employees can access the client details.

Recording messages

As a receptionist, you will be required to take messages for other members of staff. You will also need to produce evidence of this for your portfolio, so make sure you keep a copy of any messages you have passed on.

It is very important to write down the whole of the message at the time it is given to you. It is unlikely you will remember it word for word, so make a habit of writing down all the information immediately. You will need to include:

- who the message is for (there is no point taking a message if you do not know who to pass it on to!)
- the caller's name, address (if necessary) and telephone number (there may be more than one Mrs Allen, for example)
- the date and time of the call
- how important the message is – for example, it may be urgent
- a brief description of the nature of the message
- whether the caller requires a reply – in this case it is essential to have the caller's telephone number.

It is important to listen carefully and ask the caller to repeat any part of the message you did not understand or hear properly. Always repeat the message back to the caller to make sure you have all the correct details – especially contact details such as an email address or phone number.

MESSAGE

FOR Deepak

FROM Mrs Alessi

TEL. NO. 0208 321 145

TELEPHONED ✓   PLEASE RING ✓

CALLED TO SEE YOU ☐   WILL CALL AGAIN ☐

WANTS TO SEE YOU ☐   URGENT ☐

MESSAGE: Needs to speak to you asap – you can call her on the tel. no. above up to 5.30pm

DATE: 10.03.12   TIME: 9.03am

RECEIVED BY: Amber

Recording a message

Fulfil salon reception duties

How to make appointments for salon services

You have looked at the approach you need to take when dealing with clients, both face to face and on the telephone, when they enquire about their appointments or make new ones. You are now going to explore how to make appointments for clients and ensure the smooth running of the appointment system.

Good practice in dealing with appointment requests

It is usual for the appointments for each stylist to be kept on a spreadsheet if on a computerised appointment system or in a large book, usually with a column for each stylist. This allows the stylists to see at a glance what services are booked in for the day and enables them to make the appropriate preparation.

The golden rule in all salons is: have an appointments system and use it correctly. All appointment scheduling systems should be set out for several months in advance so that clients booking ahead or for special occasions (such as weddings) can make appointments with confidence. This also allows the stylist to book out time for holidays and personal appointments.

When booking an appointment, you should include the following details:

- name of client
- contact telephone number
- type of service.

Top tips

Always deal with requests from clients promptly and politely.

Top tips

If you do not allow enough time for the stylist's first appointment of the day, she will overrun, making the next appointment late. This could continue all day and the knock-on effect may be that the last client is kept waiting far too long. The stylist becomes stressed under pressure, the client may feel rushed and unhappy, and as a consequence she may not return!

Most salons have a system of coding to make life easier. For example:

- F/H Foils = Full head highlights using foil
- H/H Foils = Half head highlights using foil
- T zone = partial highlights
- D/T = dry trim
- P/W = permanent wave (perm)
- S/S = shampoo and set
- C/B/D = cut and blow-dry
- B/D = blow-dry
- W/C = wet cut.

The right way to schedule appointments

You will also need to know how long to book each appointment for. You should allow for:

- greeting the client and consultation
- client preparation during the service
- client receiving homecare and aftercare advice.

Below is a typical page taken from an electronic appointments system.

Page from a computerised appointments system

	Maeve D	Sze Kiu	Mark P
	17 Saturday	**17 Saturday**	**17 Saturday**
8am	*Checked in* **Lucy Juxton** – 01234 567890 Start time: 8am Wet cut	*Checked in* **Mr Davies** – 01345 453782 Start time: 8am Dry trim	*Checked in* **Mrs Rahim** – 07745 565758 Start time: 8am Cut and blow-dry
8.15am	*****************	*****************	*****************
8.30am	**Mrs Moorman** – 07778 981658 Start time: 8.30am Full head (foils x 2 colours)	*****************	*****************
8.45am	*****************		*****************
9am	*****************	**Mrs Adam** – 07564 271152 Start time: 9am Blow-dry	**Alexa Taylor** – 05643 272896 Start time: 9am Perm
9.15am	*****************	*****************	*****************
9.30am	*****************	*****************	*****************
9.45am	*****************	**Ms Anderson** – 01386 836775 Start time: 9.45am Cut and blow-dry	*****************
10am		*****************	**Mrs Chandler** – 07777 707777 start time:10am Cut and blow-dry
10.15am		*****************	*****************
10.30am		*****************	*****************

Some salons do not have appointment booking facilities; they rely on staff being available to receive clients who walk in off the street. The advantage of this system is that the workload can be easily distributed between staff and the manager allocates the jobs as fairly as possible. The disadvantage is that regular clients do not always get the same stylist. This type of system therefore does not suit all clients.

Task 9

1 What system does your college/salon/training institution have in place for dealing with clients who may turn up without an appointment?
2 How much time does your salon allocate for each of the different services offered?

Booking appointments

When booking an appointment in a paper-based appointment system:

- fill out the details in pencil – this allows changes, such as a cancellation, to be made without making the page messy and illegible
- use a simple code to identify any potential problems – for example, C = cancellation, L = late arrival, ✓ = client has arrived, and so on
- make sure that everyone can easily understand start and finish times
- make sure that all names and numbers are clear and legible
- allow the hard-working stylist a break for lunch – do not be pressured by a persistent client into giving a lunchtime appointment to a stylist who has no other break throughout the day
- try to stagger the stylists' lunch breaks so that there is always a stylist to cover a busy lunchtime session
- give an appointment card to the client with all the details recorded on it – they then have a record of when to come in, it confirms the appointment for the client, and cuts down the possibility of a missed appointment.

When using a computerised appointment system, a record of the appointment can be printed off and given to the client.

Always remember to double-check the appointment with the client. If a client's partner phones up to book a surprise appointment and he is not sure whether she wants a cut and blow-dry or a dry trim, how will you know how much time to book out for the appointment? What would you do in this instance?

One possible solution would be to tell the partner that you will make an appointment for the shorter service for the time being until he can confirm this later. This will ensure that the stylist is not sitting around having wasted appointment time!

When booking appointments for clients, it is important to make sure that you take all of the clients' details accurately. You need to make sure you are booking them in for the right amount of appointment time and for the service that they require.

Confirming appointments

Whenever you book an appointment for a client, always read back the appointment details to confirm that you have the right information.

Top tips

Calls may come in outside of working hours or when everyone is genuinely busy. An answer machine is a simple solution.

Top tips

When you fit in a client without a booking, always alert the stylist that the client is waiting. If the client is new to the salon, she may require hair and skin tests before certain services can be carried out. You would, therefore, need to allow more time for tests and for the initial consultation.

93

Unit

G4

Fulfil salon reception cuties

HAIR		appointments
Please retain this card for future appointments		
Date	Time	Stylist

If appointments are missed or not cancelled within 24 hours of the appointment, a charge will be applicable.

An appointment reminder card

Fulfil salon reception duties

Missed appointments and clients without appointments

Every salon should have a policy on missed appointments. Some salons have a small cancellation charge if the appointment is missed, rather like the dentist. There is usually no cancellation fee if the appointment is cancelled with 24 hours' notice. Both staff and clients need to be clear on this policy and it should be displayed in the reception area.

Be prepared to fit in a client who arrives without an appointment. You should always check the appointments system before fitting the client into a suitable slot — and then inform the stylist, who may not be aware that a client is waiting.

How to handle payments from clients

It is important that a salon has a safe and secure system for the processing of payment transactions. Most salons have an electronic or computerised till to:

- help calculate the client's bill
- help the receptionist double-check the correct amount of change
- provide a receipt for the client
- provide a till reading of the salon's daily takings
- securely hold the clients' payments and till float.

The reception area is also an excellent place to display a range of retail products, as the client may decide while she is paying for the service received to try a product that has been recommended by the stylist.

Calculating the cost of services

No matter how much a service costs, from a small child's trim to a full head colour, it is always important to treat clients in a courteous manner. The client should be treated as courteously at the end of the service as at the beginning, and they should feel that the service received was excellent value for money. You should always make clients feel important and thank them for their business.

As the receptionist, you should know which services the client has received in order to total the bill accurately. If your salon charges for extras such as tea, coffee and biscuits you should make sure that these are added to the final bill. You need to ensure clients know of any extra charges that may be added to their bill for refreshments. The stylist and receptionist should liaise to ensure the client is charged correctly.

Methods of payment

The way the client pays is very much her choice and you must be prepared and able to cope with any payment method. The main methods your client may use to pay are:

- cash
- credit card
- debit card
- cheque
- gift voucher
- loyalty card.

All are equally acceptable and should be handled with care.

Top tips

A client may visit your salon frequently and £15 adds up over the months, whereas a client spending £50 may only come to you once in a blue moon! Both clients should be valued equally.

Cash

There are several things to be aware of when a customer pays with cash. All banknotes should be checked to make sure they are genuine and not counterfeit. You confirm they are legal tender by checking for the following:

- Look for the watermark – every note has a watermark, which can be seen when the note is held up to the light.
- Look for the metallic strip which is woven into the paper – it should be unbroken.
- Compare the feel of banknote paper – often a forged note is not printed on the same quality of paper and may have a thin, papery feel.

The police often circulate a list of forged notes to be on the lookout for. The banknote numbers are on a stop list and this list should be kept near the till so that numbers can be compared.

If you are given a forged note, quietly ask the client to step away from reception, to avoid embarrassment. The client may have been given the money from another source. Ask a supervisor or the salon manager or owner to deal with the situation. You should then return to your duties at the front desk. In most cases, the client will not be aware that the note is forged, so it is not up to you to accuse her. It is important, however, that the note is removed from circulation and the police are informed.

Even when accepting money from very regular customers, it should still be checked thoroughly.

Procedure for handling cash payments

Dealing with cash involves a lot of responsibility and care must be taken to avoid errors.

- Place the client's money on the till ledge to ensure you remember what amount you have been given. Do not place the money straight into the till drawer as this may lead to confusion – was it a £10 note or a £20 note?
- Count the change required from the note and then re-count it into the client's hand.
- Place the client's money in the till drawer and close it.
- Give the client the receipt to confirm the cost of the service, how much was given to you and the change to be given.

Task 10

What security procedures does your salon use to check for counterfeit banknotes?

Top tips

- Never feel embarrassed when checking money. It will save the salon from financial loss and protect the customer.
- Payments for all services should be acknowledged, either by a handwritten receipt or a printed one from the till, regardless of which type of payment is used.
- If depositing money at the bank, avoid using a big bank bag, which advertises exactly what it is you are carrying! Never take the same route to the bank at exactly the same time every day. Someone may be watching and being a victim of a snatch robbery would be a dreadful experience. Do not be a victim – be safe!

Credit cards

Credit cards have become as common as any other payment facility. All leading banks and a variety of other financial institutions offer credit cards to those customers whom they consider creditworthy.

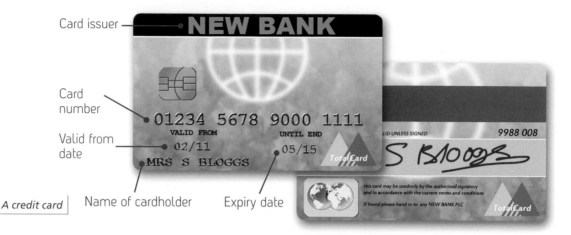

Card issuer

Card number

Valid from date

Name of cardholder

Expiry date

A credit card

So how do credit card payments work? If your salon has a contract with a credit card company, it will usually display a sign stating that credit cards are accepted. The customer's card is 'swiped' through a computerised till connected to the credit card company. Once the credit card company authorises payment, usually within a minute or two, the client keys in their Personal Identification Number (PIN) or signs the credit card receipt agreeing to make the payment. The salon must give a copy of the credit card receipt to the client and keeps one for its own records. The credit card company will then pay for the goods or services the client has bought by transferring the money electronically to the salon's bank account and the client will be billed by the credit card company at a later date. This is an efficient way for the salon to receive payment; in return, the credit card company charges the salon a handling fee of 1.5 or 2 per cent.

Debit cards

This is when payment is made electronically, transferring money straight from the client's bank account to the salon's account. This saves the client having to write a cheque. Debit cards are usually the same card as the cheque guarantee card.

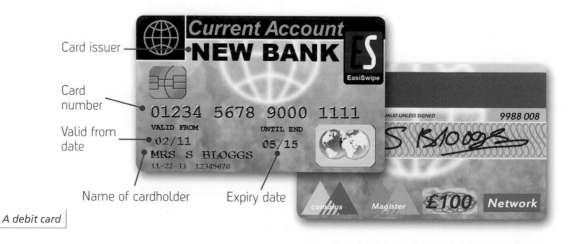

Card issuer

Card number

Valid from date

Name of cardholder

Expiry date

A debit card

To take a payment using a debit card, swipe the card through the computerised till unit using a sliding action, or put the client's card into a chip and PIN unit attached to the till. This allows the information stored on the magnetic strip on the back of the card to be read. The client then either signs a receipt or enters her PIN number into the hand-held unit. The till then produces a receipt which must be given to the client.

Cheques

A cheque is equivalent to a letter to the bank telling it to pay a certain sum to a specified person. Most banks and building societies offer a cheque service, although a debit card service is also available (see page 96). Some shops are starting to advertise the fact that they will no longer accept cheques as payment from a certain date. This is due to it becoming more costly to the business to accept cheques as a form of payment.

If a cheque payment is acceptable, certain checks and precautions need to be carried out. Always check that:

- the date is correct – day, month and year (this is especially important just after New Year!)
- the name of the salon is spelled correctly – the client could be offered a stamp with the full name pre-printed on it
- the amount is correct and that the amount in words and figures are the same
- the signature is included and that it matches the one shown on the client's cheque guarantee card.

97

Unit

G4

Fulfil salon reception duties

Is the name of the salon correct?

Is the amount of money in words and figures correct?

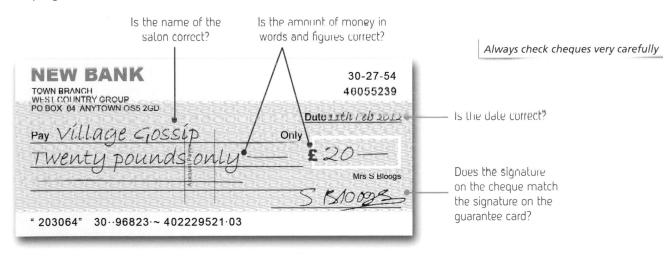

Always check cheques very carefully

Is the date correct?

Does the signature on the cheque match the signature on the guarantee card?

What is a cheque guarantee card?

A cheque guarantee card should always be provided to support a cheque payment. It has two functions:

1 It acts as proof of identity.
2 It guarantees that the bank will honour the cheque up to the limit of the card. The limit on most bank cards is £100.

There is always the exception to the rule and you may find you have a client whose limit is only £50. What happens if the total cost of the service exceeds this amount? If you have a situation where you have asked a senior member of staff for authorisation and he or she declines, how would you inform the client?

Top tips

Be careful with debit and credit cards. All the information they contain – usually the holder's account number and expiry date of card – is stored on a magnetic strip on the back of the card. If this strip comes into contact with a magnet, the information is destroyed. Even the magnetic clasp on a purse or handbag is enough to disable all information. Some retail stores use a magnet to remove security tags; this can also interfere with your debit card!

Discrepancy

A difference between items; for example, a payment discrepancy is where the payment for a service is not valid or acceptable.

Top tips

In the event of a payment discrepancy that you are unable to resolve, you should refer to the salon manager or owner. As long as you stay calm and professional and report the incident promptly to the correct person, you will have acted within the limits of your authority.

You should always check the expiry date on the cheque guarantee card – written as 03/13, for example, which is the month and year the card needs to be re-issued. You also need to check that the signatures match and that the card type is the same as the cheque. For example, an HSBC cheque is supported by an HSBC cheque guarantee card.

The cheque is then treated exactly like cash, put into the till, a receipt given and the till closed.

Salon gift vouchers

Some salons offer vouchers for clients to buy as gifts. The vouchers may be used to pay for a service or part of a service. They should be treated as cash and must be stored securely, either in the till, a locked drawer or a safe that has restricted access. It is a good idea to number gift vouchers for security purposes. When used as payment, the voucher should be placed in the till after being marked to show it has been used.

Loyalty cards

Many salons offer loyalty cards as an incentive to encourage clients to return to the salon for further services. A card is issued to the client and stamped or officially marked when the client pays for their service. Once the loyalty card is full it can be redeemed to a specific value or against a specified service. This is a very good incentive to gain client loyalty.

Task 11

If your salon sells gift vouchers, find out who has the authority to issue them and how they are processed through the till.

Handling discrepancies

Unfortunately, there may be times when payment **discrepancies** and disputes arise. They should be dealt with calmly, without causing too much embarrassment to the client. Possible problems may include:

- if the currency is invalid – perhaps a foreign note or even a forged note
- if an invalid credit/debit/cheque guarantee card is presented – it may be out of date or not match the cheque details
- if a cheque is filled out incorrectly or does not have a current cheque guarantee card
- suspected fraudulent use of a payment card – perhaps it has been put onto the stop list
- suspected fraudulent use of a loyalty card – there may be some doubt whether the loyalty card is original or copied.

Managing transactions securely

It is important to ensure the safety and security of the reception area, as this is usually a requirement of the salon's insurance policy. If money is left on show rather than safely locked in the till, it could be targeted by thieves. As the receptionist, you are responsible for the security of the salon's takings and this should not be taken lightly. It is advisable to be alert to all those who use the till to make sure transactions are correctly processed.

At the beginning of the day it is the receptionist's job to go to the bank to collect the change (daily float) for the till. It is also important to ensure that there is always sufficient change in the till. If you run out, you may need to ask a nearby shop for change. If you think you are going to run out, you should report this to a senior member of staff. It is helpful to keep some additional change in the salon to avoid this problem. However, you need to remember to replace the change when it is used.

To give you an idea of the amount of change that may be required for the day, refer to the following list.

- 3 x £10 notes
- 4 x £5 notes
- £20 in £1 coins
- £5 in 50p pieces
- £3 in 20p pieces
- £2 in 10p pieces
- £1 in 5p pieces
- £1 in 2p and 1p pieces.

It will depend on the structure of the salon's price list as to how much change your float will require. For example, if your salon's prices all end in 95p, you will need to have extra 5 pence pieces in the till.

At the end of the day's business, the till must be totalled and the takings should match the recorded amount taken, either through the till computer or a docket system. If a float has been used to provide a base of change at the beginning of the day, then it needs to be deducted. This can then be used for the next day's trading and the balance of the takings should be paid into the salon's bank account.

Most large banks offer a night-safe facility in which the takings can be deposited. It is not ideal to keep large amounts of money on the premises overnight, as there is always the risk of a burglary.

Salon life

Meeting and greeting

Poppy's story

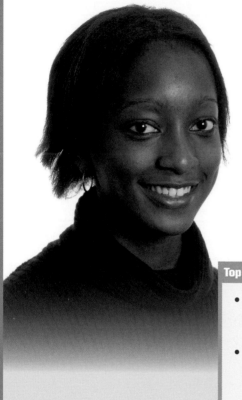

When I first joined my salon I was quite shy and nervous, and found talking to clients quite difficult. I used to try to avoid having to deal with clients at reception because I was scared in case I made a mistake and would get told off. I really didn't like having to make decisions about where to book a client in on the appointment system and I used to do anything to avoid reception duties. I was brave enough to mention this to my boss at my appraisal and she gave me extra lessons on how to book clients in and what sort of advice I should be giving to clients and this gave me more confidence. Now I can't believe I was that worried about reception and having to deal with clients. My advice to anyone new to a salon is to ask if you're not sure what to do and face your fears, because that's the only way to overcome something that's affecting you at work.

Top tips

- Always be welcoming to all clients as they enter reception. Smile and greet them warmly and don't be shy as clients may think you are being rude, even if the truth is you are very shy.
- Make sure you always stay calm at reception and don't get flustered, even if you have clients waiting and the phone won't stop ringing. The key is to be organised so you can cope at stressful times.

Ask the expert

Q   *Reception duties seem to cover so much that there is loads to learn. What do you do if you come across a problem at reception that you cannot deal with?*

A   There is always going to be something that you don't know the answer to because you are only human! If you are unsure about something, don't make an answer up as this could cause real problems. Explain to the client that you will find out the answer for them and seek guidance from a more senior member of staff.

Check your knowledge

The following questions will help you to check your understanding of this unit.
The answers can be found on page 493.

1 What is your salon's procedure for maintaining client confidentiality?

_____

_____

_____

2 What are the consequences of breaking client confidentiality?
   a) The staff in the salon will have some juicy gossip.
   b) It will give the stylists something to talk about.
   c) You could go to prison.
   d) The client could sue the salon.

3 How do you ensure cash and other payment types are kept safe and secure?

_____

_____

_____

4 Who would you refer a payment discrepancy to if you could not resolve the problem?

_____

_____

_____

5 How would you check for invalid cash payments?

_____

_____

_____

6 State what checks are necessary when a client pays by cheque.

_____

_____

_____

Fulfil salon reception duties

7 Why is effective communication important to your salon's business?

_____

_____

_____

8 State how you would deal with a client who is angry.
   a) Keep calm and do all you can to help.
   b) Pretend you know nothing about the problem and ask them to come back later.
   c) Get someone else to deal with the problem.
   d) Behaviour breeds behaviour so get angry so you know how the client is feeling.

9 How do you ensure you give clients the correct change when paying cash with a large note?
   a) Make sure you remember what note you were given by leaving it out of the till drawer until you have given the change to the client.
   b) Ask clients not to pay with large notes.
   c) Get another member of staff to deal with the payment.
   d) Ask the client if she has any other form of payment, such as credit/debit card or cheque.

10 Why is it important for the reception area to be clean and tidy at all times?
   a) So you don't have all the clearing up at the end of the day.
   b) So that everyone in the salon does some clearing up.
   c) To ensure the first impression the client has is of a well-maintained, clean and tidy business.
   d) To ensure the receptionist looks good.

Getting ready for assessment

You will be assessed using a combination of assessment methods, as described below. Remember that within each of the services you carry out with a client, you will cover different units. For example, when carrying out salon reception duties (G4), you will also have to be aware of health and safety (G20) and give clients a positive impression (G17) at all times. If you are not sure what you have covered in your service, always ask your assessor or supervisor for advice.

	NVQ	VRQ
Credit value	3	3
Guided Learning Hours	24	24

	NVQ	**VRQ**
Practical demonstrations, to be observed by assessor	Your assessor will observe you on at least three different occasions. VTCT – Simulation is not allowed for any performance evidence within this unit. C&G – Evidence from simulated activities may be used to produce performance evidence but only when naturally occurring performance evidence cannot be obtained for methods of payment range variables – cash equivalents, cheque and payment cards and handling the types of payment discrepancies listed. From the range statement you must show that you have: • handled three of the four types of people • handled two of the three types of enquiries • handled both types of appointment • obtained all the appointment details • handled all the methods of payment • dealt with all the types of discrepancy.	Your assessor will observe you on at least three different occasions. It is strongly recommended that the evidence for this unit be gathered in a realistic working environment. Simulation should be avoided where possible. All outcomes, assessment criteria and range statements must be achieved.
Service timings	There are no mandatory service times for this unit.	There are no mandatory service times for this unit.
Additional evidence	It is likely most evidence of your performance will be gathered from the observations made by your assessor but you may be required to produce other evidence to support your performance, e.g. oral questions. There is no external paper requirement for this unit.	On occasions some practical criteria may not naturally occur during a practical observation. In such instances you will be asked questions to demonstrate your knowledge in this area. Your assessor will document the criteria that have been achieved through oral questioning.

Task mapping

When you have completed the tasks in this unit, check the table below to see which Performance Criteria (purple), Range (red), Knowledge (green) and Key Skills (blue) you have covered within G4 to use as additional evidence within your portfolio. Information about which Functional Skills you have covered is available on the website.

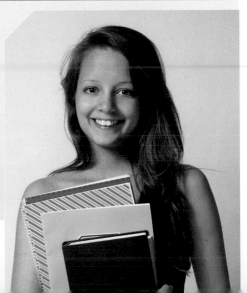

Task and page reference	Mapping to Performance Criteria, Range, Knowledge and Key Skills
1 (page 83)	Performance Criteria: Practising 2f, 3b–e, VRQ 1a, 2a Range: 2a–c, VRQ 3c, k, g, h, i, c Knowledge: 15, 16, VRQ 1g, h Key Skills: C1.2
2 (page 84)	Performance Criteria: Practising 1a, VRQ 1d, e, 2c Range: N/A Knowledge: 2 Key Skills: C1.2, C1.3, C2.3
3 (page 85)	Performance Criteria: Practising 1b, VRQ 1d Range: N/A Knowledge: 19 Key Skills: C1.2, C1.3, C2.3, N1.1, N1.2, N1.3, N2.1, N2.2, N2.3
4 (page 86)	Performance Criteria: Practising 2f, VRQ 1a, b Range: 4d, VRQ f–j, n Knowledge: 16, VRQ 1h Key Skills: C1.2, C1.3, C2.3, N1.1, N1.2, N1.3, N2.1, N2.2, N2.3
5 (page 86)	Performance Criteria: Practising 1c, VRQ 1b Range: N/A Knowledge: 5 Key Skills: C1.2, C1.3, C2.3, N1.1, N1.2, N1.3, N2.1, N2.2, N2.3
6 (page 87)	Performance Criteria: 1d, 2a, VRQ 1b Range: VRQ 1e Knowledge: 1, 2 Key Skills: C1.2, C1.3, C2.3, N1.1, N1.2, N1.3, N2.1, N2.2, N2.3
7 (page 88)	Performance Criteria: 2a, 2b, 2d, VRQ 1a–c Range: VRQ 1a–d Knowledge: 2, 4, 5, VRQ 1i, j Key Skills: C1.2, C1.3, C2.3
8 (page 89)	Performance Criteria: 2a–h, Practising 3a–e, VRQ 1a–c Range: 1a–d, 2a–c, 3a–b, VRQ 1a–d Knowledge: 1, 2, VRQ 1i, j Key Skills: C1.2, C1.3, C2.3, N1.1, N1.2, N1.3, N2.1, N2.2, N2.3
9 (page 93)	Performance Criteria: 3a–c, VRQ 2a Range: 1a Knowledge: 1, VRQ 2d, e Key Skills: C1.2, C1.3, C2.3, N1.1, N1.2, N1.3, N2.1, N2.2, N2.3
10 (page 95)	Performance Criteria: 4c, 4e, VRQ 3c Range: 5a, 6a, VRQ p–w Knowledge: 1, 2, VRQ 3d, e
11 (page 98)	Performance Criteria: 4g, VRQ 3b, c Range: 5b, VRQ r Knowledge: 1, 2, 22, VRQ 3d Key Skills: C1.2, C1.3, C2.3

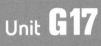

Give clients a positive impression of yourself and your organisation

Unit **G17**

Unit
G17

Give clients a positive impression of yourself and your organisation

What you will learn:

- **How to establish effective rapport with clients**
- **How to respond appropriately to clients**
- **How to communicate information to clients**

Introduction

This unit is all about communicating with clients and giving a positive impression of yourself and your salon/organisation whenever you deal with a client. Most successful salons earn their reputation through providing an excellent personal service. You are, therefore, responsible for playing your part in earning a good reputation for your salon through every client you come into contact with.

As a stylist within your salon it is your job to maintain excellent customer service to whoever walks through the salon door. This is essential to ensure the client has a good experience throughout the time spent in the salon. It is not enough to rely on a good haircut to maintain continued client loyalty as it is the 'whole salon experience' that will determine whether the client returns to your salon, or your competitor's, for future services. You need to ensure you communicate effectively and appropriately with clients however busy you are. This can be tricky when the salon is extremely busy so it is important to follow your salon's procedures to ensure you are responding to clients in the most appropriate way.

Have you ever had a poor customer service experience? It is a fact that one person who experiences poor customer service will tell at least seven other people about this negative experience. Your salon's reputation is at stake if you fail to give clients excellent service. It is therefore part of your job role to ensure you represent your salon to the highest standard possible by giving your clients outstanding customer service.

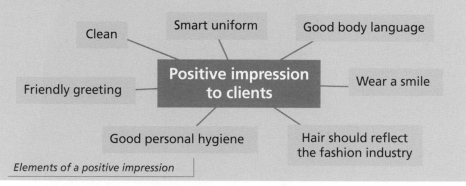

Elements of a positive impression

Clean · Smart uniform · Good body language · Wear a smile · Hair should reflect the fashion industry · Good personal hygiene · Friendly greeting · **Positive impression to clients**

Video clip

Watch video clip 'Communication skills' on the website to hear what celebrity stylist Andrew Barton has to say about the importance of great communication skills.

Rapport

A feeling of understanding or sympathy.

How to establish effective rapport with clients

When you work in hairdressing, it is very important that you are able to get on with anyone who walks through your salon's door. As a stylist, you should be pleasant, patient and helpful to everyone coming into the salon. It is only through trust and effective communication that you can start to build a **rapport** with your client, and it is vital that you start to build this from your client's first visit to your salon. It is also important to continue to build upon rapport with well-established clients. They should be made to feel special every time they visit your salon or they will try the salon around the corner; do not become complacent with well-established clients.

Appearance and behaviour

We have already discussed appearance in G20, as your appearance affects health and safety. A new client's first impression of you will be mainly visual, i.e. how you look. Therefore it is really important for you to make the right impression by making every effort to look your best while you are at work.

However, it is not just how you look that will make an impression on your client. How you behave will have a massive influence on how your client views you as a person and will reflect on your salon. As a mature adult you will be expected to act sensibly and professionally at all times so that you don't endanger anyone in the salon. This will also create the correct and positive image that your salon owner/manager will want you to help achieve.

Task 1

What are your salon's rules for stylist appearance and behaviour? Write them down and keep them in your portfolio of evidence. Why is it important to follow these salon rules?

Greeting clients

Most salons have a procedure for greeting clients, but if the salon is busy it is usually whoever is free who greets the client first. Make every effort to stop what you are doing, excuse yourself from the client you are working with, if necessary, and greet the client as soon as she walks into the reception area. The client may have entered the salon to book an appointment, to cancel an appointment, to have a hairdressing service or for a general enquiry; whatever the client's needs, she is entitled to a prompt and warm greeting.

Valuing and respecting your clients

Clients can choose from a number of different salons, all offering the same services. They choose your salon for many different reasons and can just as easily go to another salon if they do not feel **valued** or **respected**

The way you communicate with your client must always be respectful. It is not appropriate to argue with a client in the salon, even if you do not agree with her beliefs or opinions. Your client is paying for a service, not to listen to your views or opinions (unless they are asked for, of course). This is a good reason why subjects such as religion and politics should be avoided during general conversation.

Task 2

List four ways of making your client feel valued and respected.

Value

To attach importance to a client.

Respect

To hold a client in high esteem; to avoid harming, degrading, insulting, injuring or interrupting a client.

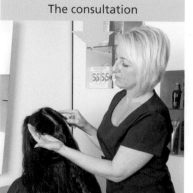

The consultation

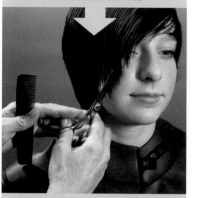

The actual service

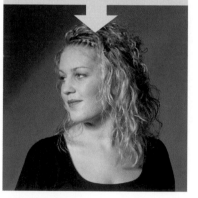

The finished result

Top tips

Hairdressers train for a long time to learn what they are doing and why they need to do it, so do not assume the client also has this knowledge!

Identifying and confirming your clients' needs

In G7 you will cover in detail client consultation and analysis of the hair and scalp. You must make sure you identify your clients' needs and also confirm their expectations, so that you are positive you know their requirements. This can only happen by effective communication.

Task 3

Sit back to back with a colleague. One of you needs a pencil and paper (the stylist). The person without pencil and paper (the client) must try to explain a hairstyle to their colleague without the use of style names, facial expressions or hand gestures. The partner must try to draw the hairstyle.

This can be quite a hard task depending on how good the communication from the client is. This is very true in real salon life.

Treating clients courteously and helpfully at all times

At many times throughout a normal salon day you will be under time pressure, from other members of staff and from clients. You need to learn how to cope with pressure without becoming stressed, as it is really important to be helpful and courteous to clients at all times. Talk to other members of the salon staff to find out how they cope with the salon's daily pressures.

Keeping clients informed and reassured

It is important to communicate effectively with your client throughout the hairdressing service. Think of the whole service as being split into three, as shown in the flowchart, left.

It is important to inform and reassure your client throughout the service, not just at the beginning. Explain what you are doing and why you are doing it, as most clients are interested in what hairdressing involves. Some clients may need less reassurance than others as they may already have some previous knowledge of hairdressing services and will understand why you have used a particular product, for example. Other clients may be totally confused by the whole process, so some explanation of what is happening during the service will be helpful.

Adapting your behaviour to respond to different client behaviour

Many different clients will enter your salon. You will need to learn how to deal with all kinds of behaviour. You will find that people have varying degrees of tolerance and understanding – unfortunately you will undoubtedly encounter some angry or confused clients during your career.

Confused clients will need a lot of reassurance and you may need to explain more than once why you are doing something, for example why you need them to hold their head in a particular position. Try to have patience and be understanding. Remember not to use technical terms, as although professional terms are useful to hairdressing professionals, they can cause confusion to clients with no technical background or understanding.

Angry clients will need to be handled very carefully. Try to establish why they are so angry and put yourself in their position — would you be angry too? A client could be angry because the result of the service is not what she had hoped or asked for. Carrying out a thorough consultation and not dismissing your client's wishes can usually avoid this. Sometimes a client may become angry because she has been kept waiting for an appointment. Even if the delay is no fault of your own, always apologise and make your client as comfortable as possible by offering refreshments and magazines. If a client becomes angry at any point during the service always remain calm, even if you are being shouted at. Getting angry yourself will not help the situation; it will just be seen as unprofessional. If you feel you cannot deal with the situation yourself, you should excuse yourself from the client and find someone experienced who can help you.

Some clients may behave unconventionally or have different needs or expectations. When faced with these types of situations it is important for you to remain calm and professional. The world is full of all different types of people and it is important to treat everyone as your equal. This may mean you need to be very tolerant by employing a great deal of patience and understanding at times, which is an excellent life skill to learn.

Personal, learning and thinking skills – Self-management

When you are working in a busy salon environment, it is important to make sure you give a good complete service if you are to promote a professional image for the salon and ensure repeat business. Think about how you manage your working day, and consider whether there are any aspects of your performance that you could improve on to help with the efficient running of the salon. This will show your manager that you have good self-management skills that will help you to plan your working day.

Video clip

Watch video clip 'Handling client complaints' on the website to hear what celebrity stylist Andrew Barton has to say about handling a client's complaint.

109

Unit

G17

Fact or fiction?

Is this statement fact or fiction?

Behaviour breeds behaviour so it is acceptable to get angry if a client gets angry with you.

To check your answer see page 494.

Give clients a positive impression of yourself and your organisation

Fact or fiction?

Is this statement fact or fiction?

If a client didn't tell you her scalp was burning during a chemical process, you are not responsible for the scarring resulting from this problem.

To check your answer see page 494.

How to respond appropriately to clients

When working in the salon, you should always be polite, assist when your clients need attention and respond promptly and positively to your clients' questions. You should always check with your clients that you have fully understood their needs and service expectations and allow them time to consider your explanations.

Responding promptly to clients' needs

When a client indicates that she needs attention, it is vital that you respond to the request immediately. Do not assume that the request is insignificant or unworthy of your time, as it may be a matter of urgency to avoid a potential incident. A client may feel colour or bleach burning her scalp which, if not treated immediately, could result in a serious scalp burn.

Choosing communication techniques

Whatever your position in a salon, you will need to communicate with others. You will come across a wide range of clientele and it is essential to identify your clients' needs and pitch your communication at the right level. For example, an elderly client may not be very interested in which nightclub you recently went to, but a teenage client might be. You may be the only person an elderly client has seen all week and she would probably welcome conversation, whereas a client booked for a relaxing scalp massage may prefer a quieter service. If your business is to be successful, you will need to communicate effectively and appropriately with all clients.

Check clients have fully understood the likely outcome

It is vital that you communicate effectively during the initial consultation to ensure you have fully understood the result or outcome the client has asked for. If this result is not possible due to factors outside of your control, e.g. the wrong hair type or texture, you must be sure your client understands this. If your client does not fully understand, you should give further explanation to help clarify the situation, otherwise this could result in unhappy and dissatisfied clients.

Responding positively and promptly to clients

Very often clients will ask questions about the hairdressing service they are having and you need to be confident in your knowledge and understanding of the service to be able to answer the questions. If you do not know the answer, be honest and try to find someone who can help straight away. This is a much more positive and pro-active way of answering a query than making it up, which can lead to disastrous and embarrassing results.

Negative reactions to questions will disappoint your client. Even if you do not think your client's suggestions for a re-style are suitable, respond in a positive way by suggesting a more appropriate style tactfully. Do not just dismiss your client's views; it is her hair after all!

Allow clients time to consider your response and give further explanation when appropriate

It is a good idea not to talk too technically about services to clients in case they misunderstand the information. It is much better to give a simplified version and know that your client fully understands the implications of the service. Also allow your client enough time to consider the information given instead of rushing her to make a decision. Experience shows that clients usually regret a hasty decision. If a client is still unsure about the service you are discussing it is worth the extra time and effort to explain further until you are confident you both agree on the final outcome of the service.

Checking clients' needs and expectations

Some clients who come into your salon will be very nervous and will say as little as possible. Make sure you know exactly how they want to look when they leave your salon before you start the service.

As a quality check after a hairdressing service you should ask yourself:

- Would I like to be treated in the same way I have just cared for the client?
- Would I pay for the service I have just given to the client?
- Did I communicate effectively with the client?
- Could I have improved upon the quality of my service?
- Was it as good as it could have been or was it rushed?
- Has the client re-booked?

How to communicate information to clients

Have you ever had your hair done and felt that the stylist did not take enough time and effort to listen properly to how you wanted your hair to look? This was probably due to lack of communication and it highlights how important it is to communicate effectively with your clients.

Communication techniques

Communication may be verbal, non-verbal or written.

Verbal communication

Verbal communication is what you say. It needs to be:

- clear
- to the point
- easily understood — using everyday language and avoiding technical terms where possible
- friendly in tone.

Eye contact with your client is important. For clients who may be hearing impaired, eye contact often reinforces the message.

111

Unit
G17

Video clip

Watch video clip 'Consequences of poor customer service' on the website to hear what celebrity stylist Andrew Barton has to say about the implications of a client receiving poor customer service.

Give clients a positive impression of yourself and your organisation

Non-verbal communication

This is another term for body language. Your body conveys messages by:

- posture
- facial expressions
- tone of voice
- gestures.

Although a client may say that she is not nervous about having a particular hairdressing service, her facial expressions, twitching or fiddling may tell you otherwise! These unconscious gestures reveal a lot more about your client than verbal communication, so the stylist should be aware of body language and develop an intuition to act upon it.

Areas of the human body that send out non-verbal messages

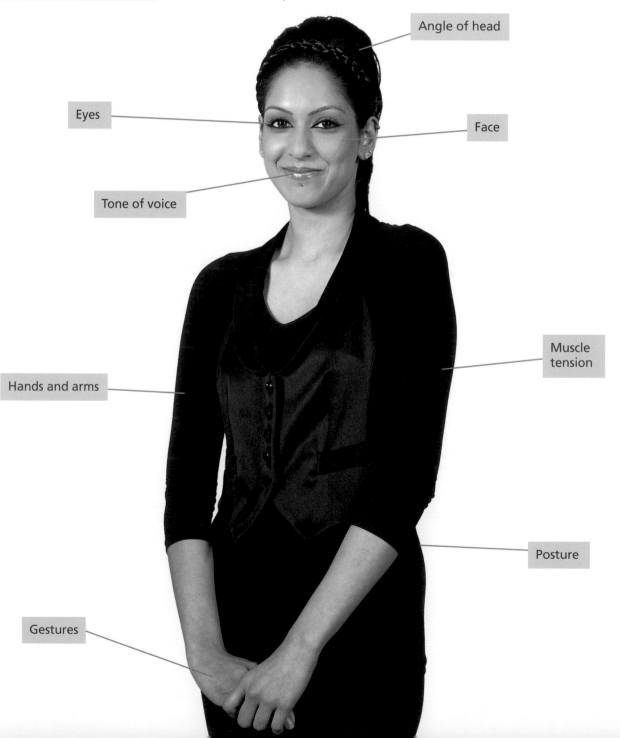

Angle of head

Eyes

Face

Tone of voice

Muscle tension

Hands and arms

Posture

Gestures

Watch for signs that understanding is not clear or that the client is not satisfied or following what you are saying. Positive body language involves expressions and gestures such as smiling, nodding in agreement, lots of eye contact and open gestures, such as uncrossed arms. Negative body language includes frowning, tension, no eye contact and closed gestures, such as crossed arms.

The ability to listen

Effective communication is a two-way process. You need to have good listening skills. This means:

* knowing when to stop talking and listen to what is being communicated
* listening with interest and understanding
* providing encouragement and confirming you have taken in the conversation, for example by nodding or agreeing with the point raised.

It is easy to talk and not really listen. Always maintain eye contact with the person who is speaking and let the speaker finish the sentence – never interrupt. Really understanding what the client is trying to say may mean you pick up on what the client is not telling you, too!

Do not plan your reply while you are being spoken to as you will not have all the facts until the client has finished.

In the early stages it is quite a compliment if the client wants to talk freely to you, but it may be some time before you fully gain the client's trust and confidence.

Task 4

Team up with a partner. One of you is the stylist and one of you is the client. The stylist must listen to the client explaining what she would like you to do to her hair for three minutes, without interrupting, cutting across the client or putting together an answer before the client has finished speaking.

This is actually very hard to do. Make notes about how you performed. What did you find difficult?

Observation skills

It is important to assess your client's body language in order to interpret if she is comfortable with any suggestions you make regarding her hair.

How to give clients information

There are many different ways to give clients the information they need about products or services offered in your salon. The most commonly used method is by talking to your client and explaining different offers you may have on products or services. Other methods could include printing information on the back of appointment cards, sending out information flyers or emails/text messages stating promotional offers, or posters in salon windows. All these methods would offer information to your client and she could then ask for further clarification from you if necessary.

Video clip

Watch video clip 'Showing you are listening' on the website to hear what celebrity stylist Andrew Barton has to say about the best way to show you are really listening to a client.

113

Unit

G17

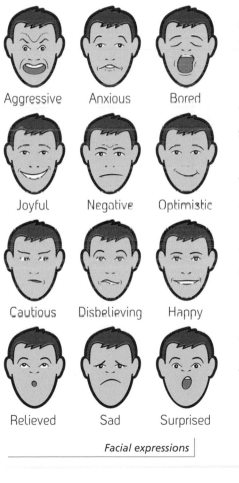

Aggressive   Anxious   Bored

Joyful   Negative   Optimistic

Cautious   Disbelieving   Happy

Relieved   Sad   Surprised

Facial expressions

Give clients a positive impression of yourself and your organisation

Top tips

Your body language conveys how you feel. You may put your client off by aggressive stances, frowning and not making direct eye contact.

Checking client understanding when information may be complicated

Clarification means checking the details given by the client to ensure the information you receive is correct. You need to do this whenever information is being passed on to you. This needs to happen at all stages of client contact. Here are some examples:

- When the client makes a telephone booking, the date, time, nature of the service and client name and phone number should be repeated back to the client as confirmation.
- When the client arrives at reception for the appointment, the time of the booking and the name of the stylist may be repeated to the client.
- When the client is having a consultation, repeating back the information you have been given allows you to clarify information. For example, you might ask: 'so, Mrs Jones, your hair has been dry for some time, is that correct?' This also gives the client opportunities to respond to your open questions and encourages a good rapport to build up.

Contraindication

Any reason that prevents a service from taking place.

Top tips

Always try to explain fully the reasons why you cannot meet your clients' needs. Always be polite and tactful in your explanation and remember to treat your clients with the utmost courtesy, otherwise you might seem rude.

Explaining to clients when their needs cannot be met

Sometimes it is not possible to carry out your client's wishes. This may be because people, systems or resources have let you down. It could also be because the client's hair is too damaged for the colour she has requested. It could be due to a **contraindication** (see G7) such as head lice, or simply because the hairstyle the client has chosen would not be achievable because her hair is too fine.

Whatever the reason, it is important for you to explain clearly and fully the reasons why you cannot carry out the service. You should be able to offer some advice to help the client's situation. Some examples are given in the table below.

Reason why service cannot be carried out	Advice to give to client
Hair too damaged for colour	Advise a course of restructurant conditioning treatments.
Head lice present	Seek medical advice from GP or pharmacist.
Hair too fine for chosen style	Help, advise and choose a suitable style more for fine hair.
Face shape not suitable for the client's chosen re-style	Advise a more suitable style to complement and enhance the face shape.
Client wants to go blonde but natural hair colour is too dark	Advise a more suitable and achievable hair colour.
Client wants to keep the length but her hair is very split and damaged	Explain that the hair will break off if the damage is not removed.
Client wants an appointment but you are fully booked	Try to accommodate your client with another member of staff.

Task 5

State how you would recognise and deal with the following clients in order to create a positive impression:

- clients who have different needs and expectations
- clients who appear angry or confused
- clients who behave unconventionally.

Salon life

We are all individuals!

Kieran's story

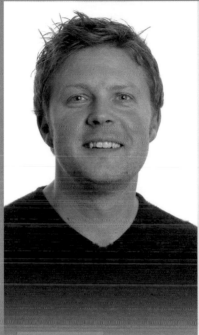

I had only just completed my training when I had a new client arrive for a cut and blow-dry. The client had severe learning difficulties and had a carer with her. I carried out the consultation and during this time it was obvious that the client was confused about what cut to have. I suggested a re-style which I felt was going to suit the client's features and the client agreed with my suggestion. It was very difficult cutting the hair as the client could not help moving. It did mean a lot of stopping and starting, which meant the cut took much longer than usual and I was really worried I might accidentally cut the client as she was moving. I was pleased when I finished the cut and blow-dry, but when I asked if the client liked it she said no and that I needed to change it. I was so disappointed as I felt I had really worked hard. The client's carer told me not to worry and that it looked lovely but sometimes my client got confused, then she paid and left. It taught me that there are many different people in the world and sometimes not everyone acts as you would expect them to, but that you have to be tolerant and patient at all times within the salon.

Top tips

- Try to have as much information as possible available for clients to read while they are at reception. This should avoid embarrassment and confusion over things like the salon's pricing structures.
- Consultation is the key – if you spend the time necessary to ensure a thorough consultation, this will help avoid angry and confused clients.

Ask the expert

Q *What is the best way to deal with confused clients?*

A You need to treat all clients as equals but you may need to adapt your method of working or how you carry out the service to your client's individual needs. If clients are confused about the suggestions you are making for their hair, try to show them examples from style books or magazines.

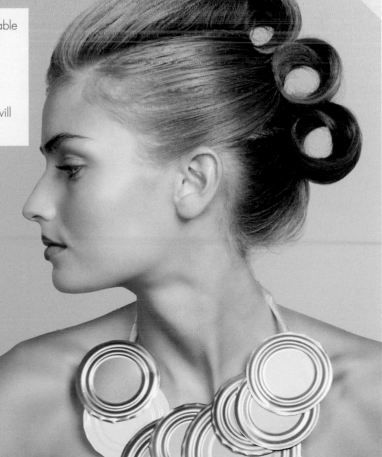

115

Unit

G17

Give clients a positive impression of yourself and your organisation

Give clients a positive impression of yourself and your organisation

Check your knowledge

The following questions will help you to check your understanding of this unit. The answers can be found on page 494.

1 Why is it important to follow your salon's rules for appearance and behaviour?

a) So you don't get the sack

b) To ensure you maintain your salon's set standards

c) To let everyone know where you work

d) To make sure no one gets picked on for not wearing the latest fashion

2 As a stylist, you should be:

a) pleasant, patient and helpful to everyone coming into the salon

b) kind to your own clients

c) kind to your bosses' clients

d) pleasant to clients that tip well.

3 What is needed to help build a rapport with clients?

a) The same interests/hobbies

b) Becoming friends on Facebook

c) An unbreakable friendship bond

d) Trust and effective communication

4 If the salon is busy, who should greet a client arriving at reception?

a) The client should be kept waiting for the salon manager

b) The client's stylist

c) The client should be kept waiting until the receptionist is free

d) Whoever is free greets the client first

5 To ensure a positive impression of the salon and yourself, the client should be made to feel:

a) valued and respected

b) clever and brainy

c) intelligent and bright

d) beautiful and fashionable.

6 You must make sure you identify your clients' needs and also confirm their expectations so that:

a) you are positive you know their requirements

b) you know the client is listening

c) you ensure you are making conversation

d) you ensure you are being polite.

7 If you find yourself in a situation you feel you cannot deal with yourself, you should:
  a) walk away and leave the client
  b) ask the client to take a seat and find someone who can help you
  c) let someone else sort it out if it's not your problem
  d) shout for help across the salon to see if someone can help you.

8 What are the three types of communication within the salon?
  a) Loud, quiet and whispered
  b) At the basin, at reception and at the workstation
  c) Friendly, unfriendly and aggressive
  d) Verbal, non-verbal and written

9 There are many different ways to give clients the information they need about products or services offered in your salon. The methods can be:
  a) talking to your client
  b) printing information on the back of appointment cards
  c) sending out information flyers, emails, text messages or posters
  d) all of the above.

10 Sometimes it is not possible to carry out your client's wishes. This may be because:
  a) the client's hair is too fine
  b) the client's hair is too damaged
  c) either a), b) or d)
  d) a contraindication is present.

Give clients a positive impression of yourself and your organisation

Getting ready for assessment

You will be assessed using a combination of assessment methods, as described below. Remember that within each of the services you carry out with a client, you will cover different units. For example, you might give clients a positive impression of yourself and your organisation (G17) when you fulfil salon reception duties (G4) or advise and consult with clients (G7). If you are not sure what you have covered in your service, always ask your assessor or supervisor for advice.

	NVQ	VRQ
Credit value	5	N/A
Guided Learning Hours	20	N/A

	NVQ
Practical demonstrations, to be observed by assessor	You must demonstrate competent performance of all practical outcomes on at least three separate occasions. Where possible, your assessor will integrate knowledge outcomes into practical observations through oral questioning.
Service timings	There are no maximum service times for this unit.
Additional evidence	Your evidence for this unit should be collected when dealing with real clients within your salon or training establishment. Simulation is not allowed for any part of this unit. You need to practise your customer service skills and then ask to be assessed when you feel ready. You should collect evidence that shows you have carried out good customer service over a sufficient period of time (a week is not enough) with different clients on different occasions in order for your assessor to be confident that you have enough competency within this unit. All outcomes and assessment criteria must be achieved (no specified range for this unit). There are no mandatory written questions required for this unit.

Task mapping

When you have completed the tasks in this unit, check the table below to see which Performance Criteria (purple), Knowledge (green) and Key Skills (blue) you have covered within Unit G17 to use as additional evidence within your portfolio. There are no ranges for this unit. Information about which Functional Skills you have covered is available on the website.

Task and page reference	Mapping to Performance Criteria, Range, Knowledge and Key Skills
1 (page 107)	Performance Criteria: 1a Range: N/A Knowledge: 1 Key Skills: C1.2, C1.3, C2.3
2 (page 107)	Performance Criteria: 1b, 1c, 1e Range: N/A Knowledge: 2 Key Skills: C1.2, C1.3, C2.3
3 (page 108)	Performance Criteria: Practising 1c, 1d, 2c, 3c Range: N/A Knowledge: – Key Skills: C1.1
4 (page 113)	Performance Criteria: Practising 2b, 2c Range: N/A Knowledge: 2 Key Skills: C1.1, C1.3
5 (page 114)	Performance Criteria: 1c, 1e, 1f, 1g, 2b, 2d, 3c, 3d Range: N/A Knowledge: 2, 5 Key Skills: C1.2, C1.3, C2.3

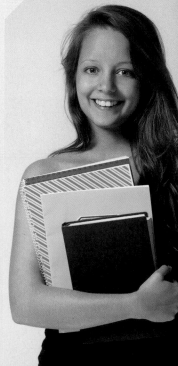

Promote additional products or services to clients

Unit G18

Promote additional products or services to clients

What you will learn:

- **How to identify additional services or products that are available**

- **How to inform clients about additional services or products**

- **How to gain client commitment to using additional services or products**

Introduction

This unit deals with the different ways you can promote the products and services offered by your salon. The promotion of additional services and products will generate extra revenue for the salon. It will also encourage clients to use the recommended home haircare products, which will help to prolong the lifespan of perms, relaxers, colours and all other hairdressing services. Hairdressing is a very competitive market and salons must continually update their marketing of products and services if they are to grow, thrive and become market leaders in the ever-changing world of fashion.

How to identify additional services or products that are available

Not all services are suitable for all clients. For example, some hair colouring services require a skin test prior to the appointment to assess the skin's sensitivity to the colouring product. If a client pays for a service that is not suitable, she will not be pleased. It is important to suggest the correct products to clients, as incorrect product advice will result in bad-hair days and unhappy clients.

Before you start to identify additional products or services for your client, ask yourself the following questions:

- Is the service you are thinking of offering suitable for your client's needs? For example, if you are trying to help a client to achieve a low-maintenance hairstyle and you suggest a perm, will this make the hairstyle last longer or will it make the hair harder for the client to blow-dry?
- Is the product you are recommending the most suitable one for your client's hair? Do not get into the habit of recommending mousse to every client, as mousse does not suit all hair types or textures. Think about the strength and the consistency of the individual products in your salon and how they can alter hairstyles to achieve different looks and effects.

Top tips

It is very important that you are fully aware of the services and products your salon offers, as business might be lost if your knowledge is not up to date. This should include awareness of service procedures and the advantages and disadvantages of each.

Task 1

List ten of the different styling and finishing products that are available in your salon and research which types of hair they are most suitable for. You could set this information out as shown in the chart below.

Product type	Suitability	Suggestions	Homecare advice
(This can be the name of the product and whether it is a styling or finishing product)	(What type of hair is this product best suited to?)	(How would you suggest the client apply this product, e.g. how much to use, should it be applied to wet or dry hair?)	(How frequently should the client use the product? What can they do to maintain the style achieved in the salon?)
Mousse (styling)			
Serum			

A worksheet containing this chart can be found on the website for you to use to record your findings.
This can then be used as additional portfolio evidence.

Updating salon information

As a member of the salon team, you are responsible for making sure all the appropriate information regarding the products and services offered by your salon is up to date. Do not leave this job to one person, as all staff benefit from this information and everyone should take an active role. This could involve checking manufacturers' and wholesalers' price lists, contacting company representatives for posters or promotional leaflets, visiting wholesalers for special offers, or simply updating the salon's price list.

Checking new product or service details

If you are unsure of a new product or service offered by your salon, you must be confident enough to ask another member of your team. It could be that new stock arrived on your day off and you are not sure whether it is suitable for your client or not.

Everyone is entitled to time off for holiday leave and often during this time new products or services can be introduced. If you have missed vital training on how to offer a new service, you should be able to arrange an in-house training session with a more experienced member of the salon team who has already carried out the service and attended the initial training.

Other ways of keeping up to date with new products and new techniques are to read industry magazines such as the *Hairdressers Journal International* and to make regular visits to trade events such as Salon International, which is held annually. Regular salon training sessions will allow company trainers/technicians to keep all members of the salon team up to date with new launches of products and equipment.

Task 2

Set yourself a challenge to discover at least three new products, tools or pieces of equipment that have just been introduced to the market place. Make up a small collage and add your own text to describe the features and benefits of the new products, tools or equipment.

Identifying individual clients' needs

Even when you are training there are opportunities to identify products or services suitable for your client. Some examples are given in the table below.

Part of service	Example of product or service you might suggest
Gowning	If you noticed your client was suffering from dandruff, you could recommend an appropriate shampoo to use at home.
Shampooing	If you noticed a build-up of styling product, you could recommend a clarifying shampoo to use at home and more appropriate styling products to help reduce the build-up. The shampooing stage may be the longest amount of time you spend with some clients, so there may also be the opportunity to discuss future services. General questions such as 'How has your hair been behaving since your last visit?' may lead to you being able to suggest a service the client is not booked in for. 'Are you having a holiday soon?' may be an opening for your client to buy some ultra-violet protective products to help protect against sun and sea damage.
Seating your client for the next service	You could talk about the products displayed on the workstation and ask if the client has tried any of the new range.

Fact or fiction?

Is this statement fact or fiction?

It is only necessary to check with manufacturers once a year for updates.

To check your answer see page 494.

121

Unit
G18

Promote additional products or services to clients

Top tips

Never be afraid to ask if you are unsure. This helps prevent mistakes from occurring in the salon.

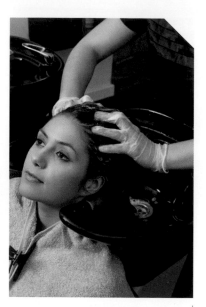

Shampooing gives you an opportunity to discuss future services

General conversation about a product may spark the client's interest and she may be encouraged to buy. Try to judge your client's body language. If you feel some helpful advice would be appreciated, try to use your verbal communication skills to their best advantage by describing all the benefits your client would get from purchasing something new, different and exciting!

If you want to obtain information from your client, use 'open' questions. These are questions that require the client to give more information than just a 'yes' or 'no' response. Try to use questions that begin with 'how' or 'what'. For example:

- How many times per week do you shampoo and condition your hair?
- What did you think of the styling product I used on your hair on your last visit?

Closed questions are questions that it is possible to answer with a simple 'yes' or 'no'. For example:

- Do you shampoo your hair every day?
- Did you like the styling product I used on your hair on your last visit?

As the client might respond with a blunt 'no', it could then become very awkward to pursue the conversation further.

Communicate confidence in your knowledge of the product or service to your client, as she will then be more likely to trust you and to follow your advice.

Spotting client opportunities

Spotting an opportunity to offer a client an additional service or product can be quite simple. If a client is waiting in the reception area and is looking at the product stand, this is an ideal opportunity for you to go over and offer your professional advice. Do not jump in with a massive sales spiel, but talk calmly and professionally to your client about her needs and requirements. You should be able to find out enough information to identify which products or services are suitable for your client's needs.

You also need to think about complementary services that your salon offers. Most salons run hairdressing and beauty therapy services alongside one another. You may have the opportunity to advise your client on services from both areas, perhaps even suggesting a manicure while a chemical process is developing (if your salon can accommodate this).

You need to be thinking all of the time what would benefit your client and increase revenue for the salon. If commission is offered for future bookings there may be a monetary incentive for you.

Personal, learning and thinking skills – Creative thinking

It is important to always be thinking of new ways in which to promote your salon and the products and services that it offers. Look at the salon displays and marketing posters to see if you can identify any missed opportunities. Think about the different types of marketing strategies that could be used, and inform your manager of your ideas. This will show that you have thought creatively about how to promote the salon in order to increase business and revenue.

Task 3

Miss Burton has arrived for her appointment. While waiting for her stylist, she asks for some advice on her hair, which has been dry since her foreign holiday two weeks ago.

Write down the advice you would give Miss Burton about:

- retail products sold in your salon
- additional services to help repair the dryness.

You should also note down the following:

- What methods of communication would you use?
- How would you check your client understands the information given?
- How would you ensure the prompt delivery of the additional services or products you have recommended?
- Who would you refer the client to if you were unable to give the appropriate information?

A worksheet for this task is provided on the website for you to complete and add to your portfolio.

Promote additional products or services to clients

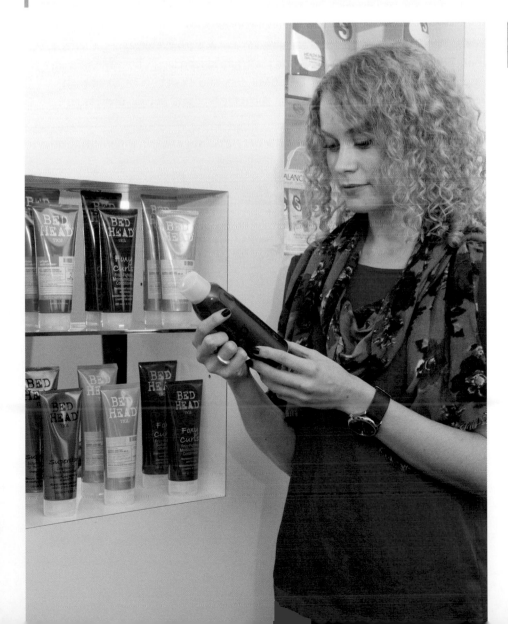

If you see a client looking at the product stand, approach her and offer your advice.

Salon life

Promoting additional products and services using good communication skills

Jess's story

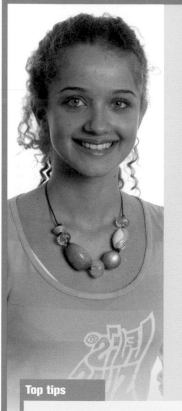

My salon manager set all staff members the task of promoting products and services, telling us that points would be earned for every product sold or additional booking made. My classmates said that as I am such a confident, chatty person, I would surely get the most points, and so they might as well not bother! It was therefore a bit of a shock when after a couple of weeks I still hadn't sold a product or made a booking. I couldn't understand it – I was friendly with the clients and chatted all the time. I told them all about the different products; we talked about everything under the sun!

I asked my friend Sammie where I was going wrong and was a bit taken aback when she said, 'Jess, you're great, a real chatterbox and always good for a laugh, but what you can't do is listen very well! You tend to talk at the client, Jess, and it can be a lot about what you've done at the weekend. You do tell them about the products, but you don't listen to their questions afterwards.'

I was hurt by what Sammie said but I knew she was right. I did just talk at my clients and never listened to a word they said! I was so embarrassed.

It's a month down the line now, and a few things have changed. I now make sure I listen to what my client is saying to me. I wait until she has finished and then I ask more questions or respond to hers. I am actually enjoying myself much more, and I realise that it takes more than one person to hold a conversation! My sales are catching up with the others and I have had clients making repeat bookings for my services.

Top tips

As well as reading information about the various products, try to use as many of them as you can. By experimenting, you will be able to see what works on different textures of hair and what your personal preferences are.

Ask the expert

Q   *I'm currently working in a salon on a Saturday, mainly on reception. The salon gives commission on products sold and all of the other staff seem to be doing really well. I have difficulty recommending the retail products, but I really want to – not only would the extra money come in handy, but I don't want to be at the bottom of the table at our weekly staff meetings. Do you have any advice you could give me?*

A   Recommending and selling products is all about having confidence in the products, but this confidence only comes when you have knowledge of the products. You need to make sure you read all of the information/leaflets and manufacturers' instructions, so that you feel able to talk to the clients about all aspects of the products.

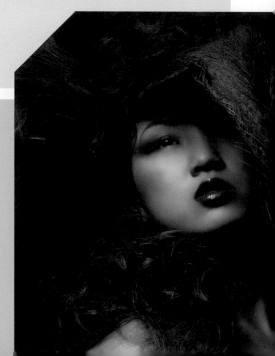

How to inform clients about additional services or products

This section deals with how to inform and advise your clients of suitable products or services that they would not usually purchase. It is important to use the correct approach when advising clients so that they can fully understand and appreciate the information you are giving them. It is not appropriate, for example, to interrupt a conversation or to pounce on a client and attempt to sell her products as soon as she enters the salon.

Appropriate timing and methods of communicating with clients

When you decide to give your client information or advice on additional products or services, timing is crucial. If a client feels hassled, she will probably not buy anything you suggest. Choose a time when your client is relaxed and there is sufficient time for her to evaluate your advice. During shampooing is an ideal time, as your client should begin to relax while being massaged.

Good times to give the client advice on additional products and services include:

- while the client is waiting for a service
- during the initial consultation
- during the shampoo process
- during waiting periods throughout the service, such as when processing a chemical service
- while the client is paying for a service.

Remember, this is only a guide and timing should be determined by your client's mood, body language and verbal signals.

Promote additional products or services to clients

Task 4

It is essential to be able to 'read' a client's body language to know if you can move the conversation on or whether to end the conversation if your client isn't showing any interest.

Complete the chart below by stating whether the following examples of body language given from a client are positive or negative buying signs. See if you can add any of your own positive or negative signs to the chart. Discuss in your groups all the various methods of communication and the benefits of each.

Client's body language	Positive?	Negative?	Continue or close?
Arms folded and legs crossed			
Not holding eye contact			
Smiling			
Fidgeting in their seat			
Feet flat on the floor with arms uncrossed			
Foot tapping and checking watch			

A worksheet containing this chart can be found on the website for you to use to record your findings. This can then be used as additional portfolio evidence.

126

Unit
G18

Promote additional products or services to clients

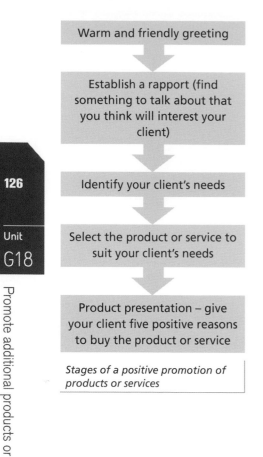

Warm and friendly greeting

Establish a rapport (find something to talk about that you think will interest your client)

Identify your client's needs

Select the product or service to suit your client's needs

Product presentation – give your client five positive reasons to buy the product or service

Stages of a positive promotion of products or services

Prosecute

Take out legal action against someone.

On the left is a flow chart to help guide you through the stages of positive promotion of products or services to your client.

Sometimes it is not possible to speak to every client individually due to the pressures of time in your salon, but you can still promote products by use of good visual aids and posters. Other ways in which you can communicate service or product information to clients is by giving them newsletters or promotional flyers before they leave the salon, or by mailing out information to existing clients. This can be done by using the clients' details stored on a computer database to mail out salon promotions at different times throughout the year. Some salons find this a very effective method of giving clients promotional deals. Some salons put promotional posters in the salon window to entice clients to ask about the latest service being offered. Whichever method you choose, make sure you make it work by being enthusiastic and motivated when a client shows interest.

Task 5

Design a promotional leaflet or poster for your salon. Decide if you are going to promote a service or a product and make it as attractive and interesting as possible to grab the attention of your clients.

When would you introduce the promotional leaflet or poster to clients? Would you leave it on reception or hand it to them upon arrival?

Think of the most appropriate times to introduce your clients to a new product or service.

Keep all of the evidence in your portfolio.

Giving accurate and sufficient information to clients

Now that you know when to give advice on products and services, you need to understand why it is important to give accurate and sufficient information to your clients.

You are governed by law when giving your clients advice and the law says you must give correct advice and not mislead your clients into buying something that is not suitable for them. This could lead to a client **prosecuting**. If your advice is accurate and sufficient, it will enable your client to make an informed decision on whether they wish to buy an additional service or product. Always have what you want to say about a product or service clear in your mind, and use simple questioning techniques to make sure your client understands the information that you have given them.

The Acts that affect the selling of services and products are:

- Consumer Protection Act 1987
- Cosmetic Products (Safety) Regulations 1996
- Trade Descriptions Act 1968 (and 1987)
- Sale of Goods Act 1979
- Supply of Goods and Services Act 1982.

(Refer to G20 for further information about the legislation for selling products.)

Service timings

The timings of services should be given accurately. Do not mislead clients or underestimate how long a service may take as they will not believe you next time. In addition, the smooth running of the salon will be disturbed if timings are not given correctly. 'Time is money' so, to be cost-effective, timing must be accurate. Standard timings help maintain the quality in the salon, so that all stylists offer the same time for each service. All clients are then treated equally and get the same value for money.

Frequency of services given should also be negotiated with the client and is dependent upon:

- time available
- financial considerations of the client
- the condition of the hair.

See pages 91–93 for a guide to filling out the appointments book. You should take into account the length of a service when booking in clients.

Prices

Prices vary from salon to salon and area to area. The salon should always display a price list where it can be seen clearly by current and potential clients. This allows clients to view for themselves the costs and may also be additional advertising!

The cost of a service given should be accurate, with no hidden extras.

Task 6

If you are employed in a salon, put the salon price list and all the advertising material the salon may have in your portfolio. Regardless of whether you can actually perform the services or not, you need to be aware of all the salon services offered. If you do not understand some of the services on the price list, ask your manager for a demonstration during staff training or ask a more experienced stylist for a full explanation.

If you are not employed in a salon, collect two price lists from salons in your area and compare the cost of services, presentation of price list and range of services offered. Discuss in class the differing services and the reasons why you think the differences occur.

The hair gallery

The Price List

	ARTISTIC DIRECTOR	DESIGN ARTIST	SENIOR STYLIST
Wet cut	£28.00	£23.00	£18.00
Cut and blow-dry	£35.00	£30.00	£25.00
Re-style	£40.00	£35.00	£30.00
Blow-dry	£20.00	£17.50	£15.00
Men's wet cut	£20.00	£15.00	£10.00
Men's cut and blow-dry	£32.00	£27.50	£20.00

Colouring:

	ARTISTIC DIRECTOR	DESIGN ARTIST	SENIOR STYLIST
Full head foils (excl. cut or blow-dry)	£60.00	£60.00	£60.00
T-zone/bar (excl. cut or blow-dry)	£25.00	£25.00	£25.00
Permanent regrowth (excl. cut or blow-dry)	£30.00	£30.00	£30.00
Full head permanent tint	£40.00	£40.00	£40.00
Individual woven or sliced packets	£2.50	£2.50	£2.50

A salon price list showing some services and prices

Special offers

If the salon has any offers to pass on to the client then the stylist needs to be aware of these. This helps promote the offer and provides a chance to sell additional services that the client may not be aware of.

There is legislation concerning sales prices, so be careful when advertising a sale in your window (see page 60).

Retail sales

Many salons offer a full retail sales service to complement the products used in a service. Be aware of what your salon sells, whether products are in stock and what the product benefits and selling points are. If your client asks for your advice before buying a product and you are unable to give it, you may lose a sale.

Product knowledge

Be sure that you give correct information to clients about the **features** and **benefits** of a product. Selling an unsuitable product just to close the sale is very bad practice and the client will lose faith in you.

Regular training and visits from manufacturers will ensure that your information is up to date and accurate. Many companies are happy to visit colleges and salons to introduce product training.

Advice

Remember that clients are paying for your skills and expertise (your knowledge) and your ability to address their particular problems. All clients should be treated with the same respect and courtesy, regardless of how trivial their questions may be. When giving advice never patronise the client. You may not know if the client has professional knowledge greater than yours.

Be both honest and realistic with the aims and objectives of the service. Remind the client that results may not be instant; for example, a course of conditioning treatments to help restore moisture and strength to the hair will take place over several weeks.

It is also important that you look professional in your appearance. If your hair is in good condition and styled well, your client will notice and may ask what products you are currently using on your hair. You will be a good advert for your salon and may have an opportunity to promote the products that you use yourself. On the other hand, if you haven't made an effort with your appearance your client may look at your unkempt hair and decide that the products in your salon must be useless!

Feature

Something that does not directly benefit the client, but does make the product look and feel attractive, such as the packaging or the smell.

Benefit

The improvements a product will make to the hair, such as adding body or shine.

Video clip

Watch video clip 'Styling products' on the website to hear what celebrity stylist Andrew Barton has to say about the importance of styling products.

How to gain client commitment to using additional products or services

The purpose of promoting additional products and services is to tell clients about something that will benefit them, help them to maintain the service given in the salon, introduce them to services that would complement their existing services, or simply to give them a new experience.

What to do if the client shows no interest

If your client is not interested in what you have to say regarding additional services and products, you need to ask yourself some questions:

- Is the information I have given relevant to my client's needs?
- Am I explaining myself clearly enough?
- Am I talking to my client at the right level, or am I being too technical?
- Is this the right time to give my client advice?

If the honest answer to these questions is 'no', you may wish to:

- make the advice more relevant to your client's needs
- make your explanations clearer to your client
- avoid technical terms when dealing with clients who have no previous background in hairdressing
- stop the conversation until the client is fully relaxed and ready to listen to your advice.

If, after trying another tactic, your client still has no interest in your advice, you should not pursue it any further as it could lead to embarrassment for both you and your client. Tactfully change the subject to something you know your client will be entertained by or interested in.

Delivery of the product or service

If, following your advice, your client has agreed to purchase something in addition to the original service, you need to check her understanding regarding delivery of the additional service or product. Is the client going to have to wait for the service, and if so, for how long? Always explain fully to avoid any misunderstandings.

You should, obviously, take responsibility for any client's order of additional products that you have dealt with. If there is a problem with delivery of the item, you should inform the client immediately to avoid misunderstandings. Ensure you do as much as possible to help the situation by knowing how to contact wholesalers, suppliers and salon representatives.

If your client has booked an additional service, it is your responsibility to do your best to arrange an appointment to suit your client's needs. This may sometimes take a little effort on your part to juggle the appointment system. A little extra effort goes a long way and will create a 'feel-good factor' for your client.

If you have sold a product or service you will also need to take payment. It is important that you understand the workings of the payment system that your salon or training establishment uses so you can close the sale.

When referral is necessary

The needs of each client will vary, so you should be able to give correct information on all additional services and products offered in your salon, even if you are not yet competent enough to perform them.

If you do not have the relevant knowledge about a particular product or service, you must be professional enough to admit this and ask a salon manager or more experienced member of staff to help. As a trainee stylist, you should be pleasant, patient and helpful to everyone coming into the salon, even if you are unable to fulfil the client's needs. Never dismiss a client and always be as helpful as possible.

130

Unit

G18

Promote additional products or services to clients

Check your knowledge

The following questions will help you to check your understanding of this unit.
The answers can be found on page 494.

1 Name the five Acts/legislation that need to be taken into account when selling additional products or services.

_____

_____

_____

2 Write a brief statement describing positive body language.

_____

_____

_____

3 What are the benefits of promoting additional services and products in your salon?

_____

_____

_____

_____

4 If you are absent when a new product is introduced at work, write a brief statement on how you would find out the relevant information on the product and who you would go to for training.

_____

_____

_____

5 Choose one product or service that your salon provides and list five positive points about it that you could discuss with a client.

_____

_____

_____

_____

_____

Getting ready for assessment

You will be assessed using a combination of assessment methods, as described below. Remember that within each of the services you carry out with a client, you will cover different units. For example, when promoting additional products or services to clients (G18), you will also have to advise and consult with clients (G7). You may also shampoo and condition hair (GH8) and set or dress hair (GH11). If you are not sure what you have covered in your service, always ask your assessor or supervisor for advice.

	NVQ	VRQ
Credit value	3	2
Guided Learning Hours	30	28

	NVQ	VRQ
Practical demonstrations, to be observed by assessor	For this unit you are required to gather evidence from a realistic working environment; simulation is not allowed for any performance evidence within this unit. The evidence must be collected over a period of time with different clients on different occasions in order for your assessor to prove your competency. The evidence must show that you: • follow salon procedures for offering additional services or products to your clients • create opportunities for encouraging clients to use additional services or products • identify your clients' requirements from discussion and spontaneous comments.	You will need to demonstrate competent performances of all practical criteria on at least three separate occasions with three different clients over a period of time. Simulation should be avoided for this unit where possible and the evidence should be gathered in a realistic working environment.
Service timings	There are no mandatory service timings for this unit.	There are no mandatory service timings for this unit.
Additional evidence	As well as face-to-face communication, you can present evidence from communication written on paper, by telephone, text message, email, intranet or by any other method you would be expected to use within your job role.	You are required to complete all outcomes, assessment criteria and range statements for this unit

Task mapping

When you have completed the tasks in this unit, check the table below to see which Performance Criteria (purple), Range (red), Knowledge (green) and Key Skills (blue) you have covered within G18 to use as additional evidence within your portfolio. Information about which Functional Skills you have covered is available on the website.

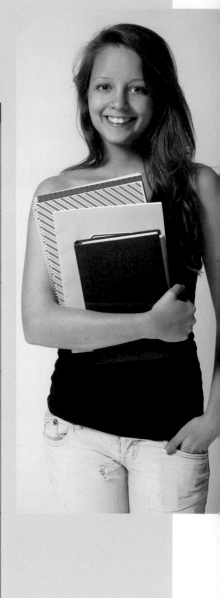

Task and page reference	Mapping to Performance Criteria, Range, Knowledge and Key Skills
1 (page 120)	Performance Criteria: 1a, 1c, 2c, VRQ 1c, 1g Range: N/A Knowledge: 2 Key Skills: C1.2, C1.3, C2.3, N1.1, N1.2, N1.3, N2.1, N2.2, N2.3
2 (page 121)	Performance Criteria: 1a, 1c, 2c, VRQ 1c, 1g Range: N/A Knowledge: 2, 4, 5, 6, VRQ 1j Key Skills: C1.2, C1.3, C2.3
3 (page 123)	Performance Criteria: 1b–d, 2a–d, 3c–e, VRQ 1a, 1b, 1c, 1d, 1e, 1f, 1g Range: N/A Knowledge: 1, 2, 5, 6, VRQ 1j, 1k Key Skills: C1.2, C1.3, C2.3
4 (page 125)	Performance Criteria: 2a, 2b, 2c, 2d, 3a, 3b, VRQ 1f Range: N/A Knowledge: VRQ 1i, 1n Key Skills: C1.2, C1.3
5 (page 126)	Performance Criteria: 1a, 1c, 1d, 2a, 2b, 2c, 2d, VRQ 1b, 1c Range: N/A Knowledge: 1, 2, 4, 5, 6, VRQ 1h, 1m Key Skills: C1.2, C1.3, C2.3
6 (page 127)	Performance Criteria: 1a, 1b, N/A for VRQ Range: N/A Knowledge: 1 Key Skills: C1.2, C1.3, C2.3, N1.1, N1.2, N1.3, N2.1, N2.2, N2.3

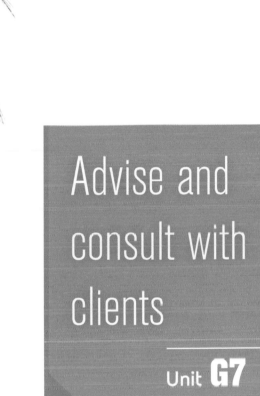

Advise and
consult with
clients

Unit **G7**

Unit

G7

Advise and consult with clients

What you will learn:

- **How to identify what clients want**
- **How to analyse the characteristics of hair, skin and scalp**
- **How to identify factors that will affect future services and product choice**
- **How to advise your client and agree services and products**

Introduction

This unit is all about getting you started as a hair stylist. Before you begin to assess any client's hair or prepare for a hairdressing service, you need to have a clear understanding of the underlying principles of what you are doing. Before any successful service comes a thorough and in-depth **consultation** with your client. During this consultation you will need to assess the hair and scalp thoroughly by looking for indications of infections or infestations and assess the condition of the hair and scalp for the intended service, while listening intently to your client's ideas and wishes and taking into account her body language. This is not easy at first and it takes some practice to get everything coordinated to achieve a successful consultation. You need to be able to consult with clients over non-technical (shampooing, conditioning, blow-drying and setting) and technical (cutting, perming, relaxing and colouring) units before you can be deemed competent by your assessor in this unit for your Level 2 qualification.

Consultation

A discussion between a stylist and a client to determine the services and products that reflect the client's requirements.

Video clip

Watch video clip 'Consultations' on the website to hear what celebrity stylist Andrew Barton has to say about the key things to find out during a consultation.

Analysis

A full assessment of the condition of the hair and scalp, by visual and manual testing, to ensure there are no factors which would prevent the service from taking place. It is also done to give the best service advice to the client.

How to identify what clients want

This unit will guide you through listening and questioning techniques that will help you to identify your clients' needs. At first, some students find it difficult to talk to clients, which makes it almost impossible to carry out a thorough consultation. It may help if you practise a **consultation** on a colleague or friend before you are faced with a 'real' client!

Assessment techniques and questioning the client

Have you ever had your hair done and felt that the stylist did not take enough time and effort to listen properly to how you wanted your hair to look? In this unit you will be given information and tips to help you to ask the right questions so that you meet the needs and wishes of the clients.

It is vital you understand the importance of consultation and **analysis** before you start the practical skills units. By learning to carry out a thorough and in-depth consultation you will have built an excellent foundation for your future career as a professional stylist.

Most successful salons earn their reputation through providing an excellent personal service. The consultation should be carried out thoroughly and the service should be free. A consultation should be carried out prior to the initial services and enables the client and stylist to meet to obtain the correct information to determine a successful service.

A good stylist will use all the skills shown in the spider diagram overleaf and observe the client's body language to help obtain the information required for an effective service plan. Both the client and stylist should agree in advance on the hairdressing service to be carried out, how much it will cost and how long it will take.

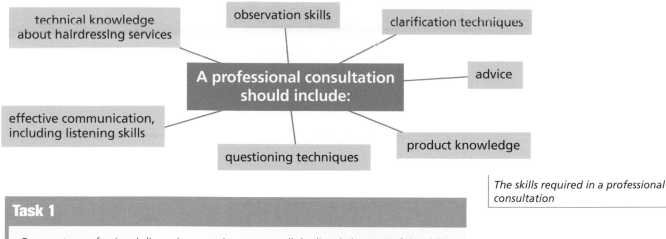

The skills required in a professional consultation

Acvise and consult with clients

Task 1

Carry out a professional discussion ensuring you use all the listed elements of the skills required for a professional consultation. Cross each skill off when you have used it.

Questioning techniques

Asking questions is a skilled task. If you really want to find out what your client thinks and needs from you, you need to ask her questions. The types of questions and how you ask them will dictate the reply you get, so it is important that you give lots of thought to your questioning technique.

The information you obtain should be included on the client's record card, which you will be filling out as you discuss details in your consultation. Use the record card as your guide. If your client is new to the salon, you will need to make a new record of her details; if your client is a regular visitor to the salon, you will need to update her client record at every visit. Computerised client record systems are commonly used and therefore client details and records of appointments are kept electronically. Any information you keep about your clients is classed as data and therefore you must follow guidelines set out by the Data Protection Act when storing it (see detailed information about this on pages 59–60).

You will need to ask the client for her personal details such as address and home/mobile telephone number. Then you have to decide which type of questioning you should use to obtain further information about the client and her needs. There are two types of questions – closed and open:

- Closed questions usually only need one-word answers. For example, 'Have you used a permanent colour on your hair?' This type of question confirms or eliminates information: 'Yes, I have' or 'No, I haven't'. Sometimes you will need to ask a closed question if you just require facts, but try to keep this type of questioning to a minimum.
- Open questions help to make the conversation flow as they require a fuller response. For example, 'How are you today?' Since open questions encourage more detailed answers, they are good to break the ice with, as the client cannot respond with a simple yes or no.

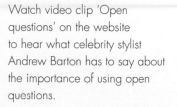

Video clip

Watch video clip 'Open questions' on the website to hear what celebrity stylist Andrew Barton has to say about the importance of using open questions.

Task 2

A professional stylist will use open, or leading, questions to help put a new client at ease. For example:

- 'What's the weather doing out there now?'
- 'Where did you manage to park the car?'
- 'How far have you come?'
- 'How did you hear about us?'

This is preferable to using closed questions, such as:

- 'Did you get the bus?'
- 'Is it still raining?'
- 'Have you been here before?'
- 'Is this your lunch hour?'

Can you spot the differences? Try making up some of your own open and closed questions then try them out within your group.

Clarification techniques

Clarification means checking the details given by the client to ensure the information you receive is correct. You need to do this whenever information is being passed on to you. This needs to happen at all stages of client contact. Here are some examples:

- *When the client makes a telephone booking* – the date, time, nature of the hairdressing service, client name and phone number should be repeated back to the client as confirmation.

- *When the client arrives at reception for the appointment* – the service booking and the name of the stylist may be repeated to the client.

- *When the client is having a consultation* – repeating back the information you have been given allows you to clarify information. For example, 'So, Mrs Laming, your hair has been dry for some time, is that correct?' This also gives the client opportunities to respond to your open questioning techniques and encourages the build-up of a good relationship.

It is also important to encourage your client to ask about any areas she is not sure about. You can usually tell by a client's facial expression or body language if she is confused.

Task 3

It may be helpful to use visual aids, for example colour charts or hairstyling magazines, to help clients with decision making. Clarification of information also gives you the chance to help clients examine their lifestyle, health and homecare routine.

Use magazines or the internet to search for images of hairstyles and colours that you think would appeal to your clients. Produce a portfolio of these images to use as visual aids when consulting with clients.

Observation techniques

It is important to assess your client's body language in order to interpret if she is comfortable with any suggestions you are making.

It is also vital to fully observe the hair's condition, growth patterns, porosity, elasticity and texture. (Refer to pages 141–44 for information on how to carry out these tests.)

Effective communication and listening skills

Communication is a two-way process. The ability to be an effective listener means:

- knowing when to stop talking
- listening with interest and understanding
- providing encouragement and confirming you have taken in the conversation, for example by nodding or agreeing with a point raised.

Listening is a good skill to develop and differs from hearing. When you hear something your brain does not necessarily process the information, whereas if you listen, you have to concentrate in order for your brain to process, make sense of and store the information in your memory. Always maintain eye contact with the person who is speaking and let the person finish her sentence.

Do not plan your reply while you are being spoken to as you will not have all the facts until the client has finished.

It is vital to your salon's business interests that all members of the team communicate effectively with clients and with each other. Clients will not return to your salon if they do not feel valued; effective communication is a way of letting your client know she is valued. Poor communication between clients and salon staff may lead to misunderstandings and potentially unhappy clients.

Say what you mean to your client clearly and use your facial expressions and body language to give meaning to the conversation. This will also show your client you are interested in the conversation. Always try to gauge your client's mood and adapt your conversation if she is in a quiet frame of mind. Some clients may not wish to discuss their feelings and you must respect this and not be embarrassed by silent pauses in the conversation. As you gain experience with clients, you will learn to listen to your client's tone of voice and be able to steer the conversation away from the topic that is causing an emotional reaction. This can be done by carefully and subtly changing the focus of the conversation to something else.

Client confidentiality

If a client is new to the salon it is quite a compliment if she wants to talk freely to you, but it may be some time before you fully gain the client's trust and confidence. When your client does confide in you, it is important to observe the rules of client confidentiality. Clients must be able to rely on you not telling anybody anything they may tell you. This includes:

- their address and telephone number
- information about illnesses or disorders
- personal confidences.

Top tips

In reality, it is easy to run out of time for a thorough consultation as 'time is money' in the salon. However, it is vital to the success of the service that you allow your client plenty of time. A client will have a 'feel-good factor' if you spend sufficient time analysing her service needs. Remember, a happy client becomes a regular client.

137

Unit
G7

Advise and consult with clients

Unit
G7

Advise and consult with clients

Video clip

Watch video clip 'Client expectations' on the website to hear what celebrity stylist Andrew Barton has to say about client expectations.

Service and client expectations

It is very important that the stylist understands the hairdressing services he or she is talking about. Do not make anything up – this is very unprofessional. Always refer to the manufacturer's instructions and product information or a more experienced member of staff if you are unsure.

Be careful not to use technical terms that your client may not understand – you will confuse and possibly concern your client by saying 'I'm just going to apply the ammonium thioglycollate to your hair', instead of, 'I'm just going to apply the perm lotion to your hair.'

How to analyse the characteristics of hair, skin and scalp

Now that you have learned how to talk to your client during the consultation, you need to know what to look for during the hair, skin and scalp analysis. In this element you will learn what to look for and how to avoid cross-infection of infestations and infections, in order to achieve a successful result.

Visual checks and tests necessary for hair, skin and scalp

Now that you know how to communicate with your client, it is time to carry out the very important client consultation. At this point it is essential to look at your client's record card to view any previous information written there that may affect the service you are about to carry out. Always remember to record all relevant information about the hairdressing service and tests you have completed for future reference.

The hair shaft differs in texture

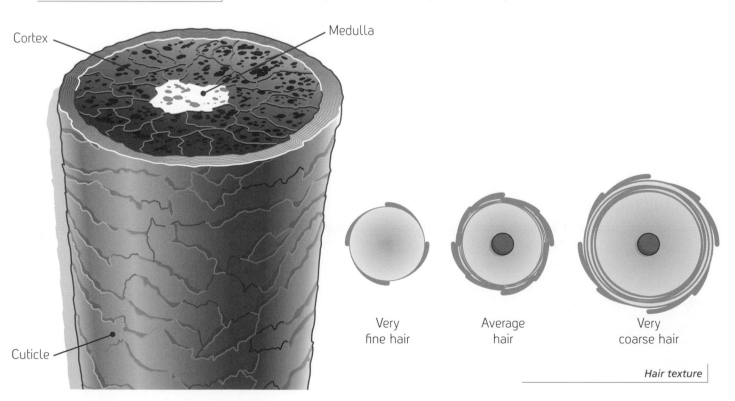

Cortex

Medulla

Cuticle

Very fine hair

Average hair

Very coarse hair

Hair texture

Visual checks are of great value to hairdressers as we are such visual people, working in a very visual industry. It is very important to look closely at the hair and scalp during the consultation and to take into account the following factors.

- *Porosity* – the condition of the cuticle scales; how smooth or rough the hair feels.
- *Texture* – how thick or fine each individual hair is (see the illustrations opposite). This will depend on the number of cuticle layers and whether there is a medulla present. Texture may affect the porosity and elasticity of the hair.
- *Density* – the amount of hair. How much hair there is per 2.5 cm^2 is important to consider when re-styling and assessing the amount of products needed. Often a client has a picture of a hairstyle on a model who has lots of thick, lustrous hair. If the client has very fine, sparse hair, you will not achieve the same look.
- *Length of hair* – is it the same length all over the head? Long hair will have been shampooed and dried hundreds of times. It may have had many chemical processes carried out on the older ends, which will affect the condition of the cuticle and the cortex.
- *Growth patterns* – the direction in which hair grows from the scalp is important to consider before many services. For example, cutting the crown area too short may produce a spiky area that is not manageable for the client.
- *Curl* – how much natural wave or curl the hair has, or whether it is permed.
- *Elasticity* – this is important to determine the strength of the cortex. Hair in good condition is springy and bouncy – this is because the hair has good elasticity. It can stretch up to one third of its length when dry (half its length when wet) and then return to its original length. Hair with poor elasticity will overstretch and then snap, for example over-bleached hair.
- *Face shape* – the shape of the face is important when looking at suitable hairstyles to maximise your client's best features (and minimise any prominent ones, for example a large nose would be accentuated by hair swept off the face). Look at the illustrations of face shapes on page 140 – these should help you to analyse your client's face shape. An oval-shaped face suits most hairstyles, and this is the face shape stylists try to create using hairstyles to minimise square jaw lines and long and round faces.
- *Previous and existing chemical services* – is there any perm, colour, bleach or relaxer on the hair? This is vital to assess correctly or there may be disastrous consequences when carrying out a further chemical process.
- *Natural hair colour* – this is important when colouring or lightening the hair. (This is discussed more thoroughly in GH9.)
- *Lifestyle* – your client needs a hairstyle that she can manage. If you create a style that is high-maintenance, the client may not have the time, energy or skills to recreate the style every day. Try to suit the needs and personality of your client by creating a style that is versatile and workable.
- *Head shape* – if a client has a flat crown area, you may need to compensate for this by leaving the hair longer on the crown when cutting or using smaller perm rods on the crown when perming.

Face shapes

You should consider your client's face shape when helping them to decide on a hairstyle (see page 139).

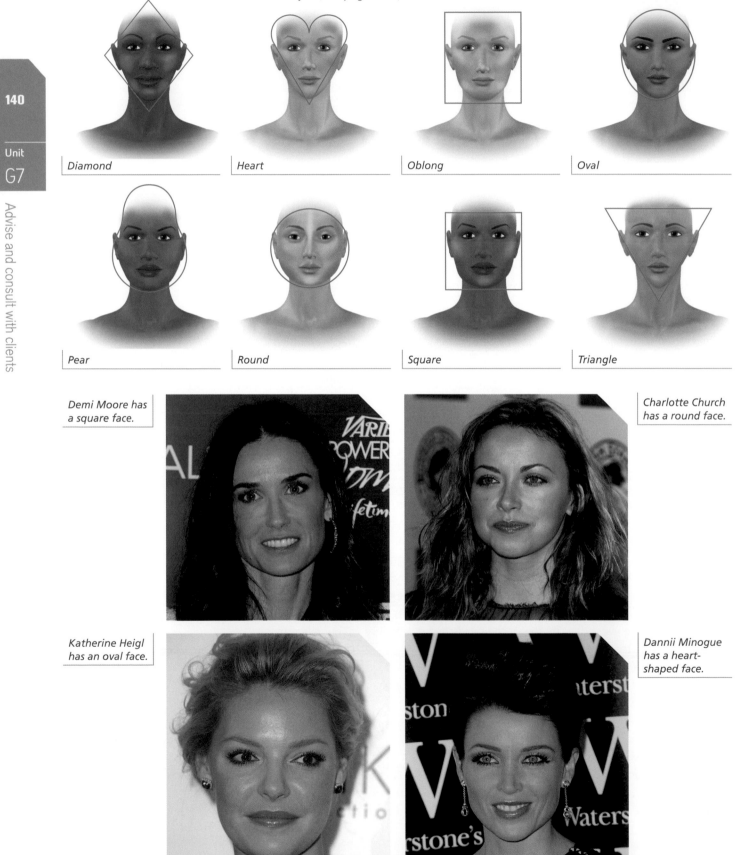

Diamond

Heart

Oblong

Oval

Pear

Round

Square

Triangle

Demi Moore has a square face.

Charlotte Church has a round face.

Katherine Heigl has an oval face.

Dannii Minogue has a heart-shaped face.

Porosity test

This tests the condition of the outer layer of the hair shaft – the cuticle (see page 3 for more information on the cuticle). **Porous** hair will absorb water and chemical products very quickly. If the cuticle scales are closed, flat and undamaged, the hair will feel smooth and look shiny. However, once the hair is chemically or physically damaged, the cuticle scales will become raised and may even be missing. Any chemical products that are then added to porous hair will be absorbed unevenly and may produce uneven curl or uneven colour results. This is why special perm lotions for tinted and highlighted hair are used. They are weaker in strength and are less likely to over-process and give a poor result.

Method

Take a strand of hair and hold it by the root (where the hair grows from) between the thumb and forefinger of one hand. Run the forefinger and thumb of your other hand from the root down to the point (where the hair has been cut). If the hair feels rough and bumpy, the cuticle scales are raised and open and this is an indication of porous hair. If the hair feels smooth, the cuticle is flat and closed and the hair's cuticle region is in good condition.

Elasticity test

This tests the internal strength of the hair. Hair that has been damaged due to chemical processes may have lost much of its natural strength. This will be due to the internal chemical links and bonds in the cortex of the hair becoming broken and damaged. Consequently, this type of hair may stretch up to two-thirds of its original length and may even break off. Therefore, it is important to carry out this test before using chemical processes. Hair that is in good condition will stretch and then return to its original length due to its good internal strength.

Method

Take one strand of hair and hold each end firmly between the thumb and forefinger of each hand and gently pull. If the hair stretches more than half of its original length and does not return to its original length, then it is over elastic and may snap or break during chemical processing.

Skin test

This test is a necessary safety precaution. It is carried out to check whether the client is allergic to colouring products. It should be carried out 24–48 hours before the colouring process.

Any colouring product which requires hydrogen peroxide to be mixed with it produces a chemical reaction that may cause some clients to have an adverse reaction such as irritation or swelling. In very severe cases, clients may have difficulty breathing due to swelling in the neck area – this is avoidable if you carry out a skin test before service.

The manufacturer's instructions will always advise if a skin test is required, so always read these carefully. Sensitivity to colour can sometimes cause an allergic reaction such as **dermatitis**. If a skin test is not carried out, you might make your insurance policy null and void, which would make you personally liable for any claim made against you.

Video clip

Watch video clip 'Porosity test' on the website to see a porosity test being carried out.

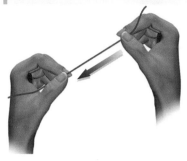

The elasticity test

Porous

The ability to absorb substances. The condition of the cuticle determines how porous the hair is. If the cuticle scales are closed or lie flat, the hair will have good porosity; if they are tightly closed, penetration of products will be more difficult. If the scales are damaged and open, raised or missing, the hair will be over-porous and absorb chemicals too easily and quickly.

Video clip

Watch video clip 'Elasticity test' on the website to see an elasticity test being carried out.

Dermatitis

Inflammation or allergy of the skin, sometimes called contact dermatitis. Usually affecting the hands of hairdressers, it causes the hands and fingers to crack and bleed due to constantly being wet and coming into contact with chemicals. Drying hands thoroughly, using a good barrier cream and always wearing gloves when shampooing and using chemicals will help avoid this condition.

141

Unit

G7

Advise and consult with clients

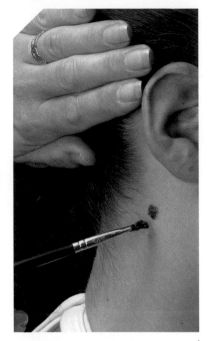

Carrying out a skin test

Incompatible

Not suitable.

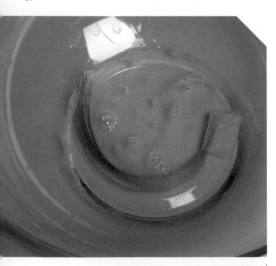

Incompatibility test being carried out

Video clip

Watch video clip 'Incompatibility test' on the website to see an incompatibility test being carried out.

Method

Use water and cotton wool or an alcohol wipe to thoroughly cleanse a small area of skin behind the ear or in the crook of the elbow. Mix together a small quantity of permanent colour (a dark shade should be used) with a few drops of 20-volume hydrogen peroxide. Apply a small amount of the colour (the size of a 5p coin) to the chosen area and allow to dry. Advise the client to leave the test on the skin for 24–48 hours unless there is any irritation and give the following client care advice.

The results will either be a positive or negative reaction:

* *Positive reaction* – redness, soreness, itching, inflammation. If any of these occur, the client should immediately wash the area clean of the colour. If the area is very sore, the client may need medical advice. If the client has a positive reaction, DO NOT proceed with the colouring process and advise her to use calamine lotion to soothe the area.
* *Negative reaction* – the skin appears normal when the test is removed and, therefore, the colouring process may proceed.

Always record the test date and outcome on the client's record.

Incompatibility test

Some chemicals do not work well together (they are **incompatible**) and may produce a bad reaction if one is used over the top of another. Some colours, for example, contain metallic salts, which are incompatible with other chemicals.

You should carry out an incompatibility test before perming, colouring or bleaching if you are unsure of the products already on the hair or if the hair has a doubtful history.

Method

Mix together (preferably in a glass bowl) 40 ml of 20-volume hydrogen peroxide and 2 ml of alkaline perm lotion. Place a small cutting of hair in the solution and wait. If heat is given off, the lotion fizzes and the hair breaks, dissolves or changes colour, then this is a positive reaction and the hair should NOT be permed or coloured with a product containing hydrogen peroxide. Always record the result.

Strand test

A strand test is taken to check the development of colouring products and relaxers while the process is being carried out.

Method

Always wear gloves to carry out this test. Remove some of the semi-permanent colour, permanent colour, bleach, colour stripper (colour reducer) or relaxer from a strand of hair with a damp piece of cotton wool. Check to see whether the product has developed properly and if you are happy with the result.

Test cutting

This is to test for the suitability of colouring products on hair and to check if the colour will have the desired result. It involves taking a small amount of hair and treating it mainly with the colouring products below:

* temporary colour – coloured setting lotion or coloured mousse
* semi-permanent colours – colour that lasts between four and twelve shampoos

- quasi-permanent colours — 12–24 shampoos
- permanent colours — colours that are mixed with hydrogen peroxide
- bleaches — used for lightening the hair's natural colour
- high lift tints.

Method

Backcomb a section of hair and take a hair cutting from this unnoticeable part of the head, placing masking tape over one end of the hair to secure. Mix a small amount of the intended product in a tint bowl and make sure the test cutting is completely covered with product. Check manufacturer's processing time instructions, but remember that there will be no heat from the scalp to help with the development of the colour. Once processing time is complete, rinse semi-permanent, permanent and bleach products (temporary colours are left on) and dry the test cutting. Examine and record the result.

Pre-perm test curl

When handling fragile, porous hair or hair with a doubtful history, it is advisable to wind, process and neutralise one or more small sections of hair. The results will be a guide to the best rod size, processing time and lotion strength to use. This test will also give a good indication of the likely condition after the perming process and will determine whether the hair is suitable for this service.

Method

It is not always suitable or possible to carry out a test curl on the head, so a cutting of hair may be taken and tested separately, but remember there will be no scalp heat to help the processing.

- Wind the hair around two or three perm rods of your chosen size.
- Apply perm lotion and leave to process for the manufacturer's specified time.
- Carry out a development test curl to see whether processing is sufficient. If so, rinse, neutralise for the time specified by the manufacturer, remove rods and evaluate and record curl result.

Development test curl

This test is carried out during the processing of the perm to check whether the desired development has been reached.

Method

- Always wear gloves to carry out this test.
- Hold the perm rod and undo the rubber fastener.
- Unwind the curler one and a half turns, holding firmly.
- Push the hair towards the scalp, allowing it to relax into an S-shape movement. Be careful not to pull the hair as it is in a very fragile state.
- When the size of the S-shape corresponds to the diameter of the perm rod, the processing is complete and should be stopped to avoid over-processing.

Always take test curls on different areas of the head as one area may be ready before another and this would cause an uneven curl result. The temperature of the salon will make a difference: perms will process more quickly on warm days than on cold days.

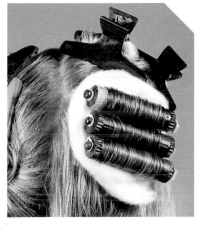

A pre-perm test curl

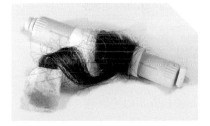

Pre-perm test result

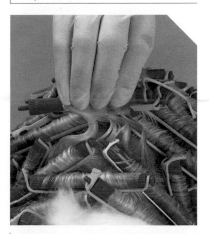

A development test curl

Pre-relaxer test

This is done to test for the suitability of products, development time and resulting condition of hair.

Method

Take a small section of hair from where the most resistant area is and pull through a slit in a piece of aluminium foil (placed as close to the scalp as possible). Apply relaxer to the strand and leave for two to three minutes.

If the test gives a satisfactory result, proceed with the service. If not, repeat the strand test, leaving the relaxer on a little longer.

Note: When carrying out subsequent processes do not re-treat this section of hair, as it will become over-processed and may break.

How to identify factors that will affect future services and product choice

A hairdressing service may be unsuitable if the client has a medical condition. This may be external and visible or it may be 'hidden' and discovered during the consultation.

Why conditions prevent hairdressing services

- If present, an **infestation**, **infection** or disease could be contagious, for example head lice, and therefore there is a risk of **cross-infection** to both stylist and other clients.
- The condition, for example open cuts or abrasions on the scalp, may be made worse by a hairdressing service.
- There may be a reaction, for example an allergic reaction to colours, which puts the client's health at risk.

A thorough consultation prior to any hairdressing service being given should reveal any **contraindications**.

A stylist should not name specific contraindications when referring a client to a GP. You do not have medical qualifications with which to make a diagnosis and it is unacceptable to cause the client concern which may be unfounded.

If the contraindication is small and localised in one area, service may take place with some adaptation. For example, eczema in its dry state may be treated, but when in its wet and open state it is a contraindication to hairdressing services.

To prevent cross-infection, follow good hygiene practices in the salon at all times.

- Maintain your own personal hygiene.
- Ensure good, effective salon hygiene.
- Maintain and clean/sterilise equipment regularly.
- Maintain client hygiene — make sure anything that comes into contact with the client, such as towels, is clean and used only for one particular client.
- Protect the salon against possible risks by taking part in training; this should include how to recognise infections and infestations and the steps to take if any are found.

Infestation

Parasites which live in or on another living creature in large numbers, e.g. head lice.

Infection

The invasion, establishment and growth of micro-organisms.

Cross-infection

The transfer of a disease, infection or infestation from one person to another.

Contraindication

The presence of a condition that makes the client unsuitable for a hairdressing service.

Fact or fiction?

Is this statement fact or fiction?

A head louse (pediculosis capitis) can live off the scalp for up to 72 hours. This means that once it has crawled off a client it can live in your brush or comb, or on your workstation, for three days.

To check your answer see page 495.

Top tips

If you treat a client and ignore the contraindication present, you are responsible and could be sued for negligence.

Protecting yourself and your client – when to refer to a trichologist

It is vital that you are able to identify the infections and infestations shown in the following chart and know what action should be taken. Cross-infection of some of these conditions can be prevented by good hygiene. Many diseases are also significantly reduced by **vaccination**. Precautions can be taken against both hepatitis B and tetanus.

It is important not to name or diagnose any medical condition you think your client may be suffering from as you are not medically trained. Instead, refer your client to their GP if you find a contagious condition or to a trichologist if you find conditions such as hair defects or scalp problems.

Vaccination

Injection with a vaccine – a tiny amount of a bacterium or virus. Vaccination is given in order that the body develops immunity (resistance) to the disease the bacterium or virus causes.

145

Unit

G7

Advise and consult with clients

Condition	Description	Cause	Treatment
Pityriasis capitis (dandruff) 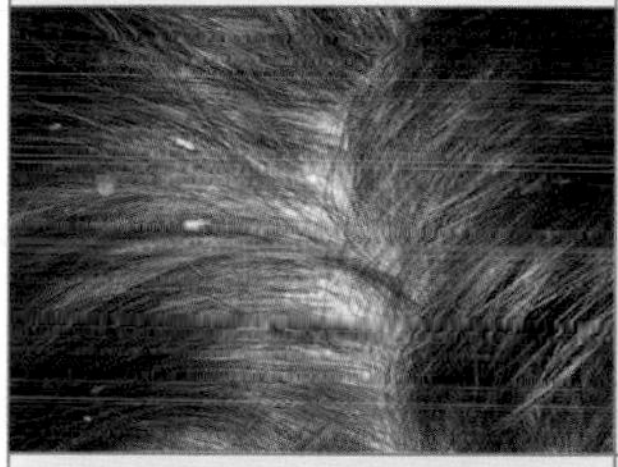	Small, itchy, dry scales (white or grey).	Overactive production and shedding of epidermal cells – stress-related.	Dandruff shampoo, e.g. selenium sulphide or zinc pyrithone; oil conditioners or conditioning creams applied to the scalp.
Seborrhoea (greasiness) 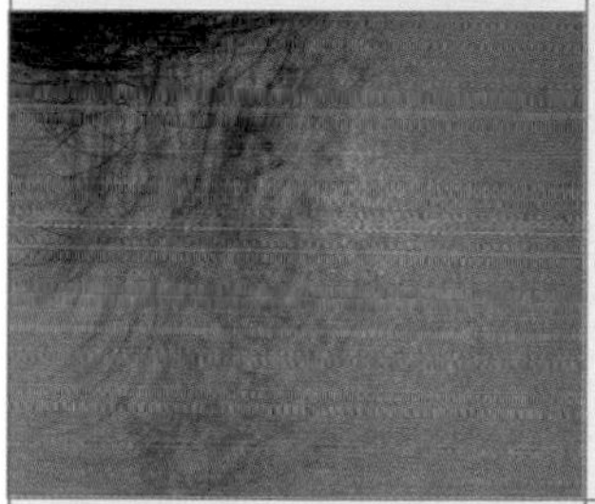	Excessive oil on the scalp.	Overactive sebaceous gland. Sometimes related to hormonal change.	Shampoos for greasy hair; spirit lotions.
Cuts and abrasions 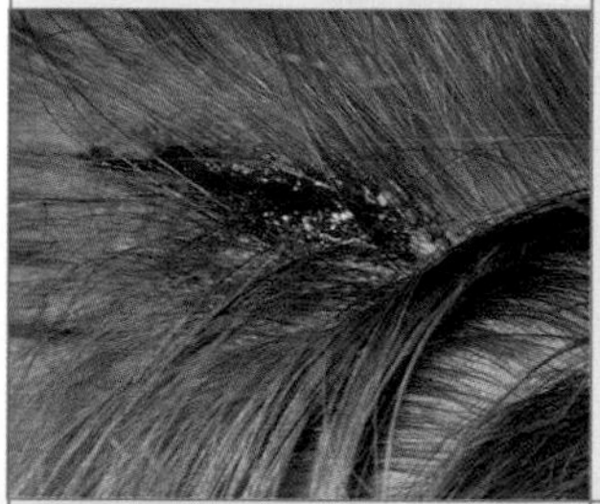	Cuts or abrasions on the scalp.	Recent injury to the scalp.	No service if wounds are open.
Cicatricial alopecia 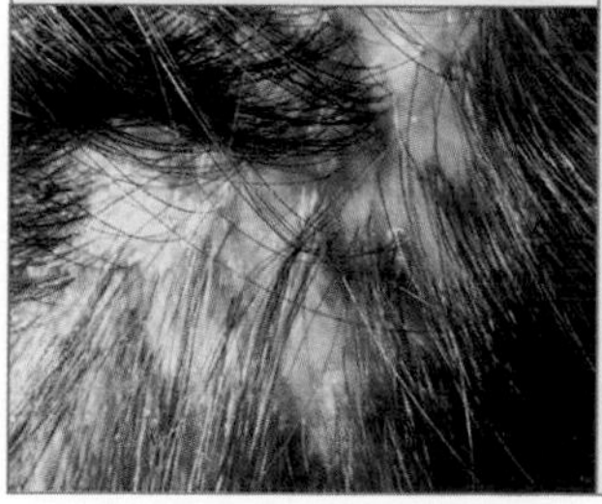	Hair loss/scar tissue.	A condition where hair follicles are destroyed and replaced by scar tissue, leading to loss of hair or baldness. This is a result of one of several scarring diseases.	Advise medical treatment.

Unit

G7

Advise and consult with clients

Condition	Description	Cause	Treatment
Psoriasis 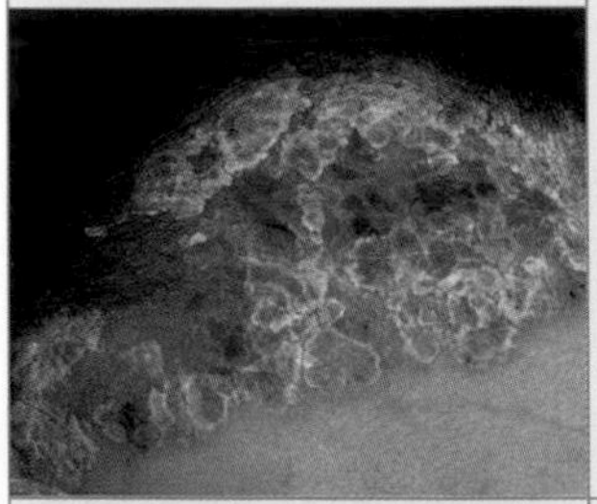	Thick, raised, dry, silvery scales; often found behind the ears.	Overactive production and shedding of the epidermal cells – passed on in families, recurring in times of stress. An auto-immune disorder.	Medical treatment; coal tar shampoo.
Male pattern baldness 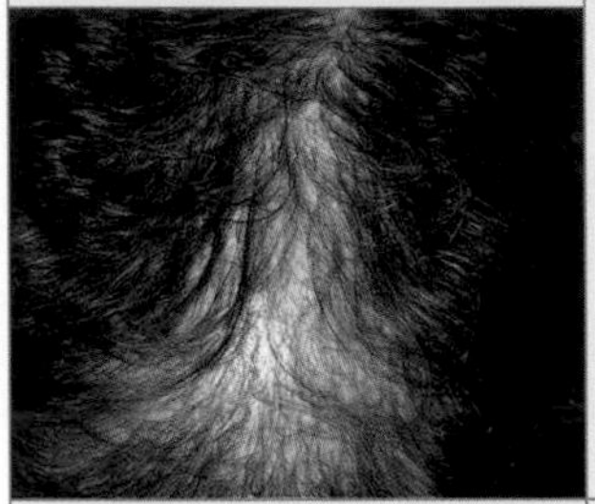	Receding hairline, thinning hair, baldness.	Hereditary, i.e. passed on in families.	Medical treatment is being developed.
Sebaceous cyst 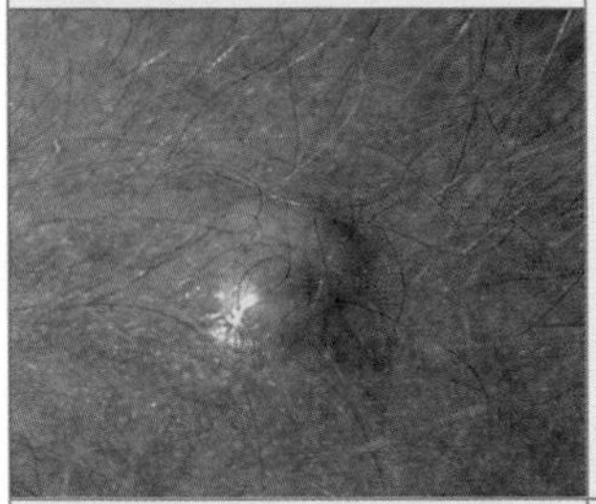	A lump either on top of or just underneath the scalp.	Blockage of the sebaceous glands and subsequent bacterial infection.	Medical treatment may be advised; treat gently during salon services.
Fragilitis crinium (split ends) 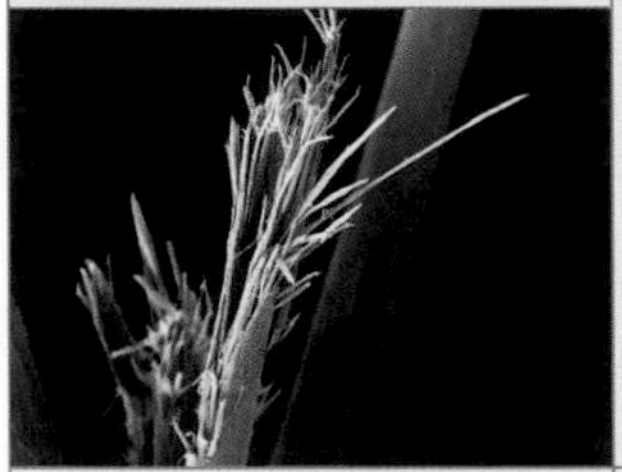	Split, dry, roughened hair ends.	Harsh treatments, chemical over-processing or general weathering of the hair.	Cutting and reconditioning treatments.
Damaged cuticle 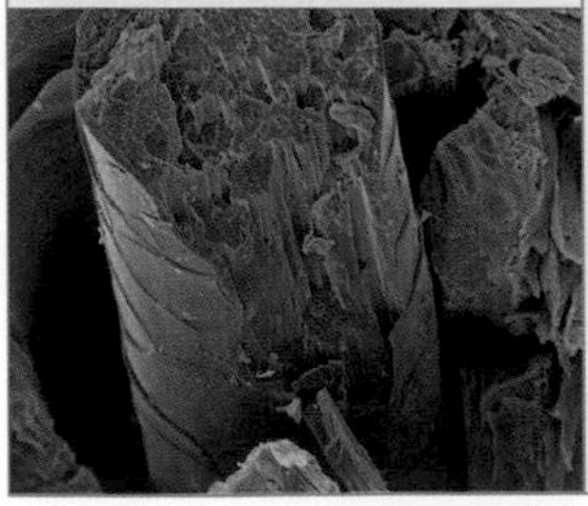	Cuticle scales toughened and damaged, dull hair.	Harsh treatments, chemical over-processing or general weathering of the hair.	Reconditioning treatments; restructurant.

Condition	Description	Cause	Treatment
Alopecia areata 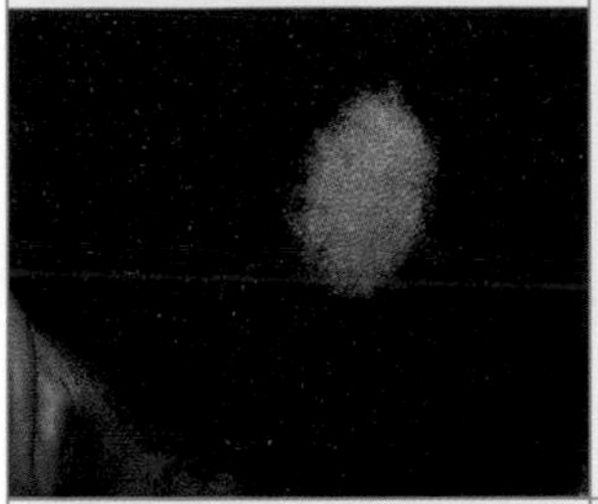 	Bald patches.	Auto-immune disorder sometimes triggered by shock. Perpetuated by stress.	Medical treatment; high-frequency service.
Trichorrhexis nodosa 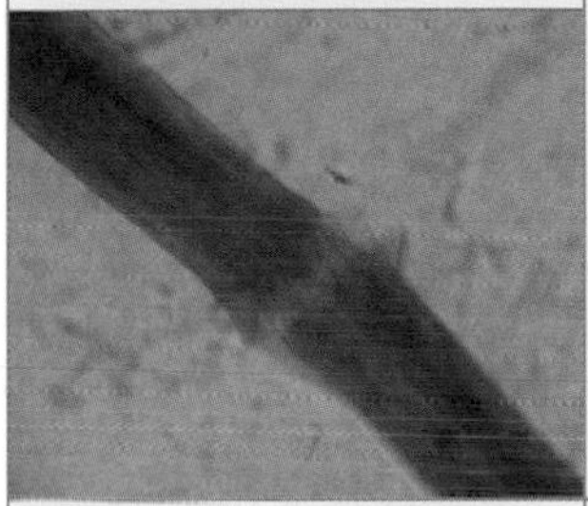 	Hair roughened and swollen along the hair shaft, sometimes broken off.	Harsh use of chemicals; physical damage.	Restructurant; reconditioning the cut hair whenever possible.
Monilethrix 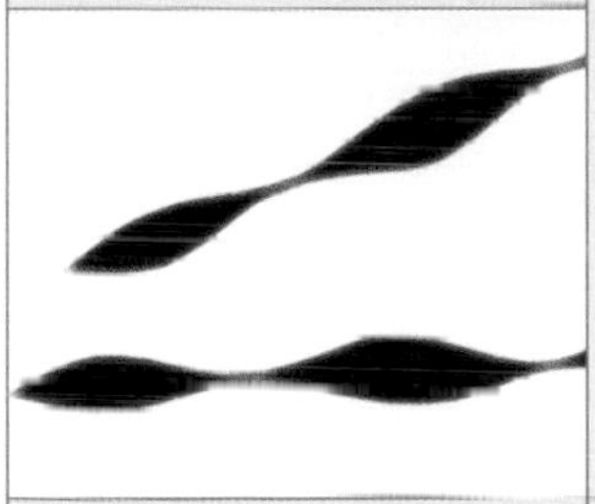 	Beaded hair – a very rare condition.	Uneven production of keratin in the follicle – hereditary.	Treat very gently within the salon.
Tinea capitis (ringworm) 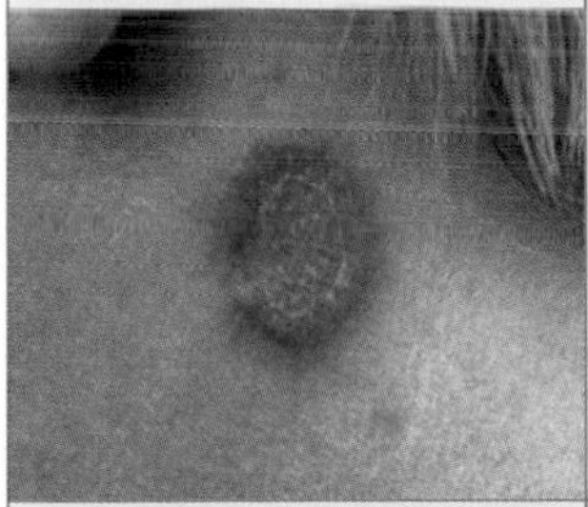 	Pink patches on scalp develop into a round, grey, scaly area with broken hairs – most common in children.	Fungus (not a worm) – spread by direct contact (touching) or indirectly through brushes, combs or towels.	Highly contagious; medical treatment required.
Impetigo 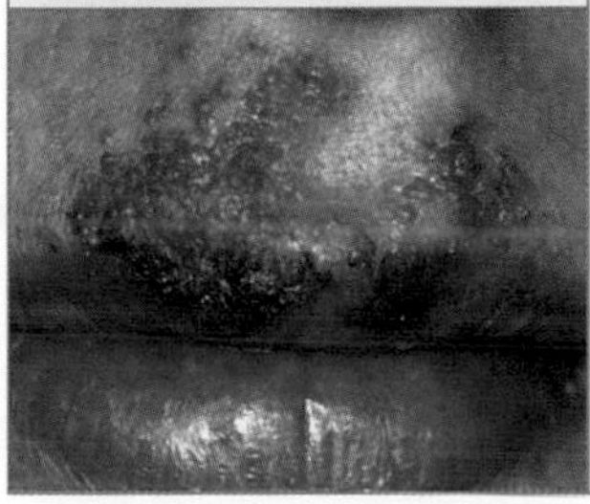 	Blisters on the skin that weep and dry to form a yellow crust.	Bacterial infection. Commonly occurring after nasal or ear infection. Spread by fingers and towels, etc.	Highly contagious; medical treatment required.

147

Unit

G7

Advise and consult with clients

Unit

G7

Advise and consult with clients

Condition	Description	Cause	Treatment
Pediculosis capitis (head lice)	White or light brown specks attached to the hair shaft close to the scalp; often at nape of neck and behind ears; itchiness — very common in children.	Small parasites (with six legs, 2 mm long), which bite the scalp and suck blood from the host. The females lay eggs (nits), which stick to the hair close to the scalp (they need warmth to survive). Cannot jump but are spread by direct contact (head to head) or indirect contact (from brushes, combs, etc.). Can live for up to 72 hours off the scalp. Once infected, lice multiply rapidly.	Highly contagious; refer to pharmacist.
Folliculitis	Small yellow pustules with hair in centre.	Bacterial infection within the hair follicle, sometimes following scratching.	Medical treatment required.
Warts	Small, flesh-coloured raised lumps of skin.	Virus spread by direct contact or touch.	Only contagious when damaged; treat with care in salon.
Scabies	Red irritating spots and lines on the skin.	Animal parasites (itch mites) burrowing in the skin.	Highly contagious; medical treatment required.
Barber's itch (sycosis)	Small yellow spots around the follicle; general irritation and inflammation; possible burning sensation.	Bacterial infection of the hair follicle; generally found in beard area.	Medical treatment required.

Conditions, infections and infestations of the hair and scalp

How to advise your client and agree services and products

In this section you will learn how to give correct recommendations to your client. It is very important to advise the proper products and services for your client to enable successful home maintenance of the hairdressing service carried out. This will promote a longer-lasting, more effective result and will encourage the client to return for further services and products, which in turn will increase the income of the salon.

How to make successful recommendations for your client

Be sure the information, benefits and effects you are claiming are true. It is also professional to ensure that the product you wish to sell to your client is in stock. Selling an unsuitable product just to close the sale is very bad practice and the client will lose faith in you.

Regular training and visits from manufacturers will ensure that your information is up to date and accurate. Many companies are happy to visit colleges and training academies to introduce product training.

Understanding salon services, products and prices

It is important to listen carefully to the information your client is giving you about the service she requires. Your clients' needs or requirements of the service must be foremost in your thoughts when you are deciding on the best way to fulfil these wishes. If you are unsure about the end result your client is asking for, you need to ask more questions or try rewording the questions so that you are sure you understand what your client is asking of you. You could use a strategy of summarising the consultation by saying, 'Okay Mrs Gerrard, so you would like a re-style but you want to keep as much of the length as possible.' You can then be sure you both have the same vision of the end result. This will help to ensure you are going to have a satisfied and happy client once you have finished.

Salon services

As a stylist, you should have an understanding of all the services offered by your salon. The needs of each client will vary and you need to be able to give correct information. If you do not know, you must be professional enough to admit this and ask your salon manager or a more experienced member of your team to help. Never make something up!

Video clip

Watch video clip 'Maintaining styles at home' on the website to hear what celebrity stylist Andrew Barton has to say about ensuring your client can maintain her hairstyle at home.

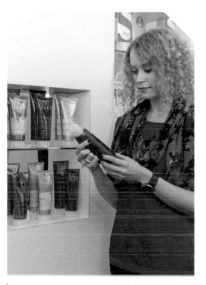

Most salons sell a range of hairstyling products

149

Unit
G7

Advise and consult with clients

Personal, learning and thinking skills – Independent enquiry

You have learned that consultation is the most important part of any hairdressing service. A thorough consultation ensures that you obtain the correct information from your client about the service they would like and that you do not miss a contraindication to the service which may have severe consequences. Your clients are your best source of information to find out if they are receiving the service they expected. Using independent enquiry, think of ways in which you can gather information to make sure you and your salon are meeting your clients' expectations.

Advise and consult with clients

Suitability of salon services

Not all hairdressing services are suitable for all clients. Some chemical processes require a skin test prior to the appointment to assess the sensitivity of the skin to hair colours. If a client has a service that is not suitable, the results can be disastrous.

Agreeing outcomes

It is important to ensure your client is fully satisfied with the outcomes of the service and products used. You must make sure you have met your client's needs fully to ensure a successful salon visit. If your client is not satisfied for any reason, this can be addressed and a note made on the record card for future reference.

Discussing cost and duration of services

Standard timings help maintain quality in the salon and ensure appointments are scheduled efficiently. It is important that all clients are treated equally and that they feel they are getting value for money.

The frequency of visits to the salon should also be negotiated with the client and is dependent upon:

- the service being booked
- the time the client has available
- financial considerations of the client
- the condition of the hair.

See page 92 for an example of a computerised appointments system. You should take into account the length of a hairdressing service when booking in clients.

Pricing structure

Prices vary from salon to salon and area to area. The salon should always display a price list where it can be clearly seen by clients and potential clients. This allows clients to view for themselves the costs and may encourage a client to enter the salon for the first time rather than walk away!

You must accurately calculate the likely cost for a service and inform your client before you start. There should be no hidden extras when your client comes to pay as this will undoubtedly cause bad feeling and will discourage your client from re-booking for future services.

See page 127 for an example of a salon price list showing salon services and prices.

Special offers

If the salon has any offers to pass on to the client then the stylist needs to be aware of these. This helps promote the offer and provides a chance to sell additional services or products that the client may not be aware of.

There is legislation concerning sales prices so be careful when advertising a sale in your window (see page 91).

Top tips

It is very important that you are fully aware of the services your salon offers, or business might be lost. This should include all salon services and the advantages and disadvantages of each.

Retail sales

Many salons offer a full retail sales service to complement the products used within a service. Be aware of what your salon sells, if it is in stock and what its benefits and selling points are. If your client asks for your advice before buying a product and you are unable to give it, you may lose a sale.

It is also important that you are aware of the legislation and guidelines that surround the retailing of products. Legislation covers how you must behave when describing products, services and their benefits to clients. The following are important Acts to be aware of:

- Supply of Goods and Services Act 1982
- Consumer Protection Act 1987
- Sale of Goods Act 1979.

See pages 60–62 of G20 for specific guidance on these Acts.

Ensuring client records are completed correctly

Good record keeping is essential to any hairdressing salon. The function of a client record system is to:

- record relevant client details (for example phone number) so that you can contact the client if necessary
- provide full and accurate information, which will ensure client safety
- ensure consistency of services regardless of who performs the service
- record the date of each service
- record changes to the service
- safeguard the salon and the stylists to prevent clients taking legal action for damages or negligence.

The client record system should be completed in full for every service the client has. It should be completed accurately and information about specific products used during the service should be included. For an example of a client record system see page 90.

A salon needs to store client records in such a way that they are accessible to the receptionist and stylist, but not so open that others can view them. A locked filing cabinet or drawer with limited access is ideal. However, many salons now keep records on a computer for safekeeping and for easy retrieval. You need to be aware of the Data Protection Act 1998, which is designed to protect individuals from misuse of the information held about them (see unit G20, page 59 for more details).

Salons generally use one of two methods to store client records.

- A computerised system which is used to book appointments and also to record client information about services carried out and products used.
- Record cards arranged in alphabetical order using the first letter of the surname — if two names begin with the same letter, then the second letter is used and so on. Where several clients have the same surname, they are filed alphabetically by their initials.

Be very careful which client is which! Always take the client's initial and full name, along with address details. Repeat the details back to the client to double-check that there is no confusion with clients of the same name.

Top tips

Information on client record systems should be kept private and confidential. If confidentiality is broken, it is an offence to the client and might lead to loss of clientele and earnings. If confidentiality is broken, it is also an offence under the Data Protection Act (see G20) and the salon or stylist may be liable to prosecution.

Unit

G7

Advise and consult with clients

The information stored on a record card

The more detailed the client record system is, the better the picture the stylist will have of the client. It also enables different stylists to work on a client knowing all possible details that may affect the service outcome.

A typical client record could include:

- the client's name, address and contact number
- the client's occupation
- contraindications, for example head lice, cuts or abrasions and so on, if present
- previous services and specific products used, and their success or problems
- services carried out and the date they were carried out
- cost and estimated time or length of a course of services, for example a course of restructurant conditioning treatments
- outcomes/results and effectiveness of salon services
- recommended aftercare
- homecare which is relevant to the client and achievable
- recommendations for further services
- purchases of products or additional services.

All these details should be checked regularly, even with a very regular client.

Task 4

Identify three problems which you might encounter during an analysis or consultation which would stop you carrying out the service the client was requesting.

- State who you would report these problems to.
- State the action you would take if they happened.

Task 5

Using the chart on the website, add the description, cause and advice/treatment needed for each of the hair and scalp conditions listed. This can then be used as additional portfolio evidence.

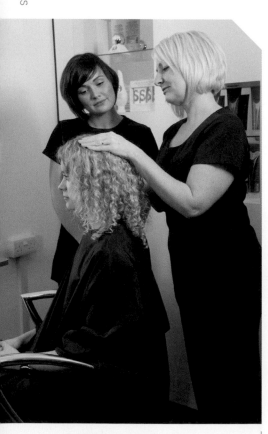

A client consultation

Salon life

Breaking the rules

Holly's story

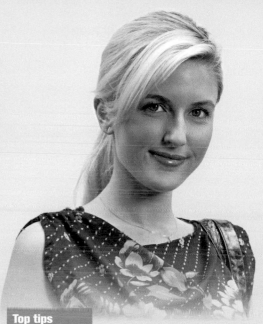

I'd been cutting a client's hair for ages and I also cut the rest of her family's hair. This particular day the client had booked her daughter in for a trim, but when she arrived she had a nasty looking sore on her face. My client explained that her daughter had impetigo but that she had had it for a week so she was no longer contagious. I said that impetigo was a contraindication in the salon and I wouldn't be able to cut the little girl's hair. My client practically begged me to do it because they were going on holiday the next day. I felt pressured so I agreed and carried out the cut.

A few days later I developed a sore on my mouth that would not go away. I went to the doctor, who diagnosed impetigo. I had to have a week off work, and lost my commission and tips for that week. I wish I'd stuck to my salon's rules. I feel I compromised my professionalism because I felt pressurised into something I knew I shouldn't do. I'll never do that again.

Advise and consult with clients

Top tips

- Never compromise your professionalism by carrying out a service when you know you should not.
- Once you have learned the fundamentals of hair facts you need to use these as a foundation to build upon all the other units, and this is vital when carrying out consultations with clients. You need to remember what you learned about the hair and skin structure, hair texture, condition, hair growth and chemical structure of hair. Everything you have learned about hair facts you need to put into practice during your consultation with clients.

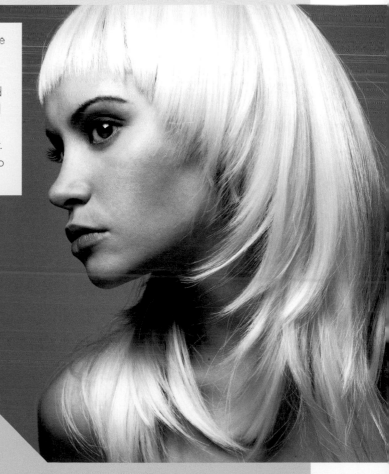

Ask the expert

Q *If you suspect your client has a condition that needs medical attention, should you tell them what you think it is?*

A If you are not medically trained you should never diagnose a client's suspected medical condition. The best thing to do is advise the client that you believe they may have something and they should seek medical advice from their GP, who would then refer them to a specialist if necessary.

Check your knowledge

The following questions will help you to check your understanding of this unit.
The answers can be found on page 495.

1 State your salon's rules for maintaining client confidentiality.

_____

2 It is important to carry out a thorough hair and scalp analysis during your client consultation to:
   a) make the service last longer
   b) assess the client's requirements and to check for any contraindications
   c) look professional
   d) seem like you are interested in your client's wishes.

3 State the seven skills required for a professional consultation.

_____

4 Which type of questioning technique is more commonly used to make conversation with your client flow?
   a) Closed questions
   b) Open questions

5 State how and when you carry out the following tests:
   a) Porosity
   b) Elasticity
   c) Skin
   d) Test cutting
   e) Incompatibility test
   f) Pre-perm test curl
   g) Strand test
   h) Development test curl

6 State the meaning of contraindication.

_____

7 Is psoriasis contagious?

_____

8 What is the cause of impetigo?

_____

9 What is pediculosis capitis?

_____

10 What is the cause of folliculitis?

_____

Getting ready for assessment

You will be assessed using a combination of assessment methods, as described below. Remember that within each of the services you carry out with a client, you will cover different units. For example, after advising and consulting with clients (G7), you may shampoo and condition hair (GH8) and set or dress hair (GH11). If you are not sure what you have covered in your service, always ask your assessor or supervisor for advice.

	NVQ	VRQ
Credit value	4	3
Guided Learning Hours	40	30 (VTCT) 60 (C&G)

	NVQ	VRQ
Practical demonstrations, to be observed by assessor	Your assessor will observe you on at least three different occasions, covering consultations for three different technical units such as cutting, perming and colouring. Simulation is not allowed for any part of the performance evidence within this unit. You must show that you have: • consulted with new and regular clients • adapted your advice to take into account the factors limiting or affecting services • used all the means of identifying clients' wishes by observing, questioning and testing • identified or can describe suspected infections and infestations needing reporting.	VTCT – Your assessor will observe you on at least three different occasions covering consultations for three different technical units such as cutting, perming and colouring. Evidence should be gathered in the workplace or a realistic working environment. Simulation should be avoided where possible. All outcomes and assessment criteria must be achieved (no specified range for this unit). C&G – Evidence should be gathered in a realistic working environment; simulation is not allowed for any performance evidence in this unit. You must demonstrate that you have met the required standard for all the outcomes and assessment criteria
Service timings	There are no maximum service times for this unit.	There are no maximum service times for this unit.
Additional evidence	You may need to produce evidence to support your performance where your assessor has not been present to witness your consultation or where evidence is not naturally occurring.	VTCT – Evidence to prove your knowledge and understanding will be provided through internally assessed workplace performance using a variety of methods. There is a mandatory written question paper required for this unit. C&G – Knowledge and understanding will be assessed by an assignment and a synoptic multiple choice test.

Unit
G7

Advise and consult with clients

Task mapping

When you have completed the tasks in this unit, check the table below to see which Performance Criteria (purple), Range (red), Knowledge (green) and Key Skills (blue) you have covered within G7 to use as additional evidence within your portfolio. Information about which Functional Skills you have covered is available on the website.

Task and page reference	Mapping to Performance Criteria, Range, Knowledge and Key Skills
1 (page 135)	Performance Criteria: 1a–f, VRQ 1a–f Range: 2a, 2b, VRQ R2a, R2b Knowledge: 20, 24, VRQ 1i, 1j Key Skills: C1.1, C1.2, C1.3, C2.1A
2 (page 136)	Performance Criteria: Practising 1b, VRQ 1a, 1b Range: 2a, VRQ R2a Knowledge: 20, 21, 24, VRQ 1i, 1j Key Skills: C1.1, C1.2, C1.3, C2.1A
3 (page 136)	Performance Criteria: 1c, 1d, VRQ 1a, 1b Range: N/A Knowledge: 21, VRQ 1j Key Skills: C1.2, C1.3, C2.3
4 (page 152)	Performance Criteria: 2d, VRQ 1d, 1e, 1g Range: 3a, 3b, 3c, 4a, 4b, VRQ R3a, R3b, R4a, R4b Knowledge: 8, 9, 10, VRQ 1h, 1n–q, 2a Key Skills: C1.2, C1.3, C2.3
5 (page 152)	Performance Criteria: 2c, 3a, VRQ 1d, 1e, 1g Range: 2b, 3a, 3b, 4a, 4b, VRQ R3a, R4a, R4b Knowledge: 8, 9, 10, VRQ 1h, 1n–q, 2a Key Skills: C1.2, C1.3, C2.3

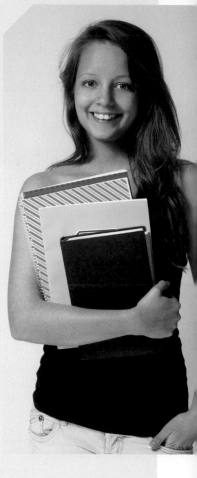

Develop and maintain your effectiveness at work

Unit **G8**

What you will learn:

- **How to improve your personal performance at work**
- **How to work effectively as part of a team**

Introduction

This unit is all about you — how to take responsibility for improving your performance at work and how to work well with your colleagues. Any personal improvement will help you make a positive contribution to the overall effectiveness of the salon. You may be asking, 'How will this help me to become a good stylist?' The answer is that being able to be objective about your own performance — that is, standing back and viewing your behaviour from the outside — will help you develop your personal and emotional attitudes, improve your relationships with your colleagues and encourage a positive working atmosphere within the salon.

It is a well-known fact in hairdressing that our industry moves at a very fast pace; there are continuously new developments in products and techniques. As a stylist it is important to continually update your knowledge of the new developments in order to have the necessary current skills and knowledge. It is important that you have the confidence to ask about new techniques and products — all the best stylists seek advice, and it is seen as a positive attribute to use your colleagues' and other professionals' strengths as an opportunity to learn and to improve your personal development. This is called **Continuing Professional Development (CPD)**. CPD also helps to build good relationships with colleagues and encourages effective teamwork within the salon. Teamwork is vital for a salon to function effectively and it is your job to ensure you assist your colleagues politely, promptly and respectfully to contribute to a harmonious working environment.

Video clip

Watch video clip 'Great training' on the website to hear what celebrity stylist Andrew Barton has to say about the importance of great training at the start of and throughout your career.

Continuing Professional Development (CPD)

Ongoing personal training which allows you to keep up to date with techniques and new trends within the hairdressing industry.

Fact or fiction?

Is this statement fact or fiction?

As a stylist you have to carry out 30 hours of CPD every year.

To check your answer see page 495.

How to improve your personal performance at work

Developing yourself as a person and your skills as a stylist are essential if you are going to play an active part within your salon. This section looks at ways in which you can improve your work by making the most of your salon's appraisal system, by working towards targets and by taking advantage of training opportunities while you are at work. It also considers the importance of keeping up to date with developments in the hairdressing industry.

Carrying out your job role to salon and National Occupational Standards

It is very important to understand your job role within the salon. If you do not understand what is expected of you while you are at work, how can you possibly fulfil all that is expected of you by managers and colleagues?

Once you have a defined job role, it is much easier to be an effective member of the salon team. As a trainee within the salon, you will be expected to assist all other members of the salon team. Once you have assisted with the services carried out in the salon, you will have an understanding of what the services involve. This will then allow you to anticipate the needs of the services and of your colleagues carrying out the services and to therefore give prompt assistance.

If you are unclear about your job role, it is vital that you approach your salon owner or manager to get clear guidelines of what you are expected to do during your working day/week. If you do not have a clear understanding of your responsibilities, your colleagues may view you as lazy when you do not carry out a task that is expected of you.

It is also important to carry out the tasks expected of you to salon and National Occupational Standards. For example, there are correct methods, techniques, sequences and timings for carrying out hairdressing tasks and these have been written into the National Occupational Standards that make up your qualification and are there for a specific reason. If, for example, you decide to neutralise a perm 'your way' instead of following your salon's guidelines and those laid down in the National Occupational Standards, you will create problems for your client, your salon and yourself.

If you always work to the highest possible standard, you will become a professional, skilled hairdresser who is known for high standards of work and is highly sought after by clients.

Task 1

Visit the HABIA website to find out how to access information on:

- the National Occupational Standards for Hairdressing
- CPD (Continuing Professional Development).

Understand how to improve your performance by identifying your own strengths and weaknesses – the appraisal system

If you keep making the same mistakes and clients complain or stop coming into the salon, something is obviously wrong! Spotting your own mistakes and then changing how you do a particular job to make sure you get it right in the future is one way of tackling this. However, it is not always easy to identify your own **strengths** and **weaknesses** and this is where a good manager will help by giving you regular work-related reviews or appraisals of your performance at work.

Many large companies provide self-appraisal forms for the employee to fill in and a joint performance appraisal form, which the manager discusses with the employee. An appraisal involves a discussion of your performance from which you as an employee will benefit as well as your employer. It is important to react in a positive way to any feedback or review. Nobody likes criticism, but it is important to listen carefully to what is said and to view any criticism constructively. If you act on your manager's comments you will become a better stylist!

Appraisal is not just about achievement within your job role or how many sales you may have completed – that is really only half the purpose of being a stylist (although an important one for the business!). It is also about your development as an individual. It opens up many areas of discussion between a manager and an employee, including future plans. It should highlight how well you as an individual are coping within your job role, whether the salon is asking too much of you, and provides you with an

Top tips

You can find a copy of the National Occupational Standards for Hairdressing on the HABIA website: www.habia.org.uk. HABIA (Hairdressing and Beauty Industry Authority) is a government-approved organisation which sets the National Occupational Standards and provides guidance on careers, business development, legislation, salon safety and equal opportunities.

Video clip

Watch video clip 'Updating skills' on the website to hear what celebrity stylist Andrew Barton has to say about constantly updating your hairdressing skills.

Strengths

These are your best personal and professional skills and attributes.

Weaknesses

The personal and professional skills and attributes that you need to develop or improve.

Top tips

You should view performance appraisals as a positive way of learning and progressing in personal growth and maintaining good working relationships.

159

Unit G8

Develop and maintain your effectiveness at work

Unit
G8

Develop and maintain your effectiveness at work

opportunity to offer your opinions on improvement. Appraisal should be viewed as a two-way discussion, not simply a reprimand for poor performance at work!

An appraisal or team review should happen regularly, perhaps once a month or every three months. However, it is common for individual appraisals to be carried out annually. Appraisals should:

- be held at a mutually agreed time
- be constructive, positive and open, not conducted in fear of job loss
- be as objective as possible
- be a review for both parties, not simply a judgement of the employee's performance
- leave the employee feeling enthusiastic, not depressed.

Self-appraisal – taking opportunities to review and set targets

A self-appraisal form used to review and set targets

⊙ssentials hair and beauty ☀

Self-assessment form for appraisal

Salon:	Date:
Position held:	Hair stylist:

Please add comments on how you feel you are progressing in each area listed.

Appearance:

Absences:

Timekeeping:

Job performance:

Sales:

Strengths:

Weaknesses:

Any areas of change:

Staff development request:

Action plan and date for next review:

Task 2

An example of a self-appraisal form is given on the website, with questions for you to answer. This worksheet can then be used as additional portfolio evidence.

A self-appraisal form includes whatever the employer/manager feels is relevant to the job role.

When identifying strengths and weaknesses, try to be honest with yourself. Do not focus only on your bad points — be constructive. Look at Masako Miyazaki's self-appraisal form (Task 2 on the website) — she balances negative with positive comments. You should have an equal balance of strengths and weaknesses.

Seeking guidance when instructions are unclear

If you have been asked to perform a specific task but are unsure what you have to do, it is important to find out more information from the relevant person to make the instructions clearer. You should, in the first instance, ask the person who gave you the task to clarify the instructions so that you fully understand what is expected of you. Only when you have a clear understanding of the task can you carry it out to the highest standard. Do not be afraid to ask — your colleagues would rather you ask for further clarification than make a mistake!

Seeking feedback on your performance

To help develop your skills, you need to identify your strengths and weaknesses. Nobody expects you to become an instant expert — you will gain more knowledge and experience over time in the salon. However, you should make sure that all the skills and knowledge you have are up to date. Regular training, reading trade journals and attending trade shows and exhibitions will help you to do this. Be enthusiastic to learn new skills and regard it as a challenge rather than a chore.

A self-appraisal form enables you to identify your strengths and weaknesses and from this you may set short-term and long-term personal targets. A joint review of your performance with your manager, assessor or tutor should then identify whether your personal targets are realistic and achievable using the SMART targets formula (see page 164).

Short-term goals are easier to measure and judge than long-term goals. Achieving these will encourage you to improve further. A short-term goal for the stylist Masako, for example, is to complete a fashion colouring course and gain her certificate. This is rewarding and achievable. A series of short-term goals can also help you achieve a long-term goal.

Long-term goals are not so easy to measure and may be harder to keep in view. They require much more dedication to achieve. A long-term goal for Masako may be to gain two more years of salon experience then apply for a job as a stylist on an ocean cruise liner.

161

Unit
G8

Develop and maintain your effectiveness at work

Top tips

Short-term goals are like the carrot dangling on the stick! They provide incentive and reward.

Unit
G8

Develop and maintain your effectiveness at work

Task 3

Look at the completed self-appraisal form below then complete the form provided on the website to review your current performance. Be as honest as possible and try to keep a good balance of strengths and weaknesses. Keep the completed form in your portfolio as evidence of self-evaluating your performance.

A performance appraisal form

the hair company

Self-appraisal

The purpose of this self-appraisal form is to help you reflect on your job performance and prepare for a performance appraisal interview. Use this form as a basis for key points you may wish to raise with your manager during the interview.

Remember, the three main objectives of an appraisal interview are to:
1   Assess past achievements/failures.
2   Consider the need for further training/development.
3   Specify ways in which future performance can be improved.

1   What parts of your job do you consider you have performed well?
    *I am confident with most services, however, I still find colouring hard and
    sometimes need help with layered cuts.*

2   What parts of your job do you feel you could have performed better?
    *I don't feel I'm very good at reception duties as I'm not very confident when
    making appointments.*

3   Comment on your overall level of job satisfaction.
    *I really enjoy my job and like assisting the other members of the team.
    Thursday is the best day as this is my 'training evening'.*

4   Indicate aspects of your work you particulary like/dislike.
    *I really like putting long hair up. I dislike setting as I find it difficult to fit the
    rollers in.*

5   What factors, if any, have made your work difficult to perform?
    *My confidence level. I need more practice with cutting and colouring.
    Perhaps a cutting/colouring course would help. More guidance needed on
    reception duties.*

Asking colleagues for help

Some people find it hard to ask others for help; however, in hairdressing you must be able to ask your colleagues for help for many different reasons. When you are training it is really important to be able to ask your colleagues to help you learn if you are finding certain tasks difficult. Remember — even the most famous celebrity hairdressers were trainees once and had to learn what you are learning. Some of you will find some parts of your hairdressing qualification harder than others, but practice makes perfect, and if at first you do not succeed, try and try again (and if you still find it hard — ask for help!).

Making and taking opportunities to learn

You may need to seek help from the relevant person in your salon if you are unable to obtain learning opportunities relating to your work. This will probably be your salon owner or manager as only she will be able to help give you the opportunity to learn if there is any cost involved. You may, however, be able to shadow another more experienced member of the team, which should provide you with a learning opportunity. Observing a talented stylist can help you to learn techniques and different methods of working. You must take every opportunity to learn, as it is very easy to sit back and think you know enough, but in our ever-changing industry there is always something new to learn!

Reviewing developments in hairdressing and related areas regularly and keeping your skills up to date

Hairdressing is a rapidly changing industry. If you wish to be a part of a busy salon that offers the latest trends and services, you will need to regularly update your skills by attending workshops and courses in cutting, colouring and so on. Various companies and suppliers, such as Wella or L'Oreal, run such courses.

You should also purchase and read trade journals. These will give you the latest information and often include step-by-step photos of new techniques. At work, you should set aside time to discuss new products that may be coming onto the market with manufacturers' representatives who may call at your salon.

You need to be aware of what is happening in the industry to enable you to offer the best and most current services to your clients. For example, if a client came into your salon with the latest copy of a fashion magazine and asked you to reproduce one of the hairstyles shown inside but you did not have the expertise to carry out this service, how would you feel? What image would you be portraying of the salon? Would the client have confidence in you and come back? Self-development and training are really important to make sure you do not become stale or lose interest or clients through poor product knowledge or skills.

All stylists should keep a record of Continuing Professional Development (CPD) to prove we have been updating our skills throughout our working life. This is important to enhance and build upon our existing skills and to ensure we do not become 'stuck in a rut' stylists. CPD also uplifts our industry to a higher level, proving that as a body of professional people we care about our industry and wish to offer the best, most up-to-date services possible to our clientele.

Video clip

Watch video clip 'Observing colleagues' on the website to hear what celebrity stylist Andrew Barton has to say about learning good customer service skills by observing your colleagues.

163

Unit
G8

Develop and maintain your effectiveness at work

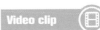

Video clip

Watch video clip 'Finding inspiration' on the website to hear what celebrity stylist Andrew Barton has to say about where he gets his inspiration.

You should keep any certificates of training courses you have attended in your portfolio of evidence for this unit.

Task 4

Research the timings you are allowed in order to be classed as commercially competent for the performance of the hairdressing services you are offering within your salon.

Agreeing and reviewing targets regularly to develop your future personal development plan

Linked into the appraisal system of monitoring performance is the setting of targets for an action plan to improve performance at work. Here are some SMART target guidelines to help you:

- *Specific* – have particular aims in mind rather than too grand an idea. Set a goal specific to you, for example 'I want to complete two assessments each week.'
- *Measurable* – make sure you are able to measure your aims with a start and a finish. You must know where you are now and where you want to be. For example, product re-sales might be on average £50 per day and a 10 per cent increase would take that to £55 per day.
- *Achievable* – aim for something that can be realised. You could have a short-term target, for example to complete a unit by a certain date.
- *Realistic* – be sensible in your aims; for example doing ten cuts per hour is not realistic.
- *Timed* – you should set a timescale in which to achieve your target, for example 'By next month I will improve my timekeeping by 50 per cent,' or, 'By December I am going to have my cutting unit ready to be signed off by my assessor.'

How often you decide to review your set targets is up to you and your salon, but short-term targets are usually easier to manage.

Top tips

You are in control of your own destiny. If you regularly review how you are doing at work you will be more focused on achieving set targets. Do not let opportunities pass you by because you are too lazy to have a development plan for your future.

Task 5

Look at the self-assessment appraisal form that you completed earlier (for Task 3).

- How would you tackle your weaknesses?
- What short-term and long-term targets could you set to develop your strengths?

How to work effectively as part of a team

Creating and maintaining good working relationships with your colleagues involves developing a variety of personal skills, including those of a good communicator, so that you can play your part in creating a happy and harmonious working environment.

Agreeing, working together and achieving objectives

Every salon will have its own working philosophy. Generally this will be to anticipate and fulfil clients' needs within a healthy and happy salon environment, thereby promoting a thriving business. In order to achieve your salon's objectives, you and your colleagues need to agree ways of working together in the salon towards a common goal. A salon team will always be made up of people with different strengths and weaknesses and it is important to make full use of everyone's strengths and try to improve the weaknesses. A team will also be made up of different personalities and it is important for everyone to get on when working together as part of a team. The team will only be effective if everyone feels they are working equally – resentment will build up if some team members are not working as hard as others. Make sure you are an effective team member by working as hard as you can. Regular team meetings (ideally weekly) will help to maintain a good working relationship, as any problems can be sorted out in a business-like forum during professional discussions.

How to be an effective team member

On joining a salon you will become part of a team and will be expected to work with other team members – your colleagues – to ensure the smooth running of the salon.

Qualities a good team should have

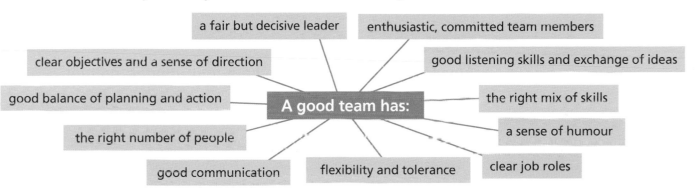

a fair but decisive leader

enthusiastic, committed team members

clear objectives and a sense of direction

good listening skills and exchange of ideas

good balance of planning and action

A good team has:

the right mix of skills

the right number of people

a sense of humour

good communication

flexibility and tolerance

clear job roles

This pie chart shows how we see one another; in other words, what we are judged upon. If we act irresponsibly, it may affect the whole team.

Team spirit can be lost:

*   if one member of the group works on her own; that is, not as part of the team
*   if there is a breakdown in communications
*   if team member(s) are unwilling to be flexible and tolerant of others' mistakes
*   when there is too much work for too few people
*   when job roles become blurred and people encroach upon areas they should not.

As a team member, it is your responsibility to know:

*   who all the staff are in the salon
*   who is responsible for what
*   who to go to for information and support.

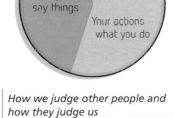

How we judge other people and how they judge us

Politely asking for help and information

Good communication between colleagues builds good relationships that will be reflected in the smooth running of the salon.

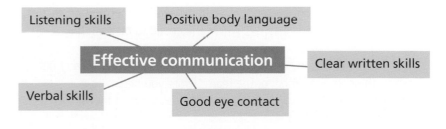

Listening skills

Positive body language

Effective communication

Clear written skills

Verbal skills

Good eye contact

Good communication involves many skills

Unit

G8

Top tips

- Treat others as you wish to be treated.
- Be professional at all times when you are in the salon.

Fact or fiction?

Is this statement fact or fiction?

You should never attempt to do a job that you have not been trained to do.

To check your answer see page 495.

Top tips

Always make sure you understand what is being asked of you – the ability to listen carefully is an important skill. Show that you understand by nodding your head, for example, or if you do not know or understand something, do not guess – ask!

Unless your colleague is telepathic or highly perceptive, she will not necessarily know that you need assistance. You should be able to ask for assistance when necessary, and perhaps next time your colleague needs assistance you can return the favour.

If you need help or information you should ask for it – politely. Stating why you require assistance will explain to other members of staff how they are helping you. Being polite and professional at all times will promote team spirit.

Responding to requests willingly and politely

When a colleague asks for your help you should respond willingly and politely to the request. If you do not, you will not be working as an effective team member and will not pass this unit of your qualification. How your colleagues perceive you at work is very important to your working professional life. You should always want to be known as a polite and willing trainee, and if you are not, you will not last very long in this industry. Salon owners, managers and other members of staff do not have to put up with unprofessional, rude trainees.

Anticipating the needs of others and offering prompt assistance

When you can see that your colleagues need your assistance it is up to you to offer help and to know whether you are capable of doing that particular job. In order to anticipate the needs of other members of your team, you need to understand your job role and responsibilities within the salon. Once you have worked in the salon for a while you will get to know when certain colleagues need your help. At first they may need to ask you for help, but you will soon learn when you are needed and this will allow you to anticipate your colleagues' needs and offer your assistance. When you know a colleague needs help it is important to stop the job you are doing (if possible) and give immediate assistance. Try to prioritise the jobs you are responsible for so that you can be as effective as possible in the salon and to all members of your team.

Being capable and competent means doing a job as well as you have been trained to do it. Do not attempt to bluff your way through a job – this could put a client or colleague at risk of harm.

Being responsible for your actions involves taking responsibility for any mistakes you may make and taking the appropriate action to minimise any further damage.

Making effective use of your working day

In a busy salon you will be asked or instructed to carry out many different services. Your job list may contain a number of items and instructions may be fired at you in quick succession. Don't panic! Here are some guidelines to help you.

- Make a list of the jobs you have been asked to do.
- Check with the relevant person that you have written them all down.
- Ask which ones are priorities, i.e. which ones need to be done first.
- Tick off the jobs/services as you carry them out.
- If you are unsure of any of the tasks that you are expected to carry out, confirm them with another member of the team before you begin.
- If a list has been left for you and you cannot understand the writing, ask a colleague to have a look.

Task 6

1 Your manager leaves you a list of jobs to do while she is away on holiday. You are not sure whether any of the jobs require immediate attention or if they are of equal importance. Who would you refer to?
2 The manager is out of the salon and you need to clarify an issue straightaway. Who would you refer to?

Task 7

Write a list of your responsibilities in your current working role. Do you have the authority to carry out these tasks? If in doubt about your responsibilities, who would you ask for confirmation? (Helpful hint: if you have a job contract, this should contain a job description.)

167

Unit

G8

Reporting problems to the relevant person

There is always a hierarchy within a salon and it is important for you to know the correct channels to go through when you experience a problem. This means you need to know who you should approach with a particular sort of predicament. For example, if it is a difficulty concerning work schedules, you may need to contact the salon manager to help you resolve the situation. However, if you have a wages problem, you may need to speak to your salon owner, who controls the salon budget. You should find out who does what in your salon so that you know who to approach with different dilemmas. If you approach the wrong person with a problem, it could make the situation even worse.

Imagine the following scenario: an angry client comes into the salon complaining that the colour you carried out over a month ago has faded and she is unhappy with the result. She demands her money back. It is not within the limits of your authority to do this, so here are some guidelines to help you handle this difficult situation:

- Be sympathetic and listen carefully to the client.
- Ask her politely to take a seat while you find someone in authority to speak to her.
- Inform your employer or the most senior member of staff that you have a client at reception who would like to discuss her last colour as there seems to be a problem. You should then explain the situation in as much detail as possible so your superior is able to talk knowledgeably to the client.
- You should be present at the following discussion so that you can see what the exact problem is and how the problem is dealt with. Only offer input to the conversation if asked.

Here are some of the things you should not do:

- Do not get angry with the client.
- Do not be rude and tell her that nothing is wrong with her hair.
- Do not lie and say there is nobody who can deal with her and ask her to come back on your day off!

In another situation, a regular client comes into the salon for a service without an appointment. You should never make a client feel unwelcome and should try to be as accommodating as possible. If it really is not possible to fit the person in at that time, make an appointment. This also applies to a client who is late for an appointment or where a stylist has been over-booked. Rescheduling appointments can work both ways. It might be as a result of staff sickness — clients may have to be juggled into other time slots. If you always deal with clients in an open, genuinely apologetic manner, most will be flexible.

When a client changes a booking, again be flexible. If time permits and the client's needs can be accommodated, then do so. The receptionist will need to be made aware so that the time slot isn't double-booked. Flexibility is the way to encourage new and repeat business.

Resolving problems with colleagues effectively

If you have a problem with another member of the team, it is important to approach that person first. You should think carefully about what you are going to say and make sure your timing and the situation are appropriate. For example, wait until you are alone with your colleague and go somewhere out of earshot of the rest of the salon. Be mature in your approach and never start shouting. Say what you need to say calmly and this should help you to resolve the situation. Listen to your colleague's point of view as well and try to get a 'win, win' situation by resolving the problem so that you can continue to work with each other without bad feeling. If you feel you cannot deal with the situation, you may need to involve your salon manager.

Task 8

Research your salon's/college's appeals and grievance procedures. Keep a record of this in your portfolio of evidence for this unit.

Task 9

How would you deal with the following relationship difficulties and conflicts within the salon? Use the worksheet provided on the website to record your answers and keep this in your portfolio of evidence.
1 One of your colleagues seems to dislike you and sometimes asks you for help in an aggressive way.
2 A colleague employed to do the same job role as you leaves everything to you and you feel she is lazy.
3 Another colleague keeps on telling you all her personal problems and sometimes this makes you feel uncomfortable.
4 A colleague is sometimes discriminatory (biased) against other members of staff and this makes you feel uncomfortable.

Understanding how to work with others by being friendly, helpful and respectful to your colleagues

Working in a commercial salon is different from working in a college or training institution. You will, however, be expected to work sensibly, responsibly and as part of a team at work and at college. There will be many instances where a colleague may require your help. This does not mean that your colleague is failing to do his or her job properly. It might be because:

- a hairdressing service took longer than anticipated
- a client may have been a few minutes late and, as a result, affected the stylist's timing
- a chemical process may have processed more quickly or slowly than anticipated
- a stylist has been inadvertently double-booked and has two clients at the same time.

Any one of these factors could contribute to a colleague needing your assistance. Here are some ways you could offer to help:

- shampoo a waiting client
- make the client a drink so that the stylist does not have to stop to do this and will then be able to begin the service straightaway
- rinse a colour or perm if it has processed more quickly than first thought
- take one of your colleague's clients if the client is agreeable.

Being part of a team means that if you are asked for assistance, you give your help willingly and courteously (politely). By being fully aware of what is happening in your working environment you will be able to anticipate your colleagues' needs. You should aim to offer assistance before being asked for it. This is called using your **initiative**.

If a job needs doing, carry it out without being asked. This will prove to your employer that you can be relied upon to work effectively and practically at all times.

Initiative

Taking the first step or action without being prompted to do so.

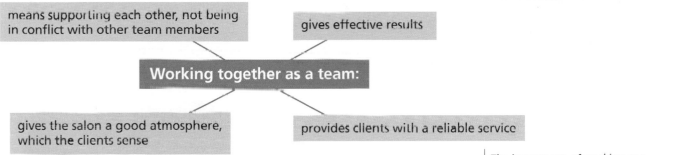

means supporting each other, not being in conflict with other team members	gives effective results

Working together as a team:

gives the salon a good atmosphere, which the clients sense	provides clients with a reliable service

The importance of working as a team

Develop and maintain your effectiveness at work

When you leave college or a training institution, you will be the newest, least experienced member of staff. It may take time to build up a regular column of clients and, as a result, you may be the person who has the most free time to be called upon. When you build up a client base and you are busy, the team will recognise this and somebody else will do the job.

When working under the guidance of a colleague, you should:

- accept that your colleague is in charge
- take instructions and act upon them
- communicate effectively
- take responsibility for your job role and do it to the very best of your ability.

Personal, learning and thinking skills – Teamwork

Being able to work as part of a team is crucial to the smooth running of the business. Within this unit, you have learned how to complete a self appraisal on your strengths and weaknesses. Now carry out an appraisal focusing on your teamwork skills. Ask for feedback from your manager and other members of the team. This will show your employer that you are conscientious and committed to being a team player within the salon.

Salon life

Making the most of appraisals

Katie's story

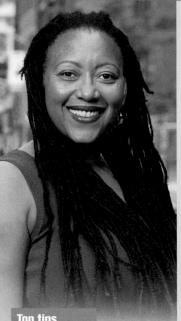

When I first started work at my salon, I was a bit worried when they said I had to fill out an appraisal form and have a meeting with my boss about my strengths and weaknesses. I found it quite hard to write down my strengths on my appraisal form as it felt a bit like I was bragging about how good I was. I managed to write down lots of weaknesses but no strengths.

When it came to the appraisal meeting I was really nervous but it went much better than I thought it would. My boss said I had lots of strengths, it was just that I didn't realise I was good at some things. We talked about my weaknesses and she gave me deadlines to complete different courses and tasks to build my confidence in these areas.

When my next appraisal was due I wasn't worried at all as I understood what was going to happen. We looked at the last appraisal form to see if I'd been on the courses identified and had done the tasks.

If I was asked to give a new employee advice on appraisals I would say, 'Don't worry, they are really helpful and nothing to be scared of. They helped me to build my confidence.'

Top tips

- Give yourself plenty of time to think about what you want to say in your appraisal. If you go into your appraisal without having prepared what you want to discuss, this will be a missed opportunity and you may have to wait a long time until your next appraisal.
- Most appraisals take place annually, but if you are unsure about your salon's procedures don't be afraid to ask your boss or salon manager.

Ask the expert

Q *Why do I need an appraisal? I don't really see the point of it.*

A An appraisal is important to assess your progress while at work. It is an opportunity to have one-to-one time with your boss or manager when they are normally very busy and may not be able to spend a great deal of time with you discussing individual matters. Try to look at your appraisal as a positive aspect of your job role where you can spend some quality time with your manager to openly talk about you!

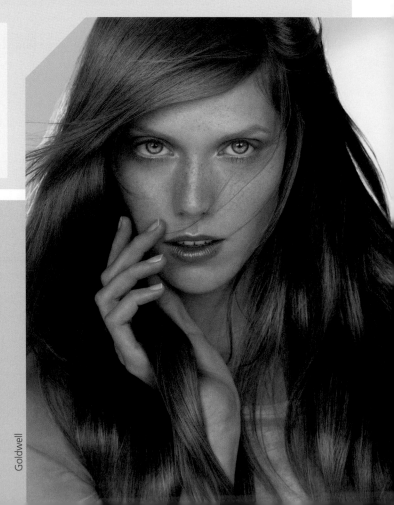

Goldwell

Check your knowledge

The following questions will help you to check your understanding of this unit.
The answers can be found on page 496.

1 How would you get information about your job, responsibilities and the standards expected of you?

_____

2 Who would you ask about information on your salon's appeal and grievance procedures?
   a) Salon owner
   b) Receptionist
   c) Junior colleague

3 How do you identify your own strengths and weaknesses?

_____

4 What does CPD mean?
   a) Continual Professional Discussion
   b) Constant Professional Discussion
   c) Continuing Professional Development

5 Who is responsible for developing the National Occupational Standards for Hairdressing?
   a) A government-approved organisation called HABIA
   b) The National Occupational Standards Organisation
   c) The National Union of Students

6 Why is it important to be aware of current and new trends and developments in hairdressing?

_____

7 If you had a difficulty with a colleague in the salon, who would you report it to?
   a) Your parents
   b) Your colleagues
   c) Your owner/manager

8 State the eleven qualities of a good team.

_____

9 State the five skills needed for effective communication.

_____

10 State why it is important for you to be a good team member of your salon.

_____

Getting ready for assessment

You will be assessed using a combination of assessment methods, as described below. Remember that within each of the services you carry out with a client, you will cover different units. For example, you will probably work as a team, helping to develop your personal effectiveness at work (G8), on a daily basis! If you are not sure what you have covered in your service, always ask your assessor or supervisor for advice.

	NVQ	VRQ
Credit value	3	N/A
Guided Learning Hours	30	N/A

	NVQ
Practical demonstrations, to be observed by assessor	Your assessor will observe your contributions to effective teamwork on at least one occasion which will be recorded, but it takes most students more than one observation to meet the necessary requirements for this unit. Evidence should be gathered in the workplace or realistic working environment; simulation is not allowed for this unit. To complete this unit you must prove that you have: • participated in all the listed opportunities to learn • agreed and reviewed your progress towards both productivity and personal development targets • offered assistance to both an individual colleague and in a group of your colleagues.
Service timings	There are no maximum service times for this unit.
Additional evidence	You will be required to collect documentary (paper) evidence for your portfolio, to prove you have participated in development activities at work. This could include evidence of your appraisal; a review/report or an action plan which has timed outcomes; certificates of training activities you have attended; and agreed and reviewed progress towards both productivity and personal development targets. There are no mandatory written questions required for this unit.

Task mapping

When you have completed the tasks in this unit, check the table below to see which Performance Criteria (purple), Range (red) and Knowledge (green) you have covered within G8 to use as additional evidence within your portfolio. Information about which Functional Skills you have covered is available on the website.

Task and page reference	Mapping to Performance Criteria, Range and Knowledge
1 (page 159)	Performance Criteria: 1f Range: N/A Knowledge: 13, 15, 16, 17, 18
2 (page 161)	Performance Criteria: Practising 1a Range: Practising 2a, 2b Knowledge: 9, 10, 11, 12
3 (page 162)	Performance Criteria: 1a, 1g–i Range: 2a Knowledge: 9, 10, 11, 12
4 (page 164)	Performance Criteria: Practising 2e Range: 2a, 2b Knowledge: 8

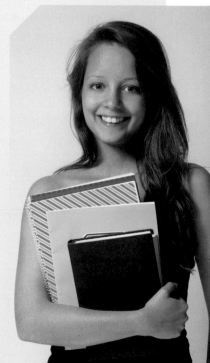

5 (page 164)	Performance Criteria: 1a, 1c, 1g–i Range: 2a, 2b Knowledge: 12
6 (page 167)	Performance Criteria: 1b, Practising 2b Range: 1a Knowledge: 2
7 (page 167)	Performance Criteria: 1b, Practising 2b Range: 1a Knowledge: 2
8 (page 168)	Performance Criteria: N/A Range: N/A Knowledge: 7
9 (page 168)	Performance Criteria: 2a, 2f, 2g Range: N/A Knowledge: 21, 23, 24

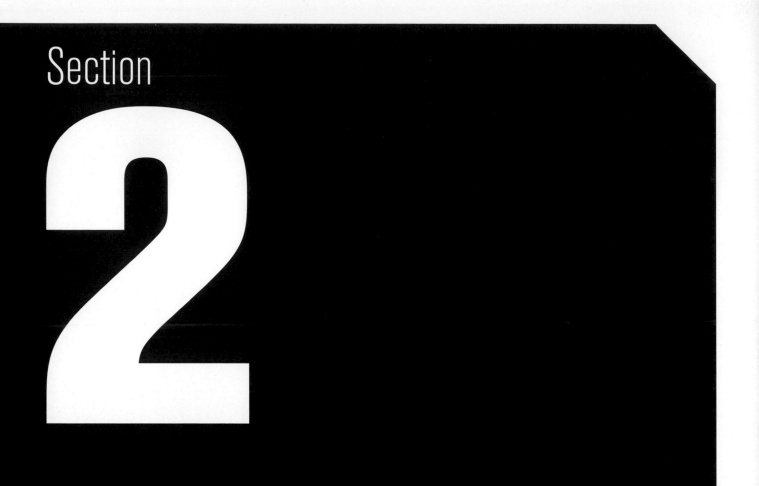

Section

2

Practical skills –

hairdressing

Shampoo, condition and treat the hair and scalp

Unit **GH8**

What you will learn:

- **How to maintain effective and safe methods of working when shampooing, conditioning and treating the hair and scalp**
- **How to shampoo the hair and scalp**
- **How to condition and treat the hair and scalp**
- **How to provide aftercare advice**

Introduction

Shampooing and conditioning are an essential part of most hairdressing services. In order to make hair more manageable for blow-drying, setting, cutting, perming, relaxing and some colouring processes, the hair must be thoroughly cleansed of all dirt, natural grease and products such as hairspray, mousse and wax. (If you need to refresh your memory, revisit 'Facts about hair and skin'.) If any of these are left on the hair before further services, such as perming, they will cause a barrier between the hair and the chemical and the service will be unsuccessful.

This is probably the first service you are going to carry out for a client and the first experience of getting your hands on the client's scalp. It is therefore very important to be able to analyse your client's hair and scalp type correctly (see G7) in order to choose the appropriate products to suit the client's individual needs. If you use the wrong shampoo, conditioner or scalp treatment, you can create problems for your client. For example, if you use a shampoo containing oil (such as coconut oil shampoo) for greasy hair, you will just add to your client's grease problem.

A good shampooing technique has the added bonus of relaxing the client – as you massage the shampoo throughout the hair and scalp, you will soothe the nerve endings and muscles within the scalp. If clients require a more intensive massage, a deep penetrating conditioning treatment will also help to improve the internal structure of the hair. Some clients regard the quality of their shampoo and conditioning massage so highly that they will return to the salon purely for the quality of the service they receive while at the basin. Some salons teach their staff a particular massage technique which is seen as a substantial added bonus to the client experience.

How to maintain effective and safe methods of working

As shampooing and conditioning are the first hairdressing services you will carry out, it is important that you understand your salon's rules and regulations on health and safety. You need to follow these rules to ensure the well-being of yourself and your client. This is the first step towards becoming a professional stylist, as the standards set by qualified staff should ensure that the quality of all services are maintained at a high level.

Carrying out a consultation and choosing suitable products

Once you have gowned the client, you should carry out a thorough consultation to assess your client's needs, choose and organise appropriate products and equipment, and think through and plan the service (see G7). It is important that you can describe the different consultation techniques you have used. Try to practise this in preparation for questioning by your assessor.

During the consultation for a shampoo and/or conditioning treatment, you should assess the following.

What to assess	Factors to consider
Hair condition	Is it normal, dry, damaged or frizzy? Does it need added moisture? Does it snap when you test its elasticity? How does the cuticle region feel?
Scalp condition	Is it dry, normal, greasy or dandruff-affected? Also ask your client if she is experiencing any scalp-related problems at the moment.
Hair type	Does it have the characteristics of Asian hair, African-type hair or European/Caucasian hair?
Hair texture	Is the hair fine, medium or coarse?
Previous chemical services	Ask your client if you are unsure what chemicals have already been used on the hair and check for any contraindications. (Refer to 'Facts about hair and skin' to refresh your memory.)
Purpose of service	Prior to a perm, for example, you must use pre-perm shampoo; if you do not, you may leave a barrier on the hair shaft which will stop the perm working properly.
Subsequent services	You may need to recommend a course of deep conditioning treatments in order to improve the hair's condition and increase its strength in readiness for other services, such as colouring, where chemicals are being used.

You will then have the information to enable you to:

- select and use products to suit the client
- organise your working area with all necessary products and equipment for the service (for example, a steamer to aid penetration of intensive conditioning treatments)
- discuss the service plan with the client
- start a record of the service
- begin the service.

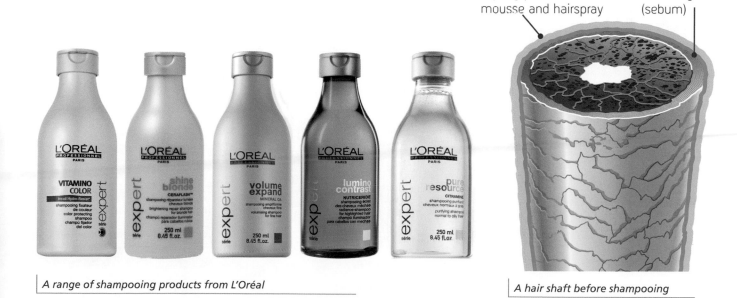

A range of shampooing products from L'Oréal

Styling products such as mousse and hairspray

Natural grease (sebum)

A hair shaft before shampooing

Shampoo, condition and treat the hair and scalp

Preparing and positioning the client for a shampoo and conditioning treatment

The client should be protected with a gown, towel around the shoulders and a disposable plastic shoulder cape secured by a sectioning clip. It is important not to place the sectioning clip too high under the client's chin or it will become uncomfortable if the client bends her head forward. The plastic shoulder cape will protect the client's clothing from becoming wet whilst you are initially practising your shampooing technique.

It is very important to position your client correctly at the basin to ensure a watertight seal around the neck. Your client should be seated comfortably in the backwash basin chair. You should guide your client back by supporting her shoulders. Position the client's neck correctly by making sure there are no gaps between the neck and the edge of the basin. If there are, your client will most certainly get wet!

Health and safety issues

Manufacturers' instructions

Before using any shampooing or conditioning product, you must read the manufacturer's instructions. These give you the information to use the product properly (as intended) and will result in the service being as successful as possible.

Top tips

If you do not follow the manufacturer's instructions when using a product and a problem occurs, the manufacturer will take no responsibility. The responsibility falls on you, as the stylist, to use a product exactly as instructed. Failure to do so might be considered negligent.

Always follow manufacturers' instructions

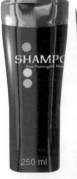

Shampoo Damaged Hair

Effect: Damaged hair is thoroughly nourished, gently cleansed and repaired. Hair is easier to comb too.
Application: Apply a small amount to damp hair and distribute evenly. Massage gently into a lather. Rinse thoroughly and repeat if necessary.
250 ml

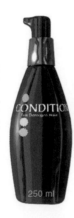

Conditioner Damaged Hair

Effect: Penetratiing deeply into the damaged hair, the nutrient complex rebuilds hair from within, leaving it easier to comb.
Application: Distribute sufficent product evenly through towel-dried hair and gently massage. Leave for 1–3 minutes. Rinse thoroughly.
250 ml

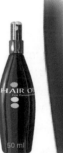

Hair Oil Damaged Hair

Effect: This highly effective formula penetrates deep into the hair structure. Regenerates and seals damaged hair shafts and ends, helping to prevent further damage.
Application: Depending on length and amount of hair, distribute and work in at least 5 pump depressions to dry hair. Do not rinse out.
50 ml

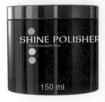

Shine Polisher Damaged Hair

Effect: The ideal preparation before styling. This highly effective complex strengthens damaged hair from within, restoring stability and shine.
Application: Apply a small amount to the palms of the hands and work into dry hair.
150 ml

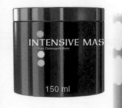

Intensive Mask Damaged Hair

Effect: Intensive, long-lasting nourishment. Repairs and cares for damaged hair, sealing the hair's structure to help protect against further damage.
Application: Apply sufficient product and distribute evenly through towel-dried hair and gently massage. Comb through and leave for approximately 5–10 minutes. Rinse throroughly.
150 ml

Water safety

It is essential that clients' safety is a priority during their time in the salon. When shampooing and conditioning, you are using water and possibly electrical equipment (such as a steamer), both of which can cause serious accidents if health and safety rules are not followed.

Workplace environment

Standard health and safety rules to follow

- The salon must always be kept clean and tidy.
- Any spillage of water or product on the floor is a potential hazard and should be wiped up immediately.
- Your work area should be kept clean and tidy throughout the service and any waste should be removed immediately after shampooing and conditioning.
- Always make client comfort an important issue and position your client carefully at the basin before you begin shampooing.
- You should position yourself to ensure good posture while working to avoid discomfort and the risk of injury.
- Any shampooing or conditioning product entering the eye should be flushed immediately with clean water, and first aid attention should be sought.
- A client suffering from an infection or infestation cannot undergo a service in the salon, as the problem is likely to cause a cross-infection to other clients, colleagues and yourself (see page 62).

Task 1

Phoebe – hairstylist

When I was a new apprentice at Eclipse Hair Salon and had only been shampooing for a couple of weeks, Will, a junior stylist, asked me to shampoo his client. I began to apply water to the hair when I noticed tiny things crawling on the top of the client's head. I was unsure what to do, so I excused myself from the client to ask Will what to do. He immediately realised that the client had head lice so no further service could take place that day. He tactfully and discreetly informed the client (who by now had wet hair) of the situation and recommended that she visit a chemist to obtain a suitable treatment to kill the parasites.

1 How could this situation have been avoided?
2 Some equipment has already come into contact with the client. What action should be taken to prevent cross-infection of the infestation to other clients and staff?

Your own safety

As mentioned in Section 1, The workplace environment, it is important to maintain correct posture throughout the working day. You should try to keep your back as straight as possible when working and if you need to bend, always bend your knees and not your back.

Another occupational hazard is dermatitis. This is a skin condition usually found on the hands, which is aggravated by the constant use of water and hairdressing products. Wear gloves when shampooing and dry your hands thoroughly afterwards. Regularly protect your skin by using a barrier cream to help prevent any dryness from occurring. You should wear **personal protective equipment**, if required, to avoid the dangers associated with skin conditions and cross-infection.

Top tips

When conditioning hair you may need to use electrical equipment to help the product penetrate. Always dry your hands before plugging in electrical equipment and make sure you have made any necessary safety checks for frayed wires. Never use equipment you have not been trained to use.

179

Unit

GH8

Shampoo, condition and treat the hair and scalp

Fact or fiction?

Is this statement fact or fiction?

Expensive conditioners can permanently repair split ends and damaged hair.

To check your answer see page 496.

Personal protective equipment

Equipment necessary to protect the skin and clothing, e.g. protective gloves.

Replenishing low levels of resources

In order to minimise any disruption to your client's service and your service plan, always replenish resources, such as clean towels and gowns, regularly throughout the day.

Reordering products

If you use the last of a shampoo, conditioner or scalp treatment during a service, you should make sure that the item is replaced. If you run out of the only product suitable for your client's needs, you will be unable to provide the client with an effective service.

You may not be responsible for the reordering of products and equipment, so make sure you know the system to follow and use it to ensure you are not the one causing an 'out-of-stock problem'.

Completing client records after shampooing and conditioning

It is important to record all service details, even for shampooing and conditioning, for future reference. This is because you are unlikely to remember which products you used on the client's previous visit to the salon. Unless you have a record of the conditioning treatment used last time, you cannot evaluate if it was successful or whether you need to change to another product.

Gianni&Jo hairdressing

Client Record Card

Name: Jasmine

Address:

Post Code:

Telephone:

Date	Treatment/Product/Perm Colour/Condition etc.	Application/Rod size/ Timing/Result	Student
25 April	Deep conditioning treatment	Good result	Alice

Gianni&Jo hairdressing

Client Record Card

Name: Jasmine Hubert

Address: 123, Russell Street
Fareham

Post Code: PO12 6JS

Telephone: 936221

Date	Treatment/Product/Perm Colour/Condition etc.	Application/Rod size/ Timing/Result	Student
25 April	Deep penetrating treatment TIGI S Factor	Good result	Alice Anderson
	Serious shampoo ⟶	shampooed twice	
	Serious conditioning treatment	⟶ massaged for 10 mins & under steamer for 10 mins	
		Successful result – hair felt smooth & shiny	
		Recommended a course of 6 treatments over next 6 weeks.	

Compare these record cards for the same client. The client says she found the conditioning treatment she had last time to be very beneficial. Which card would you prefer to use?

How to shampoo the hair and scalp

Shampooing is a very important and beneficial part of a hairdressing service. It is an essential start to many other services as it removes general dirt, natural grease and any styling and finishing products that your client may have used, such as mousse, wax and hairspray. It is probably one of the first services you will learn. It can take some time to perfect as there are many things to consider at the same time, such as trying to keep the client's face and clothing dry, using the correct products, performing a good massage, learning how to handle the hair, as well as making conversation with your client.

It is important to use the correct shampoo for the client's hair and scalp condition. You will need to learn which shampoos are suitable for specific hair and scalp conditions. Knowing the products will also enable you to give good aftercare advice so that clients benefit from using the most suitable products at home. It is also important to use the correct shampoo immediately before a chemical service such as perming. The wrong type of shampoo may affect the perm and result in an unsuccessful curl.

The massage techniques you need to learn for this unit are very important, as clients will judge the quality of their shampoo by the massage (as well as by how dry they stay!).

Preparing for shampooing

It is important to know and follow your salon's rules for preparing the client and yourself for shampooing. You should always gown the client correctly.

Shampooing fixtures and fittings

Before beginning the shampoo, decide whether to use a frontwash basin or a backwash basin.

A frontwash basin is more suitable for:

- people who have back or neck problems
- people too small to lean into a backwash basin, for example children.

A backwash basin is more commonly used because:

- it prevents water and chemicals entering the client's eyes
- it is more comfortable for most clients
- the client's clothing is less likely to get wet.

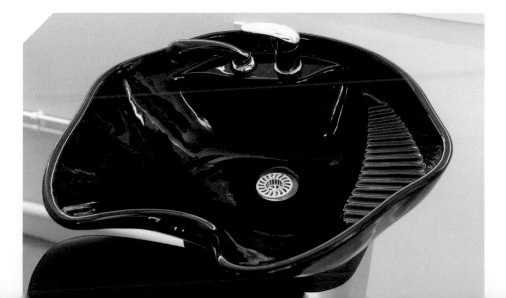

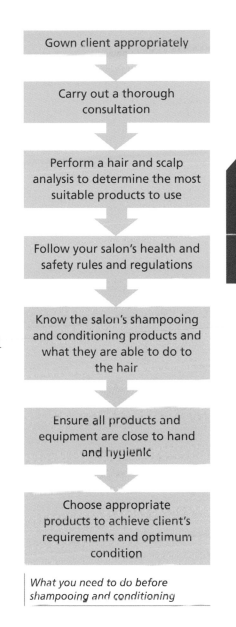

Gown client appropriately

↓

Carry out a thorough consultation

↓

Perform a hair and scalp analysis to determine the most suitable products to use

↓

Follow your salon's health and safety rules and regulations

↓

Know the salon's shampooing and conditioning products and what they are able to do to the hair

↓

Ensure all products and equipment are close to hand and hygienic

↓

Choose appropriate products to achieve client's requirements and optimum condition

What you need to do before shampooing and conditioning

A backwash basin

181

Unit

GH8

Shampoo, condition and treat the hair and scalp

Top tips

When using a frontwash basin, always give your client a towel to protect the eyes and face from chemicals or water.

Unit

GH8

Shampoo, condition and treat the hair and scalp

Medicated

Properties or substances within a specialist shampoo used to cure, heal or relieve a problem scalp.

Knowing shampoo products

Knowing the shampoo products in your salon is essential. During the initial consultation with the client, you will have checked the condition of her hair and scalp. Generally, this will be one of the following.

- chemically damaged
- heat damaged
- environmentally damaged
- normal
- dry
- oily
- dandruff-affected.
- affected by product build-up.

You will then be able to select and use the correct shampoo to suit the hair and scalp type. Your salon will have a range of shampooing and conditioning products which you will need to become familiar with but the general shampoo guide below will help you.

Shampoo	Hair/scalp type	Benefits
Coconut oil	Dry	Adds moisture.
Almond oil	Dry	Adds moisture.
Medicated	Dandruff-affected	Relieves itchiness.
Coal tar	Psoriasis	Releases scales; helps itchiness.
Strawberry (fruit)	Normal	Cleanses.
Lemon	Oily	Removes grease.
Egg and lemon	Greasy (sensitive scalp)	Removes grease; gentle on scalp.
pH-balanced	Damaged/after colour	Returns hair to natural pH.
Protein	Environmentally/heat damaged	Strengthens.
Beer	Fine/limp	Adds body.
TLS (soapless base, no additives)	All types	Leaves no residue; used for pre-chemical process (e.g. before perm).
Clarifying	Hair with product build-up	Removes product build-up.

General shampoo guide

The pH of a product is a measure of how acidic or how alkaline it is. A shampoo that is pH balanced will have a pH of 4.5–5.5, which is the same pH as the hair and skin. Because this pH is slightly acidic, pH-balanced products will automatically close the cuticle scales and promote shine and manageability.

Top tips

- When you are shampooing your client's hair, you will be in very close contact. Make sure you are 'nice to be next to' by ensuring you do not have bad- or cigarette-smelling breath or body odour.
- Always read and follow the manufacturer's instructions carefully so that the product provides the client with maximum benefit. Also give good aftercare advice by explaining fully to your client how to use shampooing and conditioning products at home.

Task 2

List each shampoo in your salon and make a note of:
- the hair and scalp type it should be used for
- the manufacturer's instructions for when and how to use it.

A worksheet for this task is provided on the websie for you to complete and add to your portfolio.

Massage techniques for shampooing

The following massage techniques should be carried out using the pads of the fingers or the palms of the hands. Never use your nails as these could scratch the client's scalp and cause an infection. If the hair is long, you will need to adapt your massage movements as long hair can become tangled very easily. Remove one hand at a time if the hair lengths start to tangle. Always remember to keep contact with the scalp with at least one hand, otherwise contact will be broken and the client may receive a jolt if they are very relaxed.

Effleurage

Using the palms of the hands:

- slow, smoothing, stroking movement
- spreads shampoo
- relaxes the client.

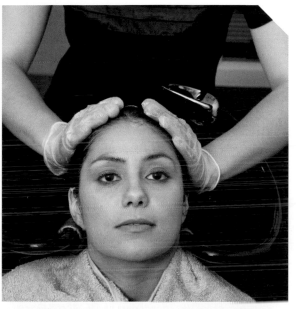

Effleurage massage

Rotary

Using the pads of the fingers:

- small, round, circular movements
- stimulates scalp
- removes dirt and grease.

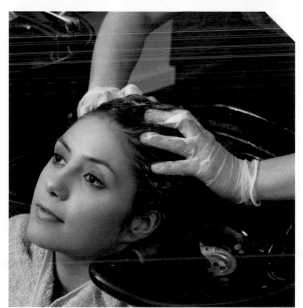

Rotary massage

Massage can be very beneficial to the client if it is carried out using the correct pressure. Always check with your client that the pressure you are using is comfortable, as some people's scalps are more sensitive than others.

Video clip

Watch video clip 'Massage techniques' on the website to see the massage techniques used during shampooing and conditioning.

Top tips

Many hairdressers believe that clients will react negatively if they wear gloves for shampooing and conditioning. Trials have shown that this is not the case, and wearing gloves will protect you from joining the 80 per cent of UK hairdressers who suffer from dermatitis during their career.

183

Unit

GH8

Shampoo, condition and treat the hair and scalp

Sebaceous glands

Glands found in the dermis of the skin, situated next to hair follicles. They secrete sebum.

Sebum

Fluid secreted by the sebaceous glands. When mixed with sweat, sebum forms the acid mantle on the skin, which offers protection against micro-organisms and infection. Over-production of sebum caused by stimulation, hormone imbalance or illness results in oily hair and scalp, giving the hair a greasy look and feel.

Adapting shampoo massage techniques

There are certain circumstances when you may need to adapt your massage technique to suit your client's needs. This may be for the following reasons:

- *Hair length* — long hair will only need rotary massage throughout the scalp. The lengths of the hair should only be massaged using effleurage as this will be effective at cleansing the hair but will not cause excessive knotting of the cuticle scales. Avoid tangling your fingers in long hair and avoid tugging the hair unnecessarily.
- *Hair density* — this is a measurement of how much hair your client has per square centimetre. If there is a lot of hair per square centimetre, it may mean that you will need to use a firmer rotary massage technique in order for your client to feel any firmness of pressure.
- *Hair condition* — hair that is very fragile, for example highly bleached hair, should be massaged with caution as it is liable to break easily.
- *Scalp condition* — scalps that are excessively oily should not be massaged vigorously using rotary shampoo massage movements. This will stimulate the **sebaceous glands** that produce our natural oil (**sebum**) to produce even more oil — not a good result for someone with an oil/grease problem.

Task 3

Mrs Ahmed is a regular client who suffers from psoriasis. During her consultation you notice that her psoriasis is very red and sore. On some parts of the scalp it appears to be open and weeping/bleeding. Mrs Ahmed is booked for a cut and blow-dry.

1 Would you be able to shampoo Mrs Ahmed with psoriasis in this state?
2 If not, what alternative service could you offer, if any?
3 What advice would you give to Mrs Ahmed?

Shampooing procedure – ensuring client comfort

Step-by-step shampooing procedure

Seat the client correctly at the basin and make sure she is comfortable. If using a backwash basin, make sure the client sits right back in the seat so that her neck fits the curve of the basin correctly without any gaps for the water to leak through. Make sure all the hair is in the basin.

1 Turn on the taps and test the water temperature on the inside of your wrist before testing on the client's scalp.

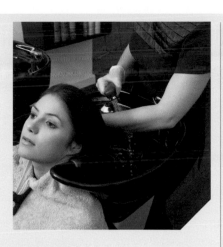

2 Check the temperature of the water with the client and then apply the water. Thoroughly wet the hair and scalp, taking extra care around the hairline so that you don't wet the client's face. Turn off the water.

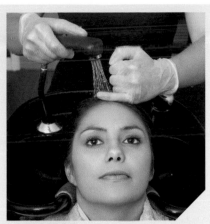

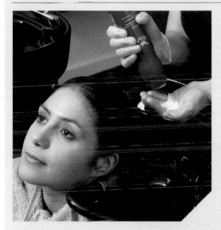

3 Dispense the correct amount of shampoo (about the size of a 2p piece) into the palm of your hand and **emulsify** between both palms. Apply from hairline to **nape** of neck using effleurage massage technique.

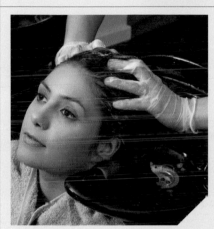

4 Start rotary massage technique from front hairline to nape, around side hairlines and then through middle sections until the whole head has been covered. Repeat until the shampoo begins to lather.

Shampoo, condition and treat the hair and scalp

5 Turn the water on and rinse thoroughly. Turn off the water. Repeat shampoo application and massage techniques. Turn the water on and rinse until the hair is clean and free of products.

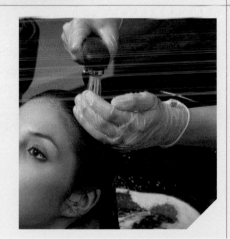

6 Turn off the water and gently squeeze hair to remove excess water. Use a towel around the head to stop any drips from the hair entering the eyes or face. The client is now ready for the next hairdressing service.

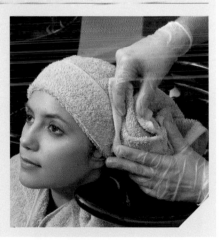

Nape

The back of the neck where the hairline starts.

Emulsify

To combine two liquids together which normally don't mix easily. In the salon, this refers to rubbing shampoo or conditioning products together in the palms of the hands to help spread the product before applying to the hair and scalp. The shampoo then emulsifies the dirt, natural grease and products in the hair. When the shampoo lather is rinsed away, the dirt, natural grease and products are removed within the lather.

Top tips

To be assessed as competent, you should take no longer than five minutes to complete the shampooing process.

Unit

GH8

Shampoo, condition and treat the hair and scalp

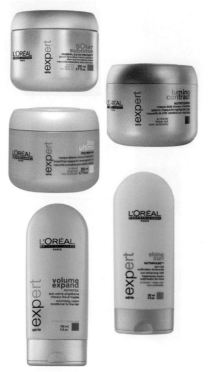

Conditioning products from L'Oréal

Smooths and coats cuticle scales

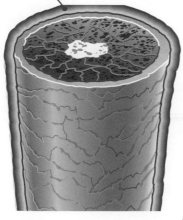

Action of surface conditioners on the hair shaft

How to condition and treat the hair and scalp

Conditioning is a very beneficial part of a hairdressing service. It not only improves the visual appearance of the hair by making it shiny, but also improves the manageability, which aids all the other hairdressing services we offer. Conditioning treatments often sell themselves as clients are usually aware if their hair is out of condition and will often ask what they can do to improve its look and feel. It is your job to assess the condition of the hair and decide which type of conditioner to use.

Preparing the hair for conditioning

It is very important to carry out a thorough consultation before you begin to condition the hair. This is because some conditioning treatments are carried out on dry hair (hot oil service, for example) and some conditioning treatment ranges include a two- or three-stage process using a shampoo, conditioner and scalp treatment, which should be used together for the best possible results. Once you have gowned the client (as for shampooing) and completed the consultation, you are ready to choose the correct products to suit the client's hair and scalp type.

Types of conditioning products

There are many different types of conditioners, but they fall into three main categories:

- surface conditioners
- penetrating and treatment conditioners
- scalp treatments.

Surface conditioners

Most surface conditioners come in cream or mousse form and work on the cuticle of the hair. They smooth and coat the cuticle scales, making the hair look shiny and manageable. They do not have the ability to go past the cuticle region and, therefore, cannot enter the cortex or re-strengthen the hair. Their function is very limited.

Where a surface conditioner is described as **anti-oxy**, it can also be used after chemical services, when its function is threefold:

- it stops the chemicals working any further (prevents creeping oxidation)
- it closes and smooths the cuticle region of the hair shaft, making the hair shiny
- it returns the hair to its natural pH value (4.4–5.5). (Refer to page 13 for more information on the pH scale.)

Types of surface conditioner include:

- hair aid or cream rinse
- herbal anti-oxy
- acid rinses, for example lemon juice or vinegar
- pre-perm services — these are specifically designed to be used before perming to even out the porosity along the cuticle region of the hair, encouraging the perm to take evenly
- conditioning mousses.

Penetrating and treatment conditioners

Penetrating conditioners work on the internal structure of the hair in the cortex because they have the ability to penetrate the cuticle region. Some have the ability to temporarily rebuild the bonds within the cortex, which give the hair its strength and elasticity, and will also smooth and coat the cuticle. If the hair has become dry or chemically damaged, these conditioners will add moisture to help improve the overall look and feel of the hair.

There are two types of penetrating conditioners:

- restructurant or protein conditioners – these will always state 'restructurant' on the packaging
- moisturising conditioners, for example henna wax or olive oil – these are used to add moisture to dry hair and help scalp problems.

Restructurant conditioning treatments help to rebuild the cortex region of the hair shaft, which gives hair its internal strength. This service is frequently carried out in salons for any of the following reasons:

- as a course of services to improve the hair's condition
- to prepare the hair and achieve optimum condition before chemical processing
- to improve hair shine and manageability
- to restore moisture and elasticity which can be lost during chemical processes such as perming, colouring, relaxing and bleaching.

If the hair is badly damaged, you may need to recommend a course of penetrating conditioners, usually between six and twelve, over a period of weeks. As the course progresses, you can analyse their effectiveness and decide if you have chosen the most appropriate conditioner in the available range.

Scalp treatments

Scalp treatment conditioners are usually two- or three-stage treatments involving a shampoo, conditioner and scalp treatment from a particular product range. They should be used together to provide the best possible conditioning results. Some scalp services claim to help regulate the production of sebum from the sebaceous glands, helping with excessive grease problems by slowing down the oil produced. They also claim to be successful when treating excessively dry scalp problems by helping to increase the production of oil from the sebaceous glands. You need to be familiar with the scalp service products in order to choose the correct product to treat your client's scalp condition.

Dry scalps can also benefit from moisturising services such as hot oil treatments. Try to think of the skin on the scalp like the skin on your hands: if your hands were dry, you would use a moisturising cream; if your scalp is dry, it also needs moisture adding to it.

Regular moisturising conditioning services will benefit a dry scalp and help to alleviate (relieve) dandruff and some milder forms of psoriasis.

187

Unit
GH8

Shampoo, condition and treat the hair and scalp

Smooths and coats cuticle scales and also penetrates the cortex to temporarily rebuild bands, helping improve hair strength and elasticity

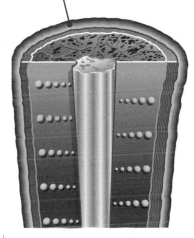

Action of penetrating conditioners on the hair shaft

Unit
GH8

Shampoo, condition and treat the hair and scalp

Massage techniques for conditioning

There are two main massage techniques used for conditioning hair. They are:

- effleurage
- petrissage.

Effleurage

This is a smoothing, stroking movement, which starts and finishes the massage routine. It uses the complete palms of the hands to apply adequate pressure evenly across the whole head.

Start at the centre front hairline and slowly work over the crown area towards the nape. Cover the whole head several times to ensure the client is used to your hands and the product is evenly distributed. It is important not to break contact with the scalp once the massage has started, so always keep one hand in contact with the client's scalp at all times. This is to ensure your client relaxes while you take the weight of his or her head in your hands – if you break contact with the head, the client may jolt her head back, which isn't pleasant or relaxing.

Petrissage

Petrissage is a deeper kneading movement which stimulates the scalp. If carried out correctly, it stimulates:

- the sebaceous glands to secrete sebum (the hair's natural moisture)
- the blood supply, which will improve the healthy growth of the hair (it will not make hair grow faster, just promote better condition).

It also loosens a tight scalp by removing tension from the muscles, improves muscle tone and ultimately relaxes the client, thereby promoting a feeling of well-being.

When carrying out petrissage, you must use the pads of your fingers and keep your elbows out at a 90-degree angle from your body in order to produce an even amount of pressure over the whole head. Use a very slow, circular movement to pick up and knead the scalp (if the client's scalp is moving, you are doing this correctly). Start at the front hairline, knead towards the crown area and then gradually work towards the nape area. Continue massaging from the nape around the side hairlines to the temple areas and then through the centre spaces, over the **occipital bone**. Make sure the whole head is covered and repeat very slowly.

Occipital bone

The bone at the lower back of the head (base) which has a prominent area (usually sticks out a little in most people).

Top tips

You should check with the client that the pressure you are using is comfortable.

Effleurage

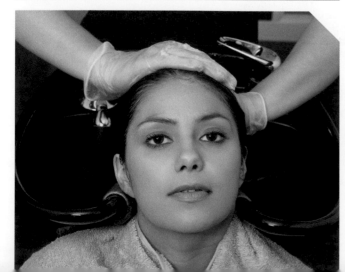

Petrissage

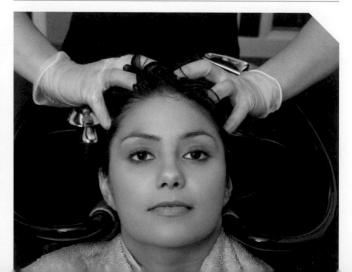
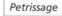

Do not massage the scalp if:

- the client feels unwell, has a temperature or is feeling tender-headed, as massaging could become uncomfortable
- the hair is greasy, as massaging will only stimulate more sebum and make the problem worse
- there are any cuts or abrasions on the scalp
- there are any contraindications such as head lice or ringworm.

Conditioning procedures

Surface conditioners

These are applied at the basin after excess moisture is removed following shampooing. They should be applied using effleurage movements and worked through the hair thoroughly using petrissage movements, and then combed through using a wide-toothed comb to make the best use of the conditioner. It is not necessary to leave the conditioner on the hair for a specified length of time, as its results are almost immediate. However, always read the manufacturer's instructions before using the product.

Comb through surface conditioner for best effect

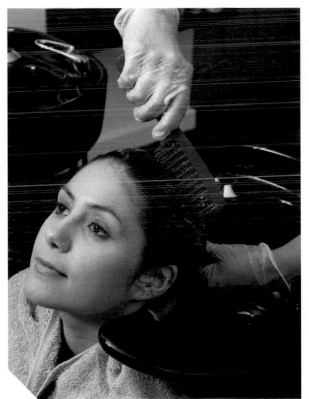

Apply conditioner cost-effectively following manufacturer's instructions

↓

Start massage using effleurage technique

↓

Continue massage using petrissage movements

↓

Complete massage with some effleurage movements

↓

Rinse thoroughly to leave hair clean and free of products

↓

Note: if using an oil conditioner, apply neat shampoo and massage before applying water

↓

Remove excess moisture from the hair

↓

Apply a towel securely to avoid drips

↓

Record products used, length of massage and results of conditioning service on the client's record for future reference

The conditioning process

189

Unit

GH8

Shampoo, condition and treat the hair and scalp

Penetrating and scalp treatment conditioners

These are usually applied using a bowl and brush method. This is a more cost-effective way of applying expensive products as you only dispense a small amount of product at a time and it ensures all the hair is adequately covered.

The client is protected with a gown, towel and plastic cape secured with a section clip (not too high under the chin). The hair is shampooed and towel-dried and the client seated at a workstation. The hair is then sectioned into four equal sections and each section secured with a sectioning clip. On your trolley you will have prepared a tint bowl with a small amount of penetrating/treatment conditioner and a tint brush. Only dispense small amounts of conditioning product, as any excess cannot be put back into the original container because of the risk of cross-contamination (your brush will have touched the client's scalp and the conditioner in the bowl).

Remove a sectioning clip and apply the conditioner to a small sub-section of hair approximately 1.25 cm wide at the top of the section. Place the completed section away from the client's face and take a new section directly underneath. Continue this procedure until all the hair has been covered. You may only wish to apply to the ends of the hair or the roots, depending on the condition of the hair and scalp and the problem you are treating. When all the necessary hair has been covered, start the scalp massage routine using effleurage and petrissage as described previously.

When the scalp massage is complete, you may decide to use heat to aid the penetration of the conditioner. Heat swells the hair and raises the cuticle scales so the penetrating/conditioning/treatment product penetrates into the cortex region more thoroughly. Moist heat is preferable as it is kinder to the hair.

Some scalp services come in tonic form and are applied to towel-dried hair directly after shampooing and conditioning. As they are the consistency of water, you must ensure your client keeps her head tipped as far back as possible to prevent the tonic entering the eyes, as this would be extremely painful. Check the manufacturer's instructions before applying. Once the scalp tonic has been applied to the whole scalp you are ready to continue drying the hair. Do not rinse out.

Types of heat used during conditioning

Steamer

A steamer produces moist heat through the evaporation of distilled water (note that tap water, especially from a hard water area, can produce a build-up of limescale). Safety checks, such as checking the water level is sufficient and checking the plug for frayed wires, must be carried out before using the steamer.

Always dry your hands before plugging the steamer in to avoid electric shocks and ensure the health and safety of yourself and the client.

A steamer takes a few minutes to warm up, so it is best to switch it on before you start to apply the conditioner.

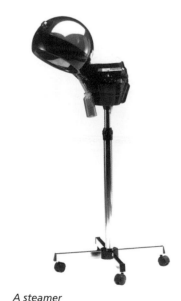

A steamer

Hot towels

This is an alternative way to apply moist heat. It is especially useful if you do not have a steamer. You need at least three towels to carry out this procedure.

Step-by-step hot towel procedure

Fold the towel lengthways in half and then lengthways again. Thoroughly wet the towel with hot water at the basin. Carefully wring out the towel as much as possible (it should not be dripping with water).

Check the temperature of the towel on your wrist before applying it to your client's hair. As you apply the towel, ask the client if the temperature is satisfactory and, if so, wrap the towel on top of the hair (the same as for shampooing).

Leave the towel on the hair for approximately two minutes or until the towel has cooled (having a cold, wet towel on your head is not pleasant, so remove it as soon as this happens). Remove the cold towel and repeat the procedure with the remaining towels.

Hood dryers and accelerators

These produce dry heat, which is not always suitable to use during a conditioning treatment. If you are treating the hair because it is dry and damaged, never apply dry heat if it is not necessary. However, the manufacturer's instructions may state this is necessary to aid the penetration of the product

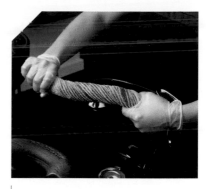

Remember that the towel must be wrung out as much as possible

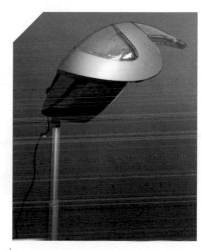

A hood dryer

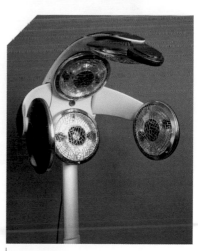

An accelerator

191

Unit

GH8

Shampoo, condition and treat the hair and scalp

Step-by-step hot oil service

This service is carried out to moisturise severely dry scalps/hair. It is best to use good-quality olive oil, as this is the most refined and purest oil with the most moisturising properties.

1 Protect your client with a gown, towel and plastic cape, then divide the hair into four equal sections and secure with sectioning clips.

Heat the oil by pouring it into a small plastic bowl, then place in a larger bowl filled with hot water.

2 Do not shampoo the hair – this procedure is carried out on dry hair. Roll a small length of cotton wool into a circular pad and test the temperature of the oil. Check the temperature with your client and apply the warm oil to the scalp/hair using the cotton wool pad (this is better than a tint brush as it makes the application of the oil less messy).

Place the completed section away from the client's face and take a new section directly underneath. Continue this procedure until all the hair has been covered.

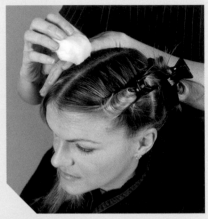

3 Start the scalp massage routine using effleurage movements.

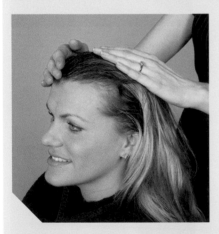

4 Continue massage routine using petrissage movements.

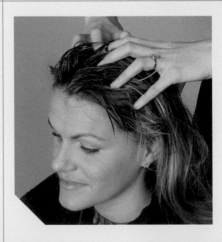

5 When the scalp massage is complete, you may decide to use heat to aid the penetration of the hot oil. The best moist heat to use for this service is the application of a few hot towels (see page 191).

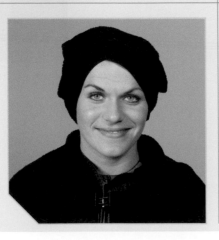

6 Apply neat shampoo and massage using rotary movements to emulsify the oil thoroughly (until the shampoo turns white) before adding any water to the hair. Repeat shampooing process.

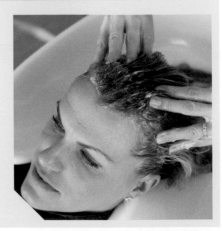

Personal, learning and thinking skills – Reflective learning

Shampooing and conditioning are essential to most hairdressing services carried out in the salon. As you have already learned, contact dermatitis is an occupational hazard for hairdressers. Therefore, it is important to understand this skin condition and how you can avoid it. Try to remember what you have already learned about contact dermatitis, and write down whether it is a viral, bacterial, fungal or non-contagious skin condition. Next, write some brief notes for yourself about how you can protect your skin from contracting dermatitis whilst carrying out shampooing and conditioning.

How to provide aftercare advice

It is important to give your client accurate aftercare advice in a constructive way. You will need to give advice on how to maintain the condition of the hair and scalp by recommending the most suitable shampooing and conditioning products to suit the client's individual needs. If you do not provide this service to your client, she may use incorrect products and techniques when managing the hair and all your hard work will be undone. You must have good knowledge of your salon's retail product range in order to recommend the correct products to suit your client's hair and scalp type. If you recommend incorrect products you could create problems for your client's hair and scalp.

Task 4

List each conditioner in your salon and make a note of:

* the hair/scalp type it should be used for
* the manufacturer's instructions for when and how to use it.

A worksheet for this task is provided on the website for you to complete and add to your portfolio.

193

Unit
GH8

Shampoo, condition and treat the hair and scalp

Salon life

Oil and water do not mix

Amie's story

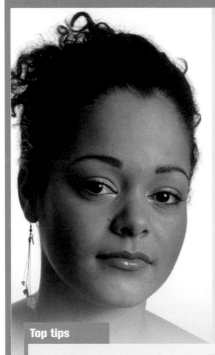

I decided to do a hot oil service to moisturise my client's dry scalp. It was the first time I'd ever done it and I had clear instructions on what to do. I heated the olive oil to the correct temperature and applied as directed. The client fell asleep during the massage and when I had finished massaging she said she had thoroughly enjoyed it.

After a few hot towels to help the oil penetrate the scalp, I took the client back to the basin to shampoo. I wet the hair and shampooed as normal. It took a while to remove the oil and then I returned my client to my workstation and started blow-drying. Halfway through the blow-dry I realised the hair was looking greasy. I stopped and asked my salon manager for advice. She told me I should have used neat shampoo first to emulsify and help remove the oil before I added water, as water and oil do not mix! I had to apologise to my client and take her back to the basin to start all over again!

My client was understanding, but it did make her late for another appointment which I felt really bad about. I certainly learned my lesson and have never made the same mistake again.

Top tips

- Try having your hair shampooed by a new and inexperienced colleague to see what your client experiences.
- Time yourself when shampooing and conditioning – a competent shampoo and surface conditioner should take no longer than 5 minutes.
- Always read your manufacturer's instructions – not all products are the same.
- Always give clear and accurate aftercare advice to enable your client to care for her hair at home. This will help promote healthy hair and scalp for your client and prolong the life of the services carried out in the salon.

Ask the expert

Q   *How will I know what shampoo and conditioner to choose for my client?*

A   You should begin your consultation by analysing and assessing the hair and scalp's condition. You also need to discuss any problems your client may be having with her hair and scalp as well as giving advice and suggestions. Once you have established these factors and discussed the service your client requires, you can then choose the appropriate shampoo and conditioner from your salon's range of products. It is important to have a good understanding of your salon's range so you have the knowledge to make the correct choices. If you are still unsure of the products to choose, ask for advice from a more experienced colleague.

Goldwell

Your questions answered

Question	Answer
Should I condition the hair before perming?	Not with a normal surface or penetrating conditioner on the same day as the perm. The hair could be given a conditioning treatment to improve the condition of the hair a few days before the perm. If necessary, a pre-perm treatment may be used immediately prior to perming, which would not interfere with the chemical action of the perming process.
Do restructurant conditioners improve the hair's condition?	Yes, they have an effect on the strength of the cortex – but only temporarily.
Can you really stimulate the blood flow, sebaceous glands and nerve endings during conditioning?	Yes, if your petrissage massage movements are deep, they will stimulate these areas within the dermis of the scalp.
Are expensive shampoos and conditioners worth the money?	Expensive shampoos and conditioners often have the same basic ingredients as 'cheaper' products, but some are more costly due to extensive research and costly ingredients such as aromatherapy oils. The only way to decide if they are worth the money is to try them, assess their results and come to your own conclusions.

The science of shampooing

Shampoo is applied to hair and emulsified. The hydrophobic (water-hating) tail of the shampoo molecule is drawn away from the water and attaches to sebum and hair products on the hair, whilst the hydrophilic (water-loving) head is attracted to the water. This 'push and pull' effect works to lift the sebum and product from the hair into the shampoo lather, which is then removed by rinsing the hair.

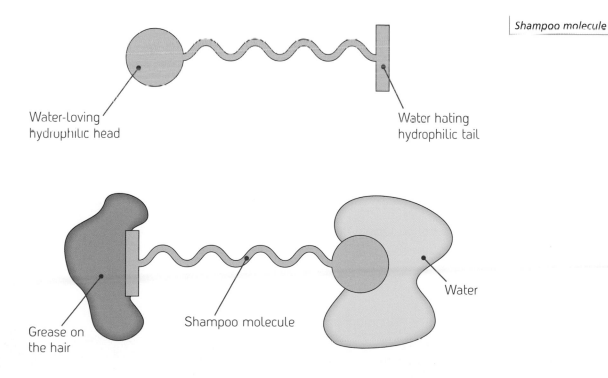

Shampoo molecule

Water-loving
hydrophilic head

Water hating
hydrophilic tail

Grease on
the hair

Shampoo molecule

Water

195

Unit

GH8

Shampoo, condition and treat the hair and scalp

Check your knowledge

The following questions will help you to check your understanding of this unit.
The answers can be found on pages 496–97.

1 Why are we recommended to wear gloves for shampooing?
   a) To allow large rings to be worn underneath gloves
   b) To avoid the risk of dermatitis
   c) To avoid chipping your nail polish

2 Which health and safety legislation covers the use of electrical equipment?

_____

3 Why is it important to carry out a thorough consultation before shampooing?

_____

4 Which health and safety legislation deals with the handling, storage and disposal of hairdressing products?

_____

5 Why is it important to have a good knowledge of the shampooing and conditioning products used in your salon?

_____

6 Which shampoo would you use before a perm in your salon?

_____

7 What effect does a surface conditioner have on the hair?

_____

8 What effect does a penetrating conditioner have on the hair?

_____

9 Which do you apply first to remove a hot oil service from the hair?
   a) Water
   b) Neat shampoo
   c) Water and shampoo

10 What types of heat are ideally used during conditioning treatments?
   a) Moist heat from hot towels or a steamer
   b) Dry heat from hairdryers and heat processors
   c) An electric current

Getting ready for assessment

You will be assessed using a combination of assessment methods, as described below. Remember that within each of the services you carry out with a client, you will cover different units. For example, when carrying out a shampooing and conditioning service (GH8), you will also have to be aware of health and safety (G20) and advise and consult with clients (G7). If you are not sure what you have covered in your service, always ask your assessor or supervisor for advice.

	NVQ	VRQ
Credit value	4	3
Guided Learning Hours	36	29

	NVQ	VRQ
Practical demonstrations, to be observed by assessor	You will be observed on at least three occasions. Within the practical element of this unit you must show that you have met the standard expected for shampooing, conditioning and treating the hair and scalp. All the practical assessments for this unit must be from work carried out with clients in the salon.	You will be observed on at least three occasions. Within the practical element of this unit you must show that you have met the standard expected for shampooing, conditioning and treating the hair and scalp. Evidence for this unit must be gathered in a real or realistic working environment. Simulation is allowed, but at least 75 per cent of 'Observation' outcomes must be on real clients.
Service timings	Shampoo, condition/treatment on hair above shoulders (excluding development time) – 10 minutes maximum Shampoo, condition/treatment on hair below shoulders (excluding development time) – 15 minutes maximum	Shampoo, condition/treatment on hair above shoulders (excluding development time) – 10 minutes maximum Shampoo, condition/treatment on hair below shoulders (excluding development time) – 15 minutes maximum
Additional evidence	There is a mandatory written paper for this unit. If you do not demonstrate all of the required knowledge in this paper, you will then be orally questioned or asked to complete a written assignment	There is one external paper for this unit. Criteria not achieved will be identified to your tutor/assessor. You will then be orally questioned or asked to produce other forms of evidence as all unit criteria must be achieved.

197

Unit
GH8

Shampoo, condition and treat the hair and scalp

Task mapping

When you have completed the tasks in this unit, check the table below to see which Performance Criteria (purple), Range (red), Knowledge (green) and Key Skills (blue) you have covered within GH8 to use as additional evidence within your portfolio. Information about which Functional Skills you have covered is available on the website.

Task and page reference	Mapping to Performance Criteria, Range, Knowledge and Key Skills
1 (page 179)	Performance Criteria: 1f, 1g, 1h, VRQ 2f Range: VRQ R5a Knowledge: 16, 17, VRQ 2p Key Skills: C1.2, C1.3, C2.3
2 (page 182)	Performance Criteria: Practising 2a, VRQ 1b, 2b, 2f Range: Practising 2a–e, VRQ R1a–e, R2a–e, R6a–e, R8b–c Knowledge: 36, 37, 38, 39, VRQ 1e, 2h, 2p, 2q Key Skills: C1.2, C1.3, C2.3
3 (page 184)	Performance Criteria: Practising 1g, 1h, 4a, 4b, VRQ 1b, 2b, 2c, 2f, 2g Range: 2c, 5a, VRQ R5a, R8c Knowledge: 16, 50, 51, 52, VRQ 1e, 2h, 2p, 2q Key Skills: C1.2, C1.3, C2.3
4 (page 193)	Performance Criteria: Practising 3c, VRQ 2b, 2g Range: Practising 2a–e, 6a–c, VRQ R1a–e, R2a–e, R6a–c, R8b–c Knowledge: 36, 37, 38, 39, VRQ 1f, 1g, 2h, 2i, 2j Key Skills: N/A

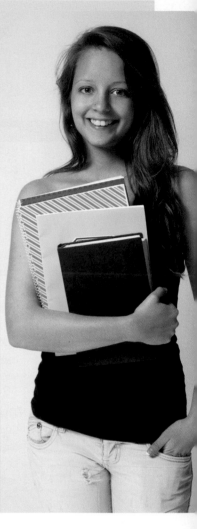

Change hair colour

Unit GH9

Goldwell

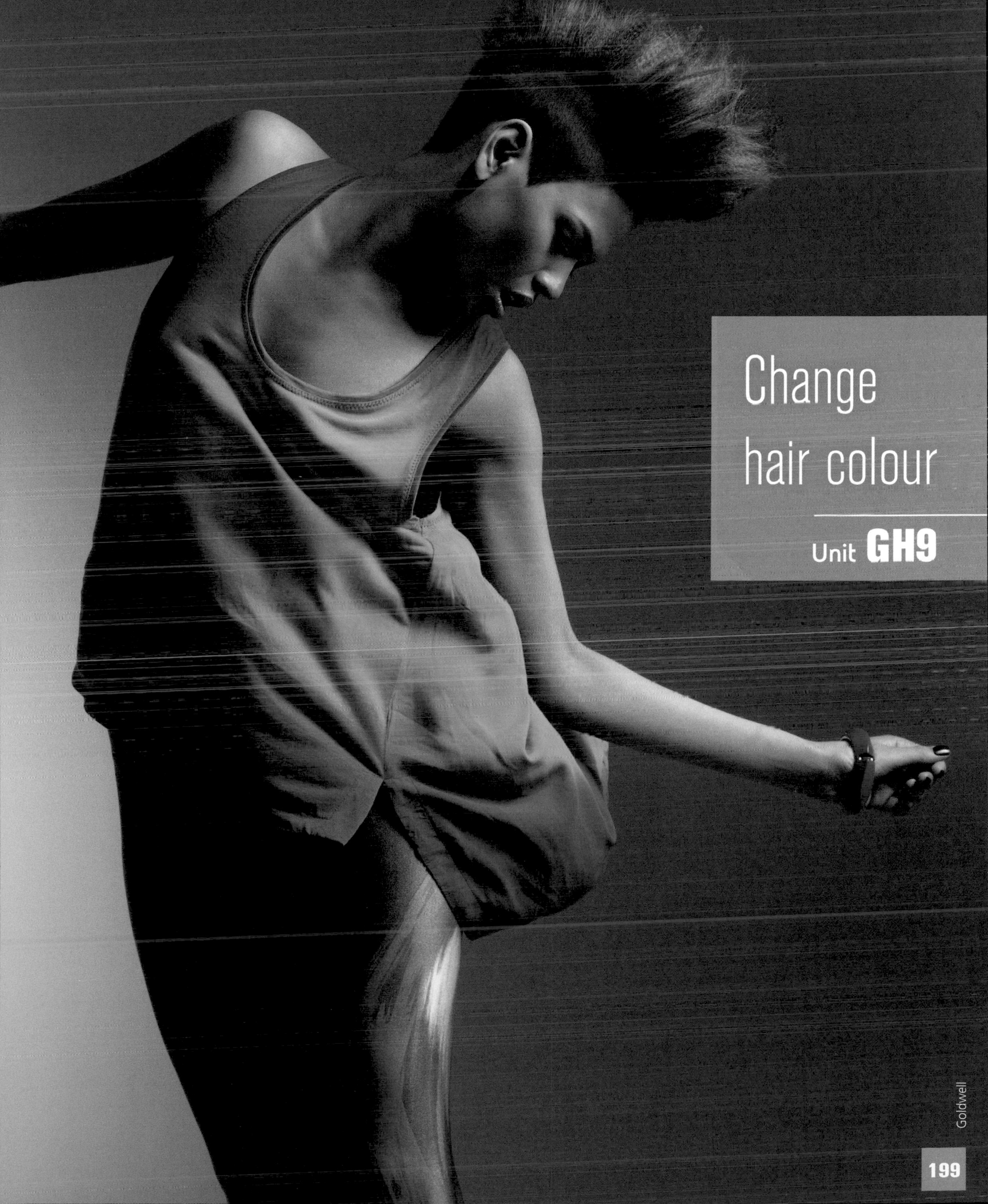

What you will learn:

- **How to maintain effective and safe methods of working when colouring and lightening hair**
- **How to prepare for colouring and lightening hair**
- **How to colour and lighten hair**
- **How to provide aftercare advice**

Introduction

Colouring can be one of the most challenging processes in hairdressing, but also one of the most rewarding and exciting. Colour aids the appearance of texture, depth and movement of the hair. There are many different levels and techniques involved in colouring, from temporary colours which will only stain the hair, to permanent colours that can be applied with foils, mesh or even combed through the hair. This unit describes the procedures and introduces the basic principles of colouring.

This is a technical unit all about changing the hair colour using a variety of colouring methods: temporary, semi-permanent, quasi-permanent, permanent and lightening. You will be required to carry out highlighting and lowlighting techniques, regrowth and full head colouring effects.

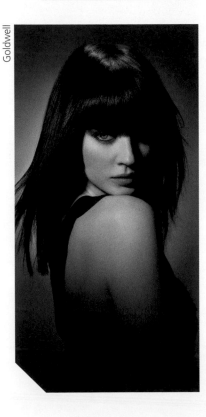

Goldwell

How to maintain effective and safe methods of working

It is important to make sure that you work in a safe manner and in a safe environment when working with colour, as you are using chemicals. You need to make sure you follow manufacturers' instructions and use the correct personal protective equipment (PPE) for both yourself and your client. You need to be aware of COSHH and risk assessment policies to ensure your working practices adhere to health and safety regulations.

Preparing the client for temporary, semi, quasi and permanent colouring services

Gowning

You should always make sure that the client is protected for any hairdressing service, but this is especially important when carrying out a colouring process. If the client is not correctly gowned, colour could fall onto the clothing and you could be held responsible for the damaged item. This is the correct gowning procedure.

- Use a chemical gown (if one is available).
- Place a plastic disposable cape around the client.
- Place a colouring towel over the top of the cape and secure. (In some training establishments/salons, a colouring towel may also be placed underneath the disposable cape for double protection.)

Using barrier cream

Barrier cream is used to prevent any tint sitting on the client's face, as dark tints will stain the skin. Some clients have very sensitive skin, which can become inflamed if a barrier cream is not used.

Top tips

Using a barrier cream that doesn't contain any perfumes will ensure your client does not have an allergic reaction to the product.

Apply the barrier cream, either with your finger or using a cotton wool bud. Make sure that the cream is evenly and thickly applied as close to the hairline as you can get without depositing any on the hair itself.

Remove the barrier cream before you shampoo the tint from the hair and before you begin the cut or blow-dry. Make sure all traces are removed, as the cream can be very greasy.

Protecting yourself

You also have a duty to ensure your own health and safety within the salon. When preparing to carry out a colouring service, your PPE should consist of:

- an apron – to protect your clothes
- gloves – to protect your hands from chemicals and staining
- sensible shoes – flat, non-slip shoes to prevent any injuries to legs and ankles.

It is important that you wear the correct PPE when colouring hair, not only to protect your clothes but also to portray a professional image to the client.

Positioning

Ensure that the client is sitting in an upright position, enabling you to work freely around the head.

You may need to adjust the position of your client while working so that you can reach the more difficult areas of the head when colouring, for example the top of the head. Do not be afraid to ask your client to tilt her head backwards or forwards so that you can apply the colour easily. Place your tools and equipment within easy reach.

You also need to consider your own posture and position when you are working at your unit. (Read back through G20 to remind yourself of this.)

Ensuring health and safety

Protecting the client

Imagine the following situation: a client comes into the salon for a regrowth colour. You get out her record card only to discover that the last time she had a colour service in the salon was over a year ago. Your first responsibility is to ensure the health and safety of the client so, for her own well-being, you have to refuse the service until you have completed a current skin test.

Applying the products

You will always need to take great care when using colouring products. Some are quite runny while others are thicker, but all require your full attention. Make sure you are aware of all health and safety rules that your salon and the manufacturers put in place when you apply these products.

Work area checks

- Put away or dispose of unwanted equipment before you receive your next client, following the COSHH regulations (see pages 56–7) if you need to.
- Check and, if necessary, mop up spillages of water or products on the floor.
- Sweep up any hair cuttings from the floor.
- Have ready the client's record card together with the appropriate equipment.
- Ensure your working area is clean and tidy to receive the next client.

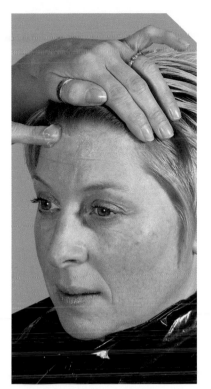

Applying barrier cream before a service

201

Unit
GH9

Change hair colour

Fact or fiction?

Is this statement fact or fiction?

PPE (personal protective equipment) only refers to towels and gowns used on the client.

To check your answer see page 497.

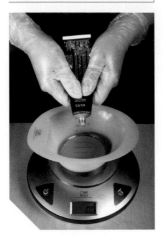

Measuring tint using scales

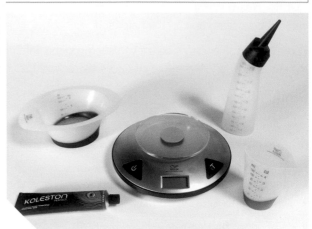

A variety of measuring equipment for colouring

Mixing colours

This should not be done by guesswork. Always prepare the colour as set out in the manufacturer's instructions. Quantities must be measured accurately – the wrong quantities may produce unwanted colour effects. It is essential to read the manufacturer's instructions to ensure that you use the product correctly. There are a variety of procedures and each is particular to the product. You will need to prepare the tint immediately before use. Do not allow it to stand for any length of time or it will lose its effectiveness.

If you are using more than one colour, mix tints together in a bowl before adding **hydrogen peroxide**. Tint tubes have measurements marked on them to ensure that the correct amount of tint can be added.

When you are working with colouring products, you may find that it is better to mix up less colour than you think you will need. You can always mix up more colour later. For example, if you are working on long hair, perhaps putting two colours through using a foil technique, the service may take you slightly longer. While your product is in the bowl it is losing its strength and you may find this could produce a different colour result. In this instance, it is advisable to mix up a small amount of product then mix up more as it is required.

Your salon will have legal requirements in place for the disposal of waste materials. Most salons will require you to dilute the product down the sink with water that is not used for any domestic services.

By law, all salons need to have risk assessment sheets on all products that are used within the salon. On these you will find all the relevant information on how to handle, store and dispose of products safely. Most salons will have these sheets located in a folder all together in an accessible location.

Hydrogen peroxide

A bleaching and oxidising ingredient, used to activate quasi-permanent, permanent and lightening products.

Top tips

When you measure out hydrogen peroxide, read the amount at eye level to be sure of an accurate measurement.

Task 1

In your salon, find out how you are expected to dispose of any waste materials left over from colouring.

Where does your salon keep its risk assessment folder?

Minimise the risk of cross-infection

As with all hairdressing services, you need to be aware of the possibility of cross-infection and infestation when you are working. To prevent the risk of either of these you will need to complete a thorough consultation to make sure that you are able to begin the service. (Refer to pages 144–48 for more information on cross-infections and infestations.)

All tools and equipment should be cleaned and sterilised regularly. Washing in warm soapy water to remove old products can clean most of the equipment used for colouring. If you discover that your client has an infection or infestation when you are halfway through the application, you will be required to complete the service. In this instance, you will need to sterilise your equipment to prevent the risk of cross-infection.

Minimising harm or injury to yourself or others

When carrying out a colouring process, you may need to use extra equipment. It is your responsibility to make sure that the equipment is in good working order.

Safety considerations

- Check that plugs and cables are in good condition.
- Do not use electrical equipment with wet hands.
- Check temperature controls before you turn on equipment.
- Check the client is comfortable while you are using the equipment.
- Always allow equipment to cool before storing.

Products

When working with chemicals, follow all of the health and safety guidelines set down by the manufacturers and your salon or training institution. Here are some guidelines.

- Complete a skin test on the client before carrying out any colouring process (apart from temporary colours).
- Mix only the amount of product that you think you are going to need – mixing too much is wasteful and uneconomic.
- Mix the product immediately before use – tint starts to **oxidise** (develop) as soon as it makes contact with the atmosphere.
- Place lids back on products as soon as you have measured out the amount that you require.
- Use the correct PPE.
- Store chemicals correctly when they are not being used – refer to manufacturers' COSHH sheets for information on the handling, storage and disposal of products, the harm they could cause and how to treat in case of an accident (see G20).

Oxidise

A chemical process that involves combining a substance with oxygen.

Using your time effectively

Each salon allows a set amount of time for the different services that it offers. Time allocation for colouring services differs depending on the method of application and the products used. For example, applying a semi-permanent colour does not take as long as applying a full head bleach.

Task 2

Find out the time allocation for the following colouring services in your salon:

- full head temporary colour
- full head semi-permanent colour
- full head quasi-permanent colour
- regrowth application permanent colour
- full head permanent colour
- highlights/lowlights with cap
- woven highlights/lowlights with mesh or foils
- partial head colour (T-zone).

A worksheet for this task is provided on the website for you to complete and add to your portfolio.

Carrying out a consultation

By completing a colouring consultation form, you will be able to answer all the following questions, allowing you to make the right choices and decisions for the colouring process.

- Identify and discuss your client's wishes.
- Is the process possible? Are there any critical influencing factors that may prevent the process, such as previous chemical services or the condition of the hair?
- Can you achieve the target colour the client wants? Is the client's natural base shade too light or dark to achieve the target colour? How much white is present in the hair?
- Decide on the products you will be using. How long does the client want the colour to last?
- What will your method of application be? Is it a regrowth colour or full head colour?

Style books and colour shade chart

During the consultation, you will find it helpful to use visual aids. A selection of style books will enable you to show the client different colouring techniques.

A colour shade chart plays a major role in your consultation. It will help your client to decide what target colour she would like and it will enable you to match up to the client's natural (base) colour. The chart will also help you to explain what can and cannot be achieved.

Most colour shade charts contain information and instructions on how to determine your colour choice, mix, application and development of the colour.

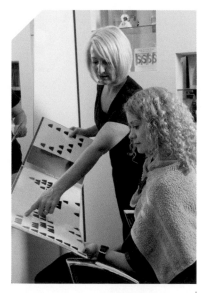

Can you achieve the colour the client wants?

Task 3

Working in pairs, complete a consultation for each other. You will need a shade chart to help determine the base you are working from and the target colour you wish to achieve.

A colouring consultation form is provided on the website for you to complete and add to your portfolio.

Choosing suitable products and equipment

When you begin a colouring service you need to take into account the type of product you will be using, as this affects how you prepare the hair for the application of the colour.

Molecule

At least two atoms in a definite arrangement held together by very strong chemical bonds.

Product type	Suitability	Effect
Coloured mousse, coloured setting lotions, hair mascara	Most hair types, but not heavily bleached or porous hair.	Deposits large **molecules** on the cuticle. Only lasts until the next shampoo. Does not lift the hair colour; it can only deposit depth and tone.
Semi-permanent	Covers up to 30 per cent white hair. Often used as a colour refresher for faded ends on fragile hair, and is a good introduction to colour as it is not mixed with any developer or peroxide.	Lasts 4–8 shampoos (depending on the brand). Does not lift the hair colour; it can only deposit depth and tone.
Quasi permanent	Most hair types. Covers a high percentage of white hair. Can produce regrowth (a band of natural hair colour at the roots, which appears when the hair grows).	Lasts 8–12 shampoos (depending on the brand). Generally does not lift hair colour and only deposits depth and tone.
Permanent	Most hair types. Covers 100 per cent white hair. Only achieves 3 levels of lift.	Grows out. Can lighten or darken the hair.
Bleach	Not suitable for over-processed, dry or damaged hair. Can be used to achieve 7 shades of lift. Suitable for dark bases when a high lift tint will not achieve the required result.	Lifts colour to lighten the hair. Grows out.
High lift tint	Suitable for a base 6 (dark blonde) and above. Not recommended on very dry or damaged hair.	Lifts colour and lightens the hair, will add tone. Grows out. Less harsh than bleach.

205

Unit
GH9

Change hair colour

Mixing and measuring

Not all colours are mixed in the same way. Different manufacturers have different mixing and measuring procedures that apply to their own specific products. Just because one permanent colour that you have used is mixed in a certain way, do not assume that all colours are the same.

- Mousses and semi-permanent colours do not require mixing; they are used straight from the container.
- Quasi-permanent colours are mixed with their own activators or developers. These usually contain only a very weak amount of hydrogen peroxide, but the same care must be used when applying them as you would use for permanent colours.
- Permanent colours are mixed with 20, 30 or 40 volume peroxide (6 per cent, 9 per cent or 12 per cent), depending on the target colour you wish to achieve.

When measuring out hydrogen peroxide and tint, make sure that you are accurate – do not guess. Read the amount in a measuring flask at eye level for accurate measurement. It is best to put the measuring flask on a flat surface, as holding it may result in an inaccurate measurement.

When mixing a quarter or a half of a tube of tint, note where the marks are on the side of the tube and only squeeze out the tint to these guidelines. Always squeeze the tube from the end as you would with toothpaste at home.

If you are using more than one colour, first mix the two tints together in a bowl before adding the hydrogen peroxide. This will ensure thorough mixing of the tints.

Prepare the tint immediately before use. Do not allow the tint to stand for any length of time or it will lose its effectiveness.

Colouring services

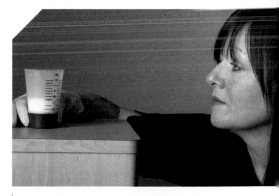

Read the amount in a measuring flask at eye level for accuracy

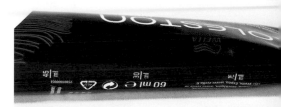

Tint tubes have guide marks to help you measure accurately

Tools and equipment

The type of colouring effect that you want will determine the equipment that you use.

Type	Suitability	Effect
Highlighting/ lowlighting cap	Short- to medium-length hair (if hair is too short, it will produce a spotty effect). Used for the application of one colour.	Strands of hair highlighted or darkened evenly over the head.
Mesh or foil	All hair lengths except very short hair (less than 5 cm). Used for the application of one or more colours.	One or more colours woven or sliced through the hair.
Block colouring	All hair lengths. Care must be taken to mask off the hair so that the colours do not run into each other.	Hair is divided into two or more sections — a solid colour is applied to one half of the head and another colour to the other half, and so on.
Wide-tooth comb	All hair lengths, but especially short hair where other techniques cannot be used.	Produces quite 'chunky' strands of coloured hair depending on the amount of tint applied to the comb.

Fact or fiction?

Is this statement fact or fiction?

You cannot carry out a highlighting/lowlighting service on hair that is below shoulder length.

To check your answer see page 497.

Reporting low levels of stock

The maintenance of adequate stock levels may not be your direct responsibility, but as part of a team it is your responsibility to report any low or missing stock items and to make sure you are prepared for the services you are giving.

In most salons and colleges/training institutions, you would report low stock levels to the person directly in charge of you. This could be your salon manager or tutor. If that person is not available, the best course of action is to leave a memo in whatever communication system you use. You would then have recorded that you identified that stock was low and notified the relevant person.

General allocation of time for colour application

As a trainee, the time allocations listed below are those you should be working towards and not what you are expected to achieve when you first begin.

Colour service	Time allocation
Temporary	These are applied as normal mousses or setting lotions, following manufacturers' instructions.
Semi-permanent	15–30 minutes for consultation, preparation and application. Development time depends on the product you are using. Always read the manufacturer's instructions.
Quasi-permanent	15–30 minutes (as above).
Permanent regrowth	30 minutes for consultation, preparation and application.
Permanent full head	45 minutes for consultation, preparation and first application, then a further 20 minutes to complete the application.
Cap highlights	30 minutes for consultation, pulling through the highlights and applying the product. Development time depends on the required end result and the product you are using.
Mesh/foil highlights/ lowlights	Usually a maximum of one hour (for hair below shoulder length). Fresh tint may have to be mixed halfway through as the product loses its strength after 30–40 minutes.

Keeping accurate and up-to-date client records

It is important to record for future reference all of the services that you carry out on a client. You should include:

- client's name, address and contact telephone number
- date of the client's last skin test
- date of last service
- products used and method of application
- cost of the service
- retail products that were bought (if any) and their cost
- aftercare advice given to the client
- comments by yourself or the client on the end result.

This information will enable you to make adjustments to colouring services, products or techniques according to the client's changing needs, or to maintain a colour if the client is happy with it.

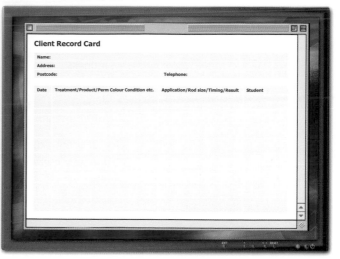

Computerised record card showing a client's colouring details

How to prepare for colouring and lightening hair

In this section you will be looking at the hair and skin tests that you need to carry out before you begin the colouring and lightening process. You will also be looking at the effect of critical influencing factors on the colouring process and the correct preparation of your products.

Carrying out and recording all hair and skin tests

Before carrying out any colouring process that will come into contact with the scalp (with the exception of temporary colours), you must carry out a skin test, sometimes called a patch test or hypersensitivity test. This is to check whether the client is allergic to the para dye (para-phenylenediamine, an artificial colour pigment) that is contained in tints. The test is a safety precaution and must be carried out 24–48 hours prior to a colouring process. However, if the colour is not going to be in direct contact with the skin, a skin test is not always required. Note: you do not need to complete a skin test for a bleaching service, but you must check that the client is not experiencing any discomfort during the process.

Method

1 Clean a small area of skin just behind the ear. Mix together a small amount of dark tint with a few drops of 20 volume hydrogen peroxide (a dark tint is used because it contains more para dye).

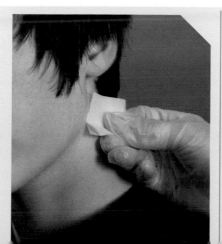

2 Using a brush or cotton wool bud, apply a small amount of tint behind the client's ear and allow to dry.

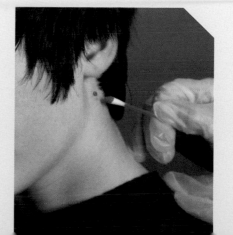

Positive reaction

Advise the client to leave the test for 24–48 hours unless there is any irritation. A positive reaction (the client is allergic to the product) would result in the following symptoms:

- redness
- soreness
- itching
- inflammation/swelling.

If your client experiences any of these reactions, do not proceed with the service. Alternative methods of colouring may be offered in which the tint does not come into contact with the scalp, such as using a cap, mesh or foil. If using foil or mesh, you must be able to confidently use these techniques without allowing colouring product to come into contact with the skin.

Incompatibility test

The purpose of this test is to see whether the client has any metallic salts (residue from metallic dyes) present in her hair. You would carry out this test only if you thought the client had been colouring the hair at home with a product that may contain metallic salts. Metallic salts are contained in hair colour restorers such as Grecian 2000, and may also be found in products that 'gradually cover'. This test should always be carried out if you are going to be using a product that contains hydrogen peroxide.

Method

- Take a small cutting of the client's hair and secure together with tape.
- In a glass bowl or container, mix together a small amount of hydrogen peroxide and alkaline perm lotion.
- Place the hair in the bowl so that the hair is covered with the mixture.
- Observe the mixture.

Positive reaction

This will normally occur within 30 minutes of the hair being placed in the mixture. You would expect to see any of the following:

- the lotion bubbles or fizzes
- the hair may change colour
- the hair may dissolve
- the solution may give off heat.

If any of these reactions occur, you should not proceed with any hairdressing process that involves using hydrogen peroxide.

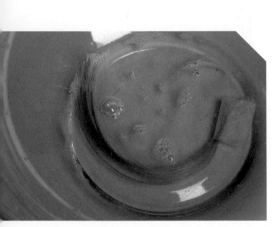

The incompatibility test

Elasticity test

An elasticity test determines the inner condition of the hair. If the elasticity is poor, the internal links and bonds in the cortex have been damaged and the hair may not be able to withstand a chemical service. Hair with poor elasticity will be further damaged by a high volume of hydrogen peroxide, so it is important to do this test to make sure that the hair can withstand the service you will be carrying out. For example, highlighting the hair involves lifting the natural colour. Generally, clients want to see a relatively high degree of lift, which requires a stronger volume of hydrogen peroxide. The elasticity test will help you determine whether it is safe to go ahead.

Porosity test

This test determines the outer condition of the hair. If the hair is very porous or unevenly porous, colour will be absorbed differently across the surface of the hair. The test will help you to work out what strength of hydrogen peroxide and what type of product to use. If the hair is in good condition, you can colour the hair with a stronger peroxide solution (if required). If the hair is over-porous, you may need to rethink your colour choice and use a weaker strength of peroxide. You may also have to adapt your application technique.

The hair's condition will affect the application and development of the colour and will determine whether you should use added heat. If the hair is in poor condition, the colour will penetrate the hair more quickly than hair that is in good condition. It will be 'active' in the cortex for a longer period of time and could cause damage to the hair if left unchecked. Using added heat helps to lift the cuticle scales to allow the colour to penetrate, but is not recommended on porous hair.

Strand test/colour test

The purpose of a strand test is to determine how well the colour is developing during the process.

Method

- Dampen a piece of cotton wool.
- Select a few strands of hair.
- Using the cotton wool, wipe off some of the tint from the hair.
- Hold the hair flat on your hand to see the colour result.

If the colour is not fully developed, leave for the further development time. If the colour is ready, rinse to remove the colour.

Recording the result

After the tests have been completed, it is important that you complete the client's record card in full. Do not leave this until later, as you could easily forget a piece of information that will be important for the client's next colouring service (look back at the record card on page 207).

Choosing products, tools and equipment, taking into account critical influencing factors

When considering your choice of colour, you have to think about any existing colour that is already on the hair, as this will affect your end result.

- If the client has colour on the hair that has faded and just wants the colour 'freshened up', you will need to match up the existing colour with the shade chart to see how much loss of depth or tone there has been from the original target colour. This will allow you to gauge the correct product choice and apply the colour following the manufacturer's instructions.
- If the client wants to tone down an unwanted red or ash tone in the hair, you will need to consult the colour wheel to find the neutralising colour and apply accordingly. You can only do this with a colour that is of the same depth or darker than the colour already on the hair. For example, if the client's hair is a base 6 and looking slightly green, and she does not wish to go any darker, you will have to apply a colour that is also a base 6 with some warm tones to neutralise the unwanted ash tones.

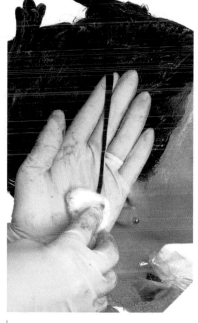

Strand test/colour test

209

Unit
GH9

Change hair colour

Virgin hair is hair that has not had any chemical service on it. You have a wide choice of colours on the shade chart although you must remember that you **cannot** lighten the hair when using temporary, semi- or quasi-permanent colours. You will be able to darken the hair or keep it on the same base and just change the tone.

The percentage of white hair that is present will also have an effect on your colour choice. When referring to the percentage of white present in the hair, we are talking about the head of hair as a whole:

- if a client's hair is completely white, it is referred to as being 100 per cent white
- if three-quarters of the hair is white, it is described as 75 per cent white
- if half of the hair is white, it is 50 per cent white
- if only a quarter of the hair is white, it is 25 per cent white.

Of course, clients will present other amounts of white in their hair. It is up to you to determine the percentage that you think is white.

Permanent base colours (International colour chart 1–10) will cover 100 per cent white hair. Fashion colours, which are all the colours that have the primary and secondary tones in them, will only cover a certain percentage of white hair if used on their own. (However, as technology is advancing, some manufacturers are now producing fashion colours that can cover 100 per cent white hair.)

If a client had 75 per cent white present in her hair and you put a bright red fashion colour on the hair, what do you think would happen? It would probably turn pink! Since all colours can be intermixed, you would still be able to colour this client's hair but you would need to introduce some base colour into the fashion colour. The base colour acts as an 'undercoat' to cover the white/grey hair. The fashion shade then acts as a 'topcoat', revealing the target shade the client wanted to see.

For example, if the client chose 7.44 as the target colour and had 50 per cent white hair, you would need to use equal quantities of base 7 with the target colour (7.44). If you did not apply the undercoat (base 7), you would be putting a very rich copper red onto white hair and it would produce a pink hue.

25% white requires $\frac{1}{4}$ tube base colour + $\frac{3}{4}$ tube fashion shade

50% white requires $\frac{1}{2}$ tube base colour + $\frac{1}{2}$ tube fashion colour

75% white requires $\frac{3}{4}$ tube base colour + $\frac{1}{4}$ tube fashion colour

This is a very simple method of deciding how much base to use and you must always check manufacturers' instructions for more detail.

Colouring porous hair

The porosity of the hair will influence the way in which you apply the colour. If the hair is porous, this may mean that the cuticle scales are damaged due to previous chemical services or environmental factors. The hair will absorb the colour unevenly and the colour result could end up uneven and patchy. Extra care needs to be taken when applying colour to porous hair.

When choosing the target colour, you will also need to take into account the following critical influencing factors:

- temperature
- existing colour of hair
- percentage of white hair test results
- hydrogen peroxide percentage by volume
- porosity of hair.

Top tips

When using added heat, always check manufacturers' instructions for development times, and check for hot or cold spots that could lead to patchy results.

Temperature

You can assist the development of the colour by adding heat. You can use:

- a climazone/accelerator – dry heat speeds up the development of permanent colours
- a steamer – moist heat is generally used for lightening products, for example bleaches, as this will stop the product from drying out.

Preparing the client and products prior to colouring and lightening

Test results

Before permanent colouring you will need to carry out:

- a skin test to determine whether the process can be carried out
- an incompatibility test (if you suspect metallic salts are present on the hair)
- porosity and elasticity tests to determine the condition of the hair.

Other preparation activities that you need to carry out before you begin the colouring service include:

- making sure that you are organised to receive the client, with client record card and colour shade chart ready
- the correct gowning procedure for the client, to protect the client's clothing
- ensuring that you have the correct PPE for yourself
- applying barrier cream to the client's skin.

Applying colour to wet hair

Always read the manufacturer's instructions, as these will tell you whether you should apply the colour to wet or dry hair. They will also give all the information that you require, including how to measure and mix your products and what peroxide strength to use.

Shampoo the hair with a soapless shampoo. A soapless shampoo (TLS – Triethanolamine Lauryl Sulphate) will not affect the pH balance of the hair as this product has a neutral pH and does not leave a residue on the hair. DO NOT use a conditioner, which would act as a barrier on the hair preventing the colour from taking.

- Towel-dry the hair to remove excess moisture.
- Section the hair (if required) to move the bulk of the hair out of the way so that you can work more easily.
- Apply the product following the manufacturer's instructions.

Colouring products applied to wet hair include:

- temporary colours, for example coloured mousses or setting lotions
- semi-permanent colours, for example Wella Colour Fresh
- some quasi colours.

Applying colour to dry hair

- Brush the hair through, removing all tangles.
- Section the hair as required, into four if a regrowth or full head application.
- Apply the colour following the manufacturer's instructions.

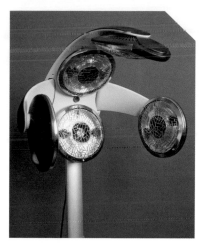

A climazone or accelerator

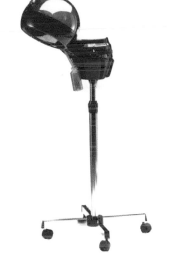

A steamer

Colouring products applied to dry hair include:

- hair mascaras and coloured sprays
- all permanent colours, for example high lift tints and bleaching products
- some quasi colours.

Adding colour to the hair means depositing colour on to the hair but not lifting (lightening) the natural colour of the client's hair.

Preparing the client for a colouring service

It is a good idea to carry out the consultation before you gown the client so that you can take into account her personality; for example, the way your client dresses is a good indication of the type of lifestyle she may lead.

You should also complete a full colouring consultation form and carry out all of the required hair and skin tests during the consultation (see pages 204 and 207–9).

Refer to a colour shade chart to enable the client to see the colour choices available. It will also enable you to match up to the client's existing colour and choose one to enhance and complement the skin tone.

When deciding whether to choose temporary or semi-permanent colours, you will need to take into account the following critical influencing factors:

- the client's existing hair colour
- the percentage of white hair
- the porosity of the hair.

The above factors will not only influence your colour choice but also the method of colour application.

Preparing the client for a permanent colouring and lightening service

The consultation

The consultation for a permanent colouring service should be slightly more in-depth than for temporary and semi-permanent colours. This is because the colour will last for a long time and so the client may find it more difficult to choose between the wide range of products available and the effects that can be achieved. For example, you can permanently:

- lighten
- darken
- change tone.

First, you should check whether the client has had an up-to-date skin test. This is to protect against any allergic reaction to the para dye that is contained in permanent colours. If the client has recently had a skin test and there was no positive reaction, you are free to continue the consultation.

Next, you should find out whether the client wants the hair to:

- go lighter than the natural base colour
- go darker than the natural base colour
- stay at the same depth as the natural base colour but add a warm or cool tone.

The target colour to be achieved will determine the strength of hydrogen peroxide that you will use.

During the consultation:

- use a colour shade chart
- match up the client's natural base shade to the shade chart
- decide whether you are lightening, darkening or adding tone
- decide on the technique that you will use
- agree with the client if it is a full head colour or regrowth colour
- check whether the client wishes to have more than one colour in the hair
- find out if the client will be able to maintain the colour
- double-check with the client that you have chosen the right colour.

Permanent tint is permanent! If the client does not like the result, she will have to grow the colour out.

As well as the colour consultation, you will need to complete the standard client consultation form, which will give you information on the hair's porosity, texture, amount of white present and previous chemical services.

Preparing the client for highlighting and lowlighting processes

As well as completing a colouring consultation form (see page 204), there are additional questions that you will need to ask the client in order to complete this specific colouring service:

- Does the client want colour added (lowlights) or the hair lightened (highlights)?
- How much colour would the client like to see — more natural hair than coloured hair, more coloured than natural hair, or equal amounts of natural to coloured hair? This will determine the size of the hook you will use and the amount of hair you pull through if carrying out a cap highlighting/lowlighting service.
- How thick or fine and how numerous does the client want the highlights/lowlights to be? (This will influence the thickness of your weaves if using mesh or foil.)
- Has the client had this procedure before? If not, you should explain the procedure.

You need to decide whether to use the highlighting cap, mesh or foils.

- Choose foils or mesh for hair that is below shoulder length and if a combination of colours is required.
- A cap should be used if the hair is too short to weave and you are using only one colour.

It is cheaper to use the cap method, as it is not so time-consuming. If the client wants foils or mesh for short hair and only one colour, that is the client's choice, but you should make her aware of the potential extra costs involved.

Select the colour the same way as in other colouring services. You will need to:

- match up the client's natural base shade to determine what depth of colour the hair is
- choose the target colour (the colour the client wants as the end result)
- determine from this if the hair is going darker than the client's natural base colour or if you are lifting (lightening) the hair
- decide how many shades you are lifting or darkening — this will determine the strength of hydrogen peroxide that you will use
- work out what percentage of white hair the client has — this will determine how much base colour (if any) you need to use.

213

Unit

GH9

Change hair colour

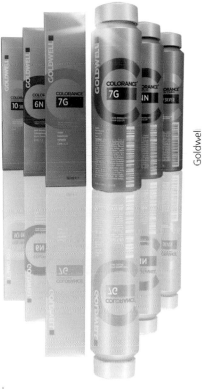

Goldwell

A range of colouring products

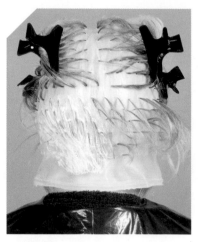

Using a highlighting cap

Gowning and hair preparation

Once you have completed the consultation, gown the client with a chemical gown, towel and plastic cape. Prepare the hair for the service.

* Brush the hair through to make sure there are no tangles.
* Make sure your highlighting cap is covered with talc; otherwise the rubber will tug the hair.
* Place the highlighting cap on the client, making sure you have parted the hair as the client wishes.
* Check the client is comfortable.

Highlighting/lowlighting procedures should be completed on dry hair. It is not recommended to use the highlighting cap on below-shoulder-length hair. The hair is likely to tangle, causing discomfort to the client. Instead, you would recommend using foils or mesh. Also, it is not recommended to use the highlighting cap on hair that is very short. This could result in the hair looking spotty (leopard spots!).

Principles of colouring

To understand how these factors will influence your colour choice, you need to have an understanding of the principles of colouring.

What is colour?

White sunlight is made up of all colours. You can see those colours in the sky when a rainbow is formed. They are known as the colours of the spectrum.

In hairdressing, indigo is not used because it is too difficult to distinguish from blue and violet. The six colours that you will use are made up of primary and secondary colours.

The primary colours are:

* red
* yellow
* blue.

These colours cannot be made by mixing other colours together.

The secondary colours are:

* orange
* green
* violet.

Mixing two primary colours together makes a secondary colour; for example red plus yellow makes orange. All other colours are made by mixing primary and secondary colours together.

The warm colours on the colour wheel are red, yellow and orange. The cool colours on the colour wheel are blue, green and violet.

A principle of the colour wheel is that opposite colours on the spectrum neutralise one another. For example, use a cool, ash tone (as ash tones contain green) to neutralise hair with too many warm red tones in it. Hair that is looking green can be made to look warmer by adding a warm tone (gold, copper or red).

The colours of the spectrum

Red
Orange
Yellow
Green
Blue
Indigo
Violet

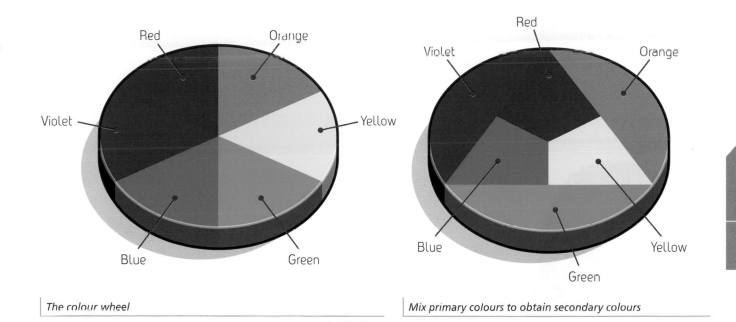

The colour wheel

Mix primary colours to obtain secondary colours

Change hair colour

Task 4

Looking at the colour wheel, list three warm tones and three cool tones.

Natural hair colour

The cortex contains all the **pigments** in the hair. These are called melanin. **Melanin** is broken down into two types of colour pigments:

- Black and brown pigments are called eumelanin – they are the cool tones in the hair (ash or matt).
- Red and yellow pigments are called pheomelanin – they are the warm tones in the hair (auburn or golden).

(Refer also to Facts about hair, pages 2–5.)

The amount of each of the four colour pigments in the hair determines the natural colour of the hair. For example, a person with a lot of eumelanin and a little pheomelanin will have medium to dark ash brown hair. A person with more pheomelanin than eumelanin would be a medium to light golden blonde.

Top tips

Colours that are opposite each other on the colour wheel will counteract each other.

Pigment

Substance that colours tissue such as hair and skin.

Melanin

The hair's natural colour pigment found in the cortex.

Salon life

The science of colouring

Dory's story

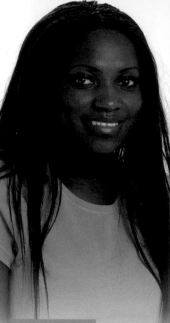

I love colouring and want to specialise in this field when I complete my course. I can do the practical side standing on my head but when it comes to the theory, I really struggle! I wasn't sure if I simply needed extra learning support with this subject because it is quite complex, or whether I just didn't get it and never would! In the end I asked my tutor for help. It was the best thing I could have done – she was so supportive and offered great advice. She even admitted that when she was training she had found the theory of colouring difficult and her lecturer had told her to use word association.

She explained: 'If you can't remember the seven colours of the spectrum, use this mnemonic to help you – Richard Of York Gave Battle In Vain. The first letter from each word is the first letter of one of the colours that make up the spectrum – Red, Orange, Yellow, Green, Blue, Indigo and Violet.'

I now use word association for all of my subjects. It's a brilliant way to help me remember the muscles and bones of the head and face (masseater = mass eating, the chewing muscle in the side of the face; trapezius = a trapeze, the muscle that allows you to tilt your head). It's a great feeling to know I have a learning strategy that I can use all by myself.

Top tips

Word association can be used and adapted to suit all lessons. For example:
- to remember that pheomelanin contains the lighter colour pigments (red and yellow), you could think of Phoebe from *Friends* who has blonde hair
- to remember that eumelanin contains the darker colour pigments (brown and black), you could think of Chris Eubank the boxer, who has dark hair.

Ask the expert

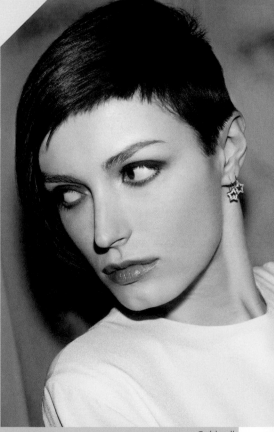

Q *I get really confused trying to work out the difference between the depth of the colour and the tone. Do you have any tips that would help me to remember?*

A The best way to remember the depth and tone of colours is first to list numbers 1 to 10 – these will be your base (depth of) colours which tell you how light or dark the colour is. These numbers stay the same for every manufacturer throughout the world, since they are the standard International Colour Chart (ICC) system, so they always relate to the same depth of colour on every colour chart. The tones can vary from one manufacturer to another, so the best way to learn these is to do the same and write the numbers down (1 to 7 usually) and learn which numbers correspond to the tones on the colour chart that your training establishment or salon works with. Once you have learned the base/depth numbers, it isn't so hard to learn the tone numbers from one colour chart to another.

Goldwell

Choosing the product and application

International Colour Chart system

The International Colour Chart (ICC) system is a guide to colouring that is used all over the world. Although each manufacturer has a slightly different colour chart, all use a similar numbering system. Base hair colours are numbered 1–10, 1 being the darkest colour (black) and 10 being the lightest colour (very light blonde). As a stylist, learning what these numbers stand for will enable you to pick up any colour chart and know exactly what depth of colour you can hope to achieve.

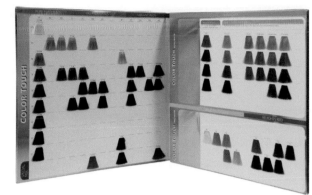

Colour chart by Goldwell

Change hair colour

The names that are given to colours, such as 'Sahara blonde' and 'Black tulip', are more for the benefit of the client, although they will help you to picture the colour in your mind when you first start colouring.

How to use the ICC system

For each colour, the first number on the chart describes its depth. For example·

- 6 = blonde
- 4 = light brown
- 2 = dark brown.

Referring to the depth of the colour is the same as referring to the base colour – that is, how light or dark the hair is.

Task 5

Write down the numbers 1 to 10. Using a shade chart, note the colour next to each number. Compare this to other shade charts and discuss any differences.

The next number on the chart after the base number tells you the primary tone of the colour. This is the dominant/strongest tone. The number assigned to each tone can differ from manufacturer to manufacturer, but here is a sample selection:

- 1 – ash/green, blue base
- 3 = gold
- 4 = red
- 5 = mahogany
- 6 = violet
- 7 = brunette
- 8 = pearl.

According to this sample, 6.3 (or 6/3) would be golden blonde. This is because the base number is 6, which tells us that the hair is blonde, and the primary tone number is 3, which tells us that the hair has golden tones.

Often there is a third number on the chart. This tells you the secondary tone. For example, 6.34 (or 6/34) would be copper gold blonde. This is because the base is blonde (6), the primary tone is gold (3) and the secondary tone is red (4). The golden tones would be stronger than the copper tones. Primary and secondary tones have nothing to do with primary and secondary colours. Sometimes colours may be

Unit

GH9

Change hair colour

Top tips

Never store diluted hydrogen peroxide solution. It is a fire hazard.

8.44 or 8/44. In these colours, the primary tone (the most intense tone) and the secondary tone (the least intense tone) are the same. This gives the colour a doubly intense tone.

There are also colours that don't have a primary tone, only a secondary tone, such as 7.03 (or 7/03). The first number after the point or slash is 0, which tells you there is no strong primary tone. The 3 following the 0 tells you that there is a weak secondary tone of gold.

Hydrogen peroxide percentage by volume

It is the oxygen in hydrogen peroxide that makes it useful for hairdressing. The strength of hydrogen peroxide is measured in percentage strength or volume strength. Percentage strength tells you how much pure hydrogen peroxide is in the solution. For example, in a 3 per cent solution, 3 per cent will be pure hydrogen peroxide and 97 per cent will be water. Volume strength tells you the amount of oxygen released from 1 ml of hydrogen peroxide solution. For example, 1 ml of 20 volume would release 20 ml of oxygen.

The higher the percentage or volume, the more oxygen is released from the hydrogen peroxide.

Hydrogen peroxide is stabilised with a mild acid to stop it releasing oxygen in the bottle, but it is very important that you put the top back on after use or it will oxidise in the bottle and lose its strength. Never pour hydrogen peroxide back into the bottle, as this will also cause the peroxide to oxidise in the bottle and therefore lose its strength.

Hydrogen peroxide softens and opens the cuticle. It can be used prior to applying permanent colour to resistant hair (known as pre-softening).

The amount of lift required determines the strength of hydrogen peroxide to be used.

- 20 volume or 6% = 0–1 shade of lift
- 30 volume or 9% = 2–3 shades of lift
- 40 volume or 12% = 3–4 shades of lift

If you have a higher strength hydrogen peroxide than you require, you may dilute it to the correct volume using distilled water. The following chart will help you check the correct ratios of water to peroxide that are needed to dilute peroxide if you ever run out. Only dilute the amount you require and never store diluted mixture.

Hydrogen peroxide by volume	Hydrogen peroxide that you may require	Quantity of peroxide to be used	Quantity of water to be added	Ratio (peroxide:water)
40	30	3 parts	1 part	3:1
40	20	2 parts	2 parts	2:2
40	10	1 part	3 parts	1:3
30	20	2 parts	1 part	2:1
30	10	1 part	2 parts	1:2
20	10	1 part	1 part	1:1

Temporary colours

Temporary colours have large molecules that coat the cuticle. They do not dramatically alter the colour of the hair but can add stronger tones. Temporary colours will not lighten the hair.

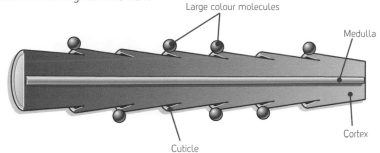

To apply to porous hair:

- shampoo the hair and divide into four sections (hot cross bun)
- pour the coloured setting lotion into a bowl and, using a tint brush, apply the lotion to the hair in sections approximately 1 cm deep. This will ensure that the lotion is applied evenly to all of the hair.

For non-porous hair, the setting lotion can be applied from the bottle and sprinkled onto the hair.

Temporary colours can be removed from the hair at the next shampoo, but if the hair is porous there may be a build-up of colour. Some sprays and paints will brush out.

Application of coloured mousses and hair mascaras

Because coloured mousses and hair mascaras stain the hair, they will also stain your hands, so always wear gloves. Shampoo the hair and towel-dry to remove excess moisture. Divide the hair if appropriate to allow ease of application.

Application of semi-permanent colours

Semi-permanent colours are available as:

- creams
- mousses
- liquids.

They have large and small colour molecules that stain the cuticle and partially penetrate into the cortex.

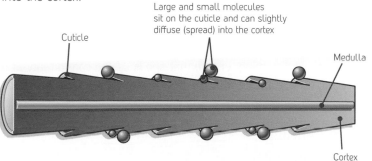

Semi-permanent colours are always applied to wet hair. They last from four to eight shampoos, but if the hair is porous there may be a build-up of colour. They cover up to 30 per cent white hair. Such products add colour to the hair but will not lighten it.

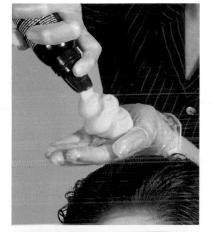

Temporary colour molecules coat the cuticle

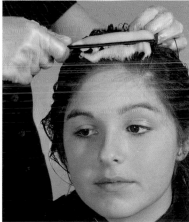

Applying mousse

Semi-permanent colour molecules stain the cuticle and diffuse into the cortex

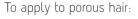

219

Unit

GH9

Change hair colour

Application of semi-permanent colours

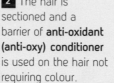 **1** Semi-permanent colours can be applied straight from the bottle. However, if you need to work precisely on specific areas of the hair, the product can be applied with a brush from a bowl.

2 The hair is sectioned and a barrier of **anti-oxidant (anti-oxy) conditioner** is used on the hair not requiring colour.

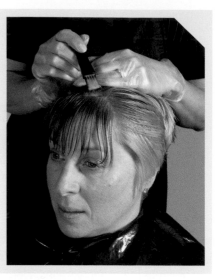

Anti-oxidant conditioner

Conditioner used after a chemical process to reduce the amount of chemical residue left in the hair. This will stop creeping oxidation, which occurs when colour continues to develop in the cortex. It will close the cuticle, add moisture to the hair and return the hair to its correct pH value (4.5–5.5).

Top tips

When applying any colouring product to the hair, make sure:
- the client is fully protected with the correct gown, towels and barrier cream
- the hair is towel-dried if the colour is to be applied to wet hair, so the colour does not drip off the hair
- the client's position is adjusted so that you can see where you are applying the tint and minimise fatigue
- any product that touches the skin is removed immediately with damp cotton wool so that it will not stain.

When the colour has been removed, check that there is no excess colour on the skin and style the hair using the correct styling and finishing products. Confirm the look with the client.

Very long hair may require two or more bottles of colour. The hair should be sectioned off and the application begun at the nape area moving up towards the crown. Always inform the client if you are going to have to use more than one application, as this will incur extra costs.

Development and removal

When applying temporary colours, there is no development time. With semi-permanent colours, read the manufacturer's instructions to check the development time, and then make a note of the time of the finished application and when the colour needs to be rinsed. In busy salons, stylists often use a timer that rings when the development time is completed.

While the colour is developing, you should make sure that the hair is not piled too tightly on the head. To help a colour develop properly, air needs to be able to circulate through the hair.

Rinsing

Once the colour has developed, take the client to the basin to remove the colour. Make sure that the client is still well protected — a towel and plastic cape should be covering the client's clothing. Ensure that she is seated comfortably at the basin. Check that you have all of her hair in the basin and that she is sitting far enough back so that you can reach to remove the tint.

Step-by-step rinsing
- Remove any barrier cream.
- Check the water temperature.
- Dampen the hair. Massage to emulsify the colour. (This means working the water into the colour to produce a slight lather that will help remove the colour more easily.)

- Rinse until the water runs clear.
- Use an anti-oxy conditioner. (If you shampooed the hair prior to colouring, there is no need to shampoo again.)
- Check that you have rinsed the entire tint from behind the ears and in the nape area.
- Towel-dry and style the hair.

The finished result

Only once you have styled the client's hair will the actual colour be fully clear to you and the client, as wet hair always looks darker. It is a good idea to take the client to a window so that she can see the colour in natural light. Let the client hold the hand mirror so that she can have a good look. Confirm with the client that she is happy with the result.

How to colour and lighten hair

When changing hair colour permanently, the world is your oyster! There is a wide variety of products and techniques, from highlighting to bold and dramatic looks, such as putting vivid, bright slices of colour through the hair.

There are additional factors to be considered when permanently colouring and lightening the hair. This is because you will be chemically changing the colour molecules in the hair. The two types of colouring methods can be combined to create both subtle and more **avant-garde** looks.

Products, techniques, application and development

Permanent colours and lightening products

All permanent colours are applied to dry hair. There are two main types:

- creams and gels – synthetic, organic
- metallic dyes – inorganic.

Synthetic dyes are known as para dyes (para-phenylenediamine). These are the dyes that are most commonly used.

Para dye facts

- They must be mixed with hydrogen peroxide to work.
- They are alkaline and so open up the cuticle and penetrate into the cortex.
- They can lighten up to 5 shades above the base colour depending on whether you are using a fashion colour or high lift tint.
- They can cover any amount of white hair.
- They can darken the hair or add tones to natural colour.
- They can cause a serious allergic reaction.

Para dyes have small molecules that allow them to enter the cortex. When they start to develop with the oxygen from the hydrogen peroxide they enlarge and become trapped inside the cortex.

Inorganic dyes

Metallic dyes contain, as their name suggests, metallic salts. They are commonly found in 'colour restorers' but are sometimes mixed with semi-permanent colour and with henna.

Video clip

Watch video clip 'Colour removal' on the website to see colour being removed.

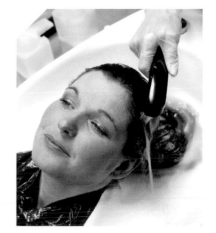

Rinsing off the colour

Avant-garde

New, exciting and unusual in style.

221

Unit
GH9

Change hair colour

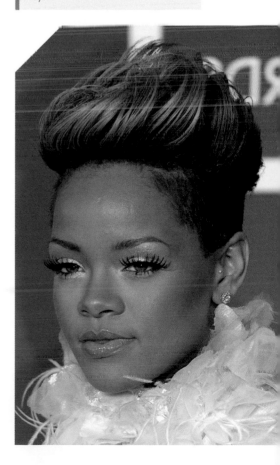

Metallic salts are not compatible with hydrogen peroxide. How bad the reaction is depends on the type of metallic salt on the hair. Some turn the hair green; others will fizz and bubble, producing enough heat to dissolve the hair. If you suspect that the client has used a colour at home that may contain metallic salts, you must carry out an incompatibility test on the hair (see page 208).

Quasi-permanent colours

Quasi-permanent colours have a lasting quality that falls between semi-permanent and permanent colourants. If used once, they will usually last between eight and twelve shampoos and then fade out, but if used regularly they will build up on the hair and can cause a regrowth.

Quasi-permanent colour molecules are small enough to enter the cortex but do not change the natural hair colour permanently

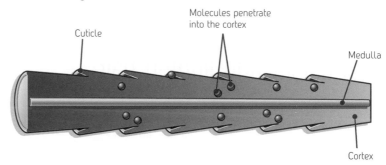

Cuticle

Molecules penetrate into the cortex

Medulla

Cortex

Most quasi-colours require a skin test to be done before they are used. You should also carry out an incompatibility test if you suspect metallic salts are present in the hair.

Most quasi-colours are mixed with a developer, which contains very weak hydrogen peroxide. They are usually mixed using 1 part colour to 2 parts developer. This makes them slightly runny, so they are often applied with an applicator flask to prevent the product from dripping. It is important to read the manufacturer's instructions, as there are no general rules for the use of these products. Quasi-colours can also be mixed as colour baths.

High lift tint

A high lift tint can lighten the hair 4–5 shades depending on the base colour of the hair (the darker the base, the less lift you will be able to achieve). High lift tints are usually recommended for use on hair of a base 6 (dark blonde) and upwards. Always check the manufacturer's instructions.

These tints are usually mixed 1 part tint to 2 parts hydrogen peroxide, for example 50 ml of tint to 100 ml of hydrogen peroxide. They usually require a longer development time (always check the manufacturer's instructions) and can benefit from the use of added heat.

Bleaches

Bleaches lighten the hair and will lift tint out of the hair. The bleaching process is one of oxidation. It is permanent. The hair must be in good condition and strong in order to withstand the bleaching process. The three most commonly used bleaches are:

- powder – used for highlights/foils
- gel – used for full head bleaching (scalp application)
- cream – used for full head bleaching (scalp application).

Fact or fiction?

Is this statement fact or fiction?

High lift tint can lighten other tints of a base 8 and below.

To check your answer see page 497.

All types of bleach are mixed with hydrogen peroxide to activate them. You must mix them in a well-ventilated room to avoid ingesting the fumes. Bleach is alkaline and so opens up the cuticle. This allows the oxygen that is released from the solution to penetrate into the cortex. Once inside, the oxygen combines with the natural hair colour pigment, melanin. This forms a new colour pigment, oxymelanin, which is colourless. The oxygen combines first with the black pigment, then the brown, then the red and lastly the yellow.

When a full head bleach is done, the colour result is often too yellow. This is because the bleach lifts out the natural colour pigments in the hair, with yellow being the last one it lifts out. If this is the case, a toner can be used to counteract the yellow tones.

Bleaches are applied to dry hair and will continue to lighten it until they are completely removed from the hair. Porosity, elasticity and possibly incompatibility tests need to be carried out prior to the process. Bleach can also be used to pre-lighten the hair if you require a strong, vibrant fashion colour and the client's hair may be too dark to achieve this with a normal tint – see the chart below.

Fashion tone required	Pre-lightening tone required
Burgundy Plum	Dark orange
True red	Orange
Auburn Bright copper	Bright orange
Warm copper	Gold
Chestnut Warm gold	Dark yellow
Sandy Gold Beige	Yellow
Ash Pinky rose	Pale yellow
Pale silver Platinum Blue Violet	Palest yellow

Choosing the correct pre-lightening tone

223

Unit
GH9

Change hair colour

Task 6

Discuss with your group why it is important not to lift the client's hair colour too much when pre-lightening.

Applying highlights/lowlights and colouring techniques

Highlighting cap

During the consultation you will have established how much colour the client wishes to see in her hair. If the client requires only one colour, you can use the highlighting cap (remember, this is only suitable on hair that is shoulder length or above). See pages 213–14 for a full explanation of how to prepare the client for the highlighting process.

Top tips

- Before placing a highlighting cap on the client, sprinkle a little talcum powder on it. This will allow the cap to slide onto the hair more easily.
- Lightening products expand as they process. Great care must be taken to ensure that the product does not seep onto the surrounding hair and create a patchy result.

When you have placed the cap on the client and have checked that she is comfortable (ears are not bent back), you can begin to pull the highlights/lowlights through. The hooks you will be using vary in size, indicated by the numbers on the hooks. Thicker highlights require a slightly bigger hook, and vice versa.

It is always best to begin at the nape area. This is because as you work up the head you will be able to see where you are going without having to hold any hair up out of the way.

1 The highlight hook needs to penetrate the hole at an angle so you don't stab the client's head! When all the hair has been pulled through, comb the hair to remove any loops at the root area.

2 Begin applying the colour at the nape area, taking sections 1 cm deep. By doing this you will ensure even coverage of all of the hair. When you have completed the application, loosen the hair slightly with the end of your tint brush to allow air to move through the hair. (This will allow the hair to develop evenly.)

3 The end result.

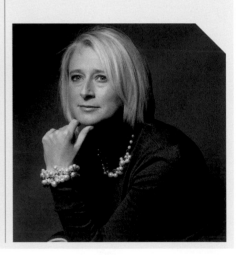

Foils

Metal that is rolled out into a thin sheet and used for various colouring techniques to separate sections of colour.

Mesh

Plastic self-adhesive packets used to secure sections of coloured hair.

Mesh and foils

If you are adding one or more colours to the hair and the hair is below shoulder length, you will have to use **foils** or **mesh**. You should ask the same questions as for the highlighting cap and prepare the hair in the same way.

When you have established the thickness of the strands of hair to be coloured, section the hair into four (hot cross bun). The amount of hair that you want to colour will determine how thickly or finely you weave out sections of the hair that are to be coloured.

As with any colouring process, gown the client correctly then mix the colours required. Beginning at the nape area, drop a fine mesh of hair about 2 cm deep. Pick up this section of hair and, using the end of a pintail comb, select the strands you wish to apply colour to.

If using two or more colours, you will need to alternate the colours as you apply them. If you require a lot of colour in the hair, weave every section. If the client does not want as much colour in her hair, leave a section in between each packet.

Top tips

When using easi-mesh, the blue band at the top of the packet is your guideline to where to apply the product. It is slightly sticky and secures the packet when closed. If you apply the product over the top of the band it will not secure the hair. Some products also expand on development; by using the band as a guideline you will prevent seepage of the product onto the rest of the hair.

Slicing using foils

1 Cut the foil to the required length and place as close as possible to the root. Place the colour on the section of the hair, making sure you allow for the expansion of the colour so it does not seep out of the packet.

2 Fold the foil in half using your comb.

3 Fold in either side of your packet to secure the packet to the head.

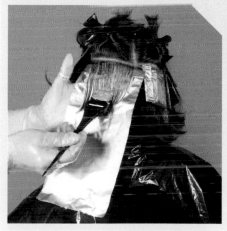

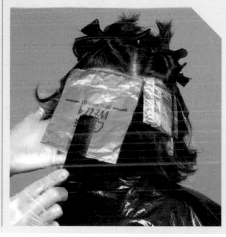

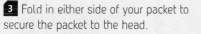
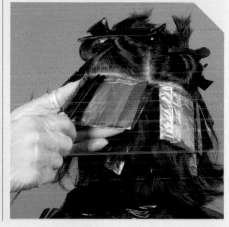

225

Unit

GH9

Change hair colour

Step-by-step weaving using foils

1 Determine the thickness of the hair to be coloured and weave the hair accordingly using the pintail comb. Fold the top of the foil over the metal tail of your comb and push up underneath the weaved hair to the root area.

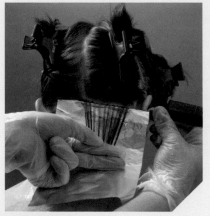

2 Slide your comb out, ensuring you don't pull the packet away from the root area. Apply the tint, leaving a very small gap to allow expansion of the product. Ensure enough product is used for even colouring.

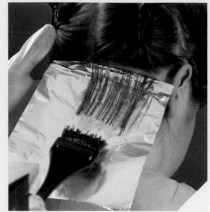

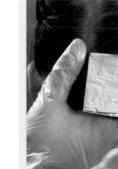

3 Fold your packet in half and then fold the sides in to anchor the packet in place.

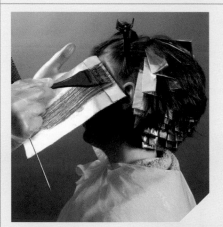

4 Continue to work up the back to the crown area in your chosen pattern. Move to the side sections just above the ear. The hair is taken at an angle to prevent obvious colour banding at the root.

5 Make sure all packets are in place, and your infill colour (if one is required) is completed. Place your client under heat (if required), checking the manufacturer's development times.

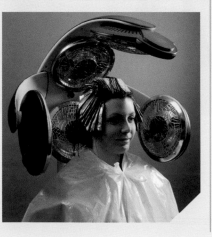

6 Check your client is happy with the finished result and offer the appropriate aftercare advice.

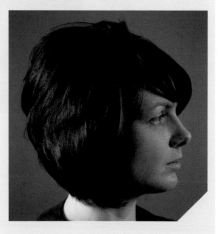

Critical influencing factors

When deciding on the product and technique to use, you will need to take into account the following critical influencing factors:

- temperature
- existing colour of hair
- percentage of white hair
- porosity of hair
- length of hair
- test results.

Temperature

When colouring the hair, there are 'hot spots' in the nape area and the top of the head that you need to be aware of. In the case of a full head of foils, where you begin at the nape area, this hair will start to process as soon as you apply the product to the hair. By the time you reach the front of the head, the first section of hair may be near to the end of its development time. If this is the case, you need to apply the product quite quickly and you may need to think about using added heat on the last packets applied. You may need to remove developed packets using a water spray and cotton wool.

A climazone offers an excellent way of adding heat only where you require the heat to be directed. Because you turn off the arms that you do not require on the climazone, you can process specific parts of the hair, allowing the hair on other parts of the head to 'catch up'.

When completing a highlighting/lowlighting service with a cap, a plastic disposable hat should be placed over the top. This will trap the body heat of the client, which will assist the development of the colour.

If using a product such as bleach, and the hair colour is not lifting as much as you would want, place the client under a steamer to help the bleach to develop.

Existing colour of hair

When deciding on the target colour for the client, you should know the following:

* Tint will not lift tint.
* You can only achieve 3 shades of lift with a fashion colour.
* High lift tint will give you 4–5 shades of lift if on a base 6 or above.
* If going darker than the base colour, it is only advisable to go 3 shades darker so that the colour will still suit the client's skin tone.

Percentage of white hair

The amount of white hair present will determine the strength of peroxide you use and if a base colour needs to be added to the hair.

If the client wishes to go darker or stay at the same depth as her natural colour to cover white hair, you will be adding colour not lifting it. However, you will still need to use hydrogen peroxide to open the cuticle and allow the tint into the cortex.

Porosity

The porosity of the hair determines how well the colour takes. If hair is in good condition, the cuticle scales lie flat and the colour will coat the hair evenly, reflecting the light back to show healthy, shiny hair. If hair is in bad condition, the cuticle scales may be open. This means that the colour will not take evenly and the light will bounce off in all directions, making the hair look flat and dull.

Length of hair

As discussed in Preparing the client for highlighting and lowlighting processes (page 213), the length of hair plays an important part when deciding which technique and method of application to use. Also, the longer the hair is, the older it will be, and therefore it is more likely to be porous. This may not be from chemical services but from day-to-day wear and tear.

Test results

If the client has hair that has poor elasticity, you need to carefully consider the choice of products you will use.

Top tips

A hood dryer can dry out bleach, so a steamer is a better option if one is available. When using added heat, always carry out health and safety checks.

Application of products

Basic techniques

There are many techniques that you can use when applying colour to hair.

Step-by-step regrowth application

1 Consult with your client on their requirements. Carry out all hair and skin checks and tests.

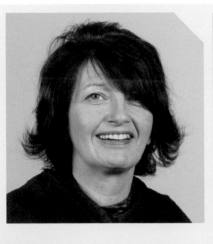

2 Begin your application at the greyest area if darkening the hair. Only apply to the regrowth area, ensuring you don't overlap onto previously coloured hair.

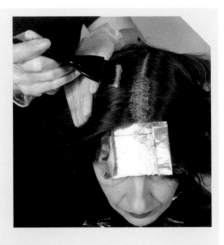

3 Continue to work through the regrowth sections ensuring that you don't overlap onto previously coloured hair.

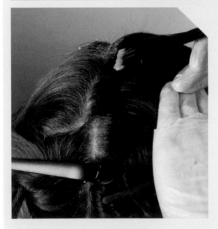

4 Once you have completed all of the regrowth area, check the manufacturer's instructions for development times.

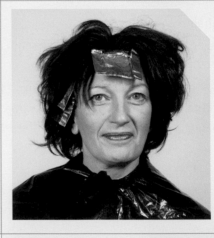

5 Confirm your client is happy with the end result and give the appropriate aftercare advice.

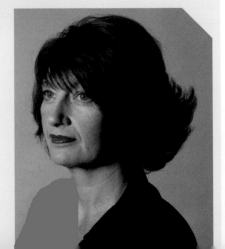

Application of permanent tint or bleach to virgin hair

In order to get an even colour result, you need to take into account:

- the length of the hair
- the porosity of the hair
- body heat.

On hair that is over 2.5 cm long, colour at the roots will develop more quickly than at the ends of the hair. This is because heat that escapes from the scalp speeds up the development time. Colour on the hair that is furthest away from the scalp takes longer to develop because it does not have the benefit of body heat. Colour on hair that is more porous will develop more quickly than colour on hair that is in good condition.

On long hair, the ends will be more porous than the mid-lengths (because the hair is older) and therefore the colour will develop more quickly at the ends.

Full head tint or bleach should be applied to the hair in the following order:

1 mid-lengths
2 ends
3 roots.

When using lightening products, do not allow one application to overlap the other. This can cause breakage to the hair, as you are effectively double-processing the hair. Overlapping may also cause a banding effect, whereby the hair that has had a double application of product on it will develop into a different colour.

Step by-step application of full head tint

1 Wearing the correct PPE, mix the product, making sure you measure out the quantities correctly.

2 Section the hair into four and begin to apply the tint mixture to the darkest area of the hair if lightening or the lightest area if darkening. Apply the colour up to 2.5 cm from the roots, to the mid-lengths only.

3 Continue to apply all of the tint, making sure that the root area is left, and develop following the manufacturer's instructions.

4 Check the manufacturer's instructions for application to the rest of the hair (ends and roots).

5 Carry out a strand colour test by removing some of the product with damp cotton wool. Check the colour match from roots to ends and in several different places on the head.

6 Remove the product with tepid (lukewarm) water, not massaging too vigorously. Shampoo with TLS shampoo (see page 182) and use an anti-oxy conditioner. Style the hair in the appropriate manner using the correct styling and finishing products.

Changing tone

To change the tone of the hair and achieve a rich colour result, you could use a quasi-colour. Because quasi-colours have a small amount of hydrogen peroxide in the developer, they allow the colour molecule to diffuse into the cortex and deposit some of the tone.

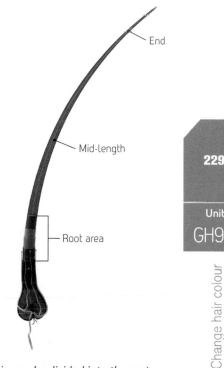

Hair may be divided into the root, mid-length and end

End

Mid-length

Root area

229

Unit

GH9

Change hair colour

Step-by-step changing tone

1 Consult with your client to choose the desired colour, holding the colour swatches against the skin to give an impression of the colour choice.

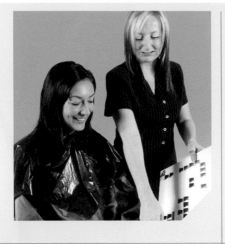

2 Gown yourself and the client. Apply barrier cream to the hairline area.

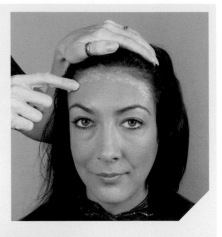

3 Apply the colour directly from the applicator flask to the hair, working from roots straight through to the ends of the hair.

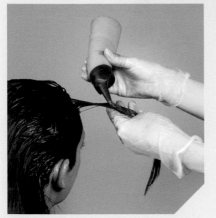

4 Check the development of the colour halfway through its development time by removing some of the product with damp cotton wool. When ready, rinse the colour from the hair until the water runs clear.

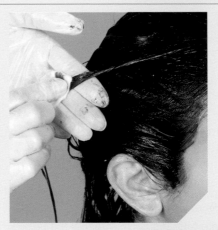

5 The finished result. Check the colour result with the client and style as desired. Provide the appropriate aftercare advice.

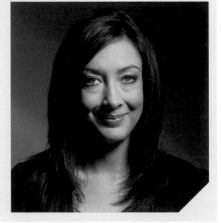

Applying colour

When mixing, make sure you use the correct quantities so that the mixture is of the right consistency and will not drip on the client's face or clothing, and so that you achieve the correct colour result.

When applying any colour to the client's hair, make sure that you use the correct protective equipment and take great care when applying the colour. Do not apply any tint beyond the barrier cream.

When developing the colour, you should complete a strand test (see page 209) halfway through the development time. This will enable you to determine how well the colour is developing and if added heat is required.

When using added heat:

- check the temperature controls before you put the client under a heat source
- do not allow the product to dry out (this is especially important with bleaches and it is best to use a steamer for this reason)
- use a timer
- monitor the development at regular intervals.

Product removal

When the colour is fully developed and you are happy with the result, remove the colour from the client's hair using the following method.

1   Take the client to the basin.

2   Moisten the hair with warm water and gently massage to loosen and emulsify the tint. Pay particular attention to the front hairline and nape area. Tint removes tint, so this is the best way of doing it.

3   Rinse the tint until the water runs clear.

4   Shampoo the hair twice using a TLS shampoo, again checking that you have removed all traces of tint from the nape area, behind the ears and the front hairline.

5   Condition with an anti-oxy conditioner to stop further oxidation and return the hair to its natural pH.

Development and removal for highlighting effects

Once you have finished applying the colour, check the following.

- Are the protective towel and cape still in place and not covered in tint? If they are covered in tint change them.
- Is there any product spilt on the trolley you have been using? If so, clean it up.

If using a highlighting cap, lift up the front so the client can see again and secure with a pin curl clip (make sure that it is to the side of the head so that it does not mark the skin). If using foils or mesh, you should secure any that are around the client's face with a pin curl clip.

Check the manufacturer's instructions for development times. You should monitor the development process all the way through. Take regular strand tests to check that the colour is developing evenly all over the head.

Step-by-step product removal for highlighting effects

1 When the colour has processed, take the client to the basin and rinse the product from the cap. Make sure you ask the client to close her eyes or shield her face with your hand to protect from splashes.

2 To remove the cap, apply some anti-oxy conditioner to the hair and gently ease the cap from the client's head, checking that there is no discomfort.

3 If the hair does not want to come away from the hat freely, use your fingers to ease the hair out.

Coping with problems

Problem	Possible causes	Action
Uneven result 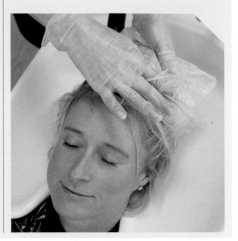	• Porous hair • Uneven application • Incorrect use of heat • Wrong product choice	Spot colour the required areas.
Scalp irritation	• Allergy to product • Peroxide strength too high • Added heat	Remove product with lukewarm water.
Coverage not good, especially on white hair	• Resistant hair • Uneven application • Incorrect choice of colour	Pre-soften with peroxide. Use a double base colour or a higher proportion of base colour to the fashion shade.

Problem	Possible causes	Action
Hair breaking	• Hair in poor condition • Peroxide too strong • Incorrect application of product • Too much heat	Remove product and use restructuring conditioning treatments.
Too yellow	• Wrong choice of product or peroxide • Not developed for long enough • Natural tones not taken into account	Reapply bleach or use a violet toner to neutralise yellow tones.
Seepage of product	• Incorrect masking of area not to be coloured • Incorrect mixing of product • Incorrect use of foils or mesh • Product too runny	Spot recolour on problem areas.
Colour fade	• Porous hair	Look at using a semi/quasi colouring product to restore depth and tone.

Task 8

Choosing from the table, can you identify the colouring problems that you could confidently deal with on your own? Which of the problems would have to be referred to a senior member of staff or lecturer?

A worksheet for this task is provided on the website for you to complete and add to your portfolio.

If you identify a colouring problem but are unable to correct it, you should seek advice from the person in charge, either the salon manager or your lecturer. Explain the problem and the course of action that you may have already taken. The manager/ lecturer will then be able to help you deal with the situation. If the problem resulted from the condition of the client's hair and was unforeseen, you will need to make a note on the client's record card so that future stylists will be aware of potential difficulties. If the colouring problem was caused by you, the experience will help you to see that all services must be followed in a logical order with great care and attention to detail, and hopefully you will not repeat the same mistake in the future!

Coping with problems when highlighting

If some areas are processing slower than others, use added heat. When using foils or mesh, if you find that part of the hair has processed more quickly than another, remove the product from the part that has developed while leaving the rest to continue developing.

Removing foils and mesh

It is important that you remove the foils and colour from the hair without disturbing the rest of the colouring process. To do this, you will need:

- damp cotton wool – to remove the colour from the hair
- sectioning clips – to hold the packets out of the way as you work
- the correct personal protective equipment
- a bin close at hand – to dispose of the cotton wool and foils/mesh.

1   Section the hair away from where you will be working so that you can get to the packets that need to be removed.

2   Open up the packets. Making sure you have a towel across your hand, spray the packets with a water spray and gently slide them out.

3   Using damp cotton wool, wipe away the colour from the hair. Do not over-wet the hair, as it will drip (think health and safety!).

4   Continue in this way until you have removed all of the packets that have developed. Leave the rest of the hair to carry on processing, checking at regular intervals.

Confirming and recording the end result

You should be able to tell from your client's reaction whether she is pleased or not with the result, but you also need to ask such questions as:

- 'That's a really good result, what do you think?'
- 'Shall I book you in for a root regrowth colour in five weeks?'

As soon as possible, fill in the client's record card. For the service, you will need to make a note of:

- how long the bleach took to develop fully (if bleach was used)
- the number of colours used and in what order for full head foils
- any extra costs incurred for using more than one colour
- any problems encountered during the service
- what colours and peroxide strength were used
- what method and techniques were used
- whether added heat was used.

Personal, learning and thinking skills – Effective participation

There will be times within your day when you will have the opportunity to observe other stylists as they work. Through appearing eager and enthusiastic, you may be able to turn this into an opportunity to become actively involved in the task they are carrying out. Think of all the ways in which you could participate effectively during a colouring process, without actually carrying out the service yourself. Not only will you gain more experience from a hands-on approach, you will also benefit the salon and aid in its cost-effectiveness.

How to provide aftercare advice

When you carry out any hairdressing service it is important to give your client the most suitable and appropriate aftercare advice on how to maintain the service you have provided. This is especially important with a colouring or lightening service because it will give the client knowledge of the best way to preserve the colour at home, and will ensure repeat business for the salon.

The type of aftercare advice given will depend on the colouring or lightening service that has been carried out.

Suggested advice

Temporary colours

These will only last until the next shampoo, so you could suggest that the client purchases the product to use at home to be able to maintain the colour. Another good selling point is that coloured mousse can also be used on dark bases of 6 and below to blend a very small percentage of white hair in between other colouring services. You need to advise your client to wear gloves when applying the colour and avoid getting any on the skin — remember, coloured mousse stains the hair so it will stain skin and clothes as well! You should not recommend this product on hair that has a high percentage of white or is pre-lightened because you will not achieve a true colour result.

Semi-permanent colours

You need to check your manufacturer's instructions, but as a general guide most semi-permanent colours will last between four and eight shampoos. You can advise a client that this is a good conditioning product that can be used to refresh faded mid-lengths and ends of a permanent colour. It is also a good introduction to colour. Because the colour gradually washes out, the client should expect to see colour loss each time she shampoos the hair. You should be recommending a colour-saver shampoo and conditioner as this will prolong the life of the colour. Some manufacturers sell coloured shampoos to maintain the colour at home.

Quasi-permanent colours

Again, always check the manufacturer's instructions as products do vary from one company to another. These products contain a small amount of hydrogen peroxide in the developer which allows the colour molecules to enter into the cortex. They last between eight and twelve shampoos and will produce a slight root regrowth if used continually. These products are good for clients who have a small percentage of white hair that doesn't yet require the use of a permanent colour. You would recommend that a client return to the salon every four weeks to have their colour refreshed.

Permanent colours and lighteners

Both of these services have to grow out so require a great deal more maintenance. A good colour-saver shampoo and conditioner should be advised. You should give advice on maintaining the general condition of the hair, as permanent colouring and lightening products can be more drying to the hair because they may be used with a high-strength hydrogen peroxide. If a client has a full head of foils/mesh, you could suggest that the top T-zone section is recoloured every other visit. This may prove more affordable to your client, prevent a build-up of colour and help the condition of the rest of the hair.

With all of the colouring services provided, a good colour-saver shampoo and conditioner should be advised. If the client goes swimming on a regular basis, then a swimming hat should be worn to protect the hair from fading as a result of the hair coming into contact with chlorine (bleaching agent). If a client spends a lot of time in the sun or perhaps goes sailing, a hat should be worn. This will not only protect the hair colour from fading but will also help to keep the hair in good condition.

You should recommend that a heat-protective spray is applied before using heated appliances, as repeated use of heat will damage the condition of the hair, making the cuticle raised and roughened. This will impact on the next colouring service and cause the colour to fade more quickly

It is always a good idea to discuss with your client how fast their hair grows. Most heads of hair will grow on average 1.25 cm per month, but some heads of hair will be quicker or slower. By determining the rate of growth for your client you will be able to advise how often they should return to the salon for a retouch.

Check your knowledge

The following questions will help you to check your understanding of this unit.
The answers can be found on page 497.

1 The purpose of a skin test is to determine:
   a) what colouring product can be used on the client's hair
   b) whether the client is allergic to a colouring product
   c) how long a colouring product can safely be left on the skin
   d) how much staining will occur if the colouring product comes into contact with the skin.

2 Barrier cream is used to:
   a) stop colour from dripping onto the client's face
   b) give you a guide to work towards when applying regrowth applications
   c) prevent the tint from coming into contact with the skin and staining
   d) allow you to apply tint to the root area.

3 Quantities of colour and developer/peroxide should be mixed accurately:
   a) to make the colouring product last longer
   b) to ensure the target colour is achieved
   c) because manufacturers' instructions tell you to
   d) to make the colouring product runny enough to work with.

4 The highest strength of peroxide that is used in hairdressing is:
   a) 40 volume
   b) 9 per cent
   c) 20 volume
   d) 3 per cent.

5 A colour that sits on the cuticle and can slightly diffuse into the cortex is known as:
   a) permanent colour
   b) temporary colour
   c) a lightening product
   d) semi-permanent colour.

6 What colours are mixed on the colour wheel to obtain violet?
   a) Red and yellow
   b) Yellow and blue
   c) Blue and red
   d) Blue, red and yellow

7 Using the ICC system, the second number of a colour after the point or slash is:
   a) the depth of the colour
   b) the primary tone
   c) the base shade
   d) the secondary tone.

8 Opposites on the colour wheel will:

   a) complement one another

   b) neutralise one another

   c) contrast

   d) hide one another.

9 Quasi-permanent colours have the ability to:

   a) lighten the hair up to 3 levels of lift

   b) lighten the hair up to 2 levels of lift

   c) add depth and tone

   d) lighten the hair by 1 level of lift.

10 The best type of added heat to use during a bleaching service is:

   a) a steamer

   b) a climazone

   c) a hand-held hairdryer

   d) any of the above.

11 An incompatibility test is to determine whether:

   a) there are any styling products on the hair

   b) the hair can withstand the service

   c) the hair is in good condition

   d) there are any metallic salts present in the hair.

12 A skin test should be carried out:

   a) 12 hours before the service

   b) 24–48 hours prior to the service

   c) a week before the service

   d) every 6 months.

13 Application of tint to virgin hair should begin at:

   a) the root, mid-lengths then ends

   b) the ends, roots then mid-lengths

   c) the mid-lengths, ends then roots

   d) the ends, mid-lengths then roots.

14 What action should you take if the hair is too yellow?

   a) Reapply the bleach or use a violet toner

   b) Comb the tint through and use a quasi-permanent tint

   c) Pre-soften the hair

   d) Pre-pigment the hair

15 How many levels of lift can be achieved with bleach?

   a) 3–4

   b) 5

   c) 5–6

   d) 7

16 Products need to be mixed in a well-ventilated room because:
a) in natural daylight you can see the target colour better
b) some products need air in order to work
c) this will prevent breathing problems
d) the smell can be strong.

17 What are the three primary colours on the colour wheel?
a) Red, orange, yellow
b) Violet, blue, green
c) Red, yellow, blue
d) Green, red, yellow

18 What colour should be used to neutralise unwanted yellow tones in the hair?
a) Violet
b) Green
c) Red
d) Orange

19 What is meant by the 'depth' of a colour?
a) How bright the colour is
b) How light or dark the colour is
c) The tone that is present
d) How much build-up of colour there is on the hair

20 It is important to use an anti-oxy conditioner after a colouring service in order to:
a) prevent creeping oxidation and return the hair to its natural pH balance
b) prevent creeping oxidation and remove the smell of the colour
c) prevent creeping oxidation and put a barrier on the hair
d) prevent creeping oxidation and leave the hair with a high alkaline pH balance.

Getting ready for assessment

The assessment for the colouring hair unit is similar whether you are doing the NVQ or VRQ. You will be assessed using a combination of assessment methods, as described below. Remember that within each of the services you carry out with a client, you will cover different units. For example, when carrying out a colouring service (GH9), you will also have to be aware of health and safety (G20) and advise and consult with clients (G7). You may also shampoo and condition hair (GH8) and set or dress hair (GH11). If you are not sure what you have covered in your service, always ask your assessor or supervisor for advice.

	NVQ	VRQ
Credit value	11	10
Guided Learning Hours	105	91

	NVQ	VRQ
Practical demonstrations, to be observed by assessor	At least seven. You must cover all of the points listed in the range for this unit. Observations should include: • one regrowth application of permanent colour • one full head application of permanent colour • two applications of woven highlights and/or lowlights, one of which must be carried out on a full head • use of three out of the four colouring products listed in the range.	At least seven. You must cover all of the points listed in the range for this unit. Observations should include: • one regrowth application of permanent colour • one full head application of permanent colour • two applications of woven highlights and/or lowlights, one of which must be carried out on a full head • use of three out of the four colouring products listed in the range • performance of all tests • providing all types of aftercare advice.
Service timings	To achieve a competent assessment you will be required to complete the performances within a specified timescale. However, your tutor/salon manager can use their discretion if the head of hair you are working on is more 'challenging', i.e. extremely long or thick hair. • Regrowth application of permanent colour – 25 minutes • Partial head pulled-through highlights and/or lowlights covering at least 20 per cent of the head – 15 minutes • Full head pulled-through highlights and/or lowlights – 35 minutes • Full head woven highlights and/or lowlights – 75 minutes	• Regrowth application of permanent colour – 25 minutes • Partial head pulled-through highlights and/or lowlights covering at least 20 per cent of the head – 15 minutes • Full head pulled-through highlights and/or lowlights – 35 minutes • Full head woven highlights and/or lowlights – 75 minutes
Additional evidence	You will be required to complete a written independent paper to prove your understanding and knowledge. Other documentary (paper) evidence will need to be gathered to support your performances.	It is strongly recommended that all range items are practically demonstrated. Where this is not possible, other forms of evidence may be produced to demonstrate competence.

Task mapping

When you have completed the tasks in this unit, check the table below to see which Performance Criteria (purple), Range (red), Knowledge (green) and Key Skills (blue) you have covered within GH9 to use as additional evidence within your portfolio. Information about which Functional Skills you have covered is available on the website.

Task and page reference	Mapping to Performance Criteria, Range, Knowledge and Key Skills
1 (page 202)	Performance Criteria: 1g Range: N/A Knowledge: 4, 8, 16, VRQ 1o, 1q, 2o Key Skills: C1.2, C1.3
2 (page 204)	Performance Criteria: 1m Range: VRQ R5a–e Knowledge: 2 Key Skills: C1.2, C1.3, C2.3, N1.1, N1.2, N1.3, N2.1, N2.2, N2.3
3 (page 204)	Performance Criteria: 1j, 2a–d, 2h, VRQ 1b, 2a Range: 2a–f, 3a–e, 4a–i Knowledge: 28–34, 40, 47, VRQ 1g, 1i, 1j, 1k, 1m, 1o, 1p, 2m, 2n, 2o, 2p Key Skills: C1.1, C1.2, C1.3, C2.3
4 (page 215)	Performance Criteria: N/A Range: N/A Knowledge: N/A Key Skills: C1.2
5 (page 217)	Performance Criteria: 2h Range: 4b, 4c, 4h Knowledge: 35, 36, 37, VRQ 1k Key Skills: N1.1, N1.2, N1.3, N2.1, N2.2, N2.3
6 (page 223)	Performance Criteria: 2k, 3d–g, 3j, 3k Range: 1c, 1d Knowledge: 17, 19, 36, VRQ 1g, 1i, 1j, 1l Key Skills: C1.1, C1.2, C1.3, C2.1A, C2.2B
7 (page 228)	Performance Criteria: 1i, 2e, 3l Range: VRQ R3c, R3b, R4d, R4f Knowledge: 5, 6, 33, 61, 62, VRQ 1g, 1h, 2m Key Skills: C1.1, C1.3
8 (page 233)	Performance Criteria: 3m, VRQ 2m Range: 2a–f, VRQ R4a–i Knowledge: 5, 6, 35–41, 55, 56, 58, 60–63 Key Skills: C1.2, C1.3, C2.3

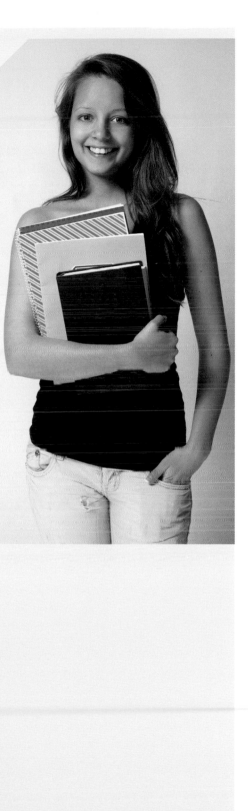

241

Unit

GH9

Change hair colour

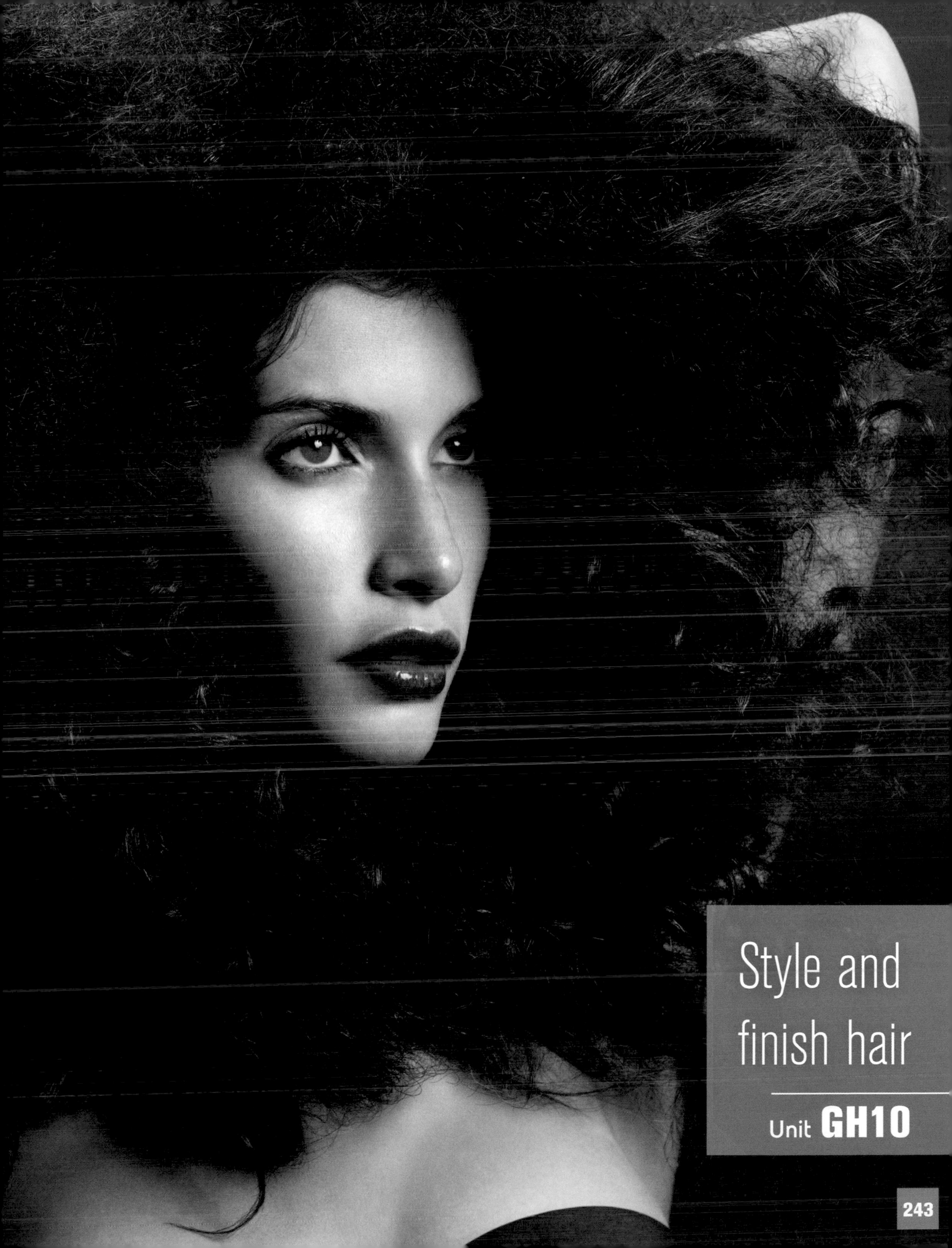

Style and
finish hair

Unit **GH10**

243

What you will learn:

- **How to maintain effective and safe methods of working**
- **How to blow-dry and finger-dry hair into shape**
- **How to dress and finish hair**
- **How to provide aftercare advice**

Introduction

In this unit you will be looking at the different techniques that can be used to style and finish the hair. This unit is important because every stylist has to be able to present the client with a satisfactory finished result.

You will learn about the properties of the hair that enable you to manipulate and work the hair into different styles. You will also learn how to blow-dry and finish the hair to achieve a variety of looks on long and short hair, using a range of tools and heated styling equipment. You will also find out about the products you will be using to carry out services while maintaining a high standard of health and safety as you work.

How to maintain effective and safe methods of working

You must ensure the health and safety of your client and yourself at all times. In this section you will learn about:

- preparing the client for blow-drying and finishing the hair
- choosing suitable products, equipment and tools
- following health and safety measures at work
- organising your working area and time effectively.

Preparing your client for blow-drying and finishing the hair

Gowning and positioning

Client comfort is always important. You must take care of your client when gowning and positioning her for a service.

- Make sure you have not tied the gown too tightly around the client's neck — she still needs to breathe!
- Always secure the towel with a clip so that it does not slide off the client.
- Remember when shampooing to use a disposable plastic cape on top of the towel for double protection.
- Make sure that the client is positioned correctly at the basin so that she is comfortable and the water cannot drip down her neck.
- Do not be afraid to reposition the client. If she is not sitting correctly, you cannot perform the service properly.
- Try not to let the client sit up in the chair before you towel-dry the hair.
- Remove the plastic cape and allow the client to dry her neck and ears.
- When you seat the client at your workstation, remove and replace the towel with a dry one and comb the hair through with a wide-toothed comb.

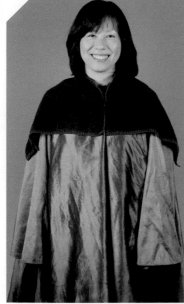

Make sure the client is gowned correctly

Task 1

In your training establishment or salon, find out what the correct gowning procedure is and compare this with your colleagues' to see if there are any differences. Discuss the benefits of each method.

When you seat your client in the chair at your workstation, it is important that the client is sitting squarely in front of the mirror with both feet flat on the floor or footrest. This is to enable you to move freely around your client and also to ensure that you get an even balance to the hairstyle.

Standing in the most comfortable and effective way

It is important to make sure that you position yourself correctly alongside your client while you are working. All your working positions should feel natural. The more comfortable you are, the less tired you will become.

Your work area

Your work area must be clean and tidy before you receive your client. This means putting away any electrical equipment that you will not be using and making sure that your work area is free from spillages, trailing wires or anything else that might cause harm to you or your client.

Potential hazards include:

- products such as wax or serum which may have dropped onto the floor – mop them up immediately
- tongs and hot brushes; if left on, these may pose a risk to your client.

It is also important to keep mirrors clean and wipe down work surfaces regularly. You need to be particularly careful if a client brings children into the salon.

Choosing suitable products, equipment and tools

Personal, learning and thinking skills – Independent enquiry

New products and tools are introduced to the hairdressing market on a regular basis. Your salon may work with a specific manufacturer and will be informed of their new products and tools. It is important to be up to date and knowledgeable across a wide range of products. This will enable you to answer clients' questions and ensure you are getting value for money. By carrying out some independent enquiries of your own, find out what new products and tools other companies are offering. Compare these with the range available in your own salon, and report the information to your manager.

Using products without being wasteful

For successful services, you need to know the effects of different products on all hair types. There is a wide range of products available, from those that protect the hair from the effects of atmospheric moisture, to products that make the hair easier to shape.

You need to know how, when and why you are using these products and the amount of product that you should be using. If you are wasteful when using products, you will be 'eating into' your salon's profits. It is always better to use a small amount

Fact or fiction?

Is this statement fact or fiction?

If a client sits with her legs crossed for the hairdressing service, you could end up with a lopsided result.

To check your answer see page 497.

245

Unit
GH10

Style and finish hair

Style and finish hair

and then apply a little more rather than squeezing too much out of the bottle or tube and having to throw it away. The following table will help you understand what the different types of products are used for.

Product	Application	Suitability	Comments
Gel (wet or dry look)	Apply to wet hair at the roots and spread through.	Firm hold – gives support to short, spiky styles.	Ideal for short, textured styles.
Mousse	Apply to wet hair and comb through evenly.	Medium to firm hold – gives body and bounce to hair.	Ideal for most hair types, but not very thick hair.
Glaze	Apply evenly to towel-dried hair.	Firm hold – dries hard.	Ideal for slicking back unruly hair.
Dressing cream	Apply small amount evenly with hands.	Light hold – large amounts will produce a slicked-back look.	Leaves hair sticky to touch.
Setting lotion	Sprinkle or spray from bottle onto towel-dried hair.	Light to firm hold – use with rollers for a firm result.	Good for all hair types; can leave the hair a little hard to the touch.
Blow-drying lotion	Apply before blow-drying.	Gives hair a softer look and feel.	Some contain chemicals that protect hair from heat.
Hairspray	Apply sparingly onto styled hair from a distance of 20 cm.	Holds finished style in place.	Brushes out; can have drying effect on hair; overuse may give the appearance of white flakes in the hair.
Hair gloss	Apply small amounts on wet hair.	Reduces frizz and increases shine.	Ideal for African-type hair.
Moisturiser	Apply to hair before styling.	Makes hair soft and shiny; loosens tangles.	Useful for conditioning African-type hair.
Activators	Apply to wet or dry hair.	Used to maintain curl or replace moisture in permed or naturally curly hair.	Defines curl; adds moisture and shine to hair.
Heat protectors	Apply to dry hair before using heated styling equipment. Many styling products contain their own heat protector.	Will coat the hair with a protective layer to stop the natural oils drying out of the hair.	Excessive amounts may give the hair an oily appearance.
Serum	Apply to either wet or dry hair where required.	Ideal for naturally dry, brittle hair and hair that has had excessive use of lightening products or heated styling equipment on it.	May weigh down very fine hair. If used on the root area when not required could produce an oily effect.
Waxes	Apply small amounts to dry hair	Used to create a textured look in the hair and give a degree of hold.	Some wax needs to be softened in the hands before applying. Overuse of wax can result in making the style heavy and cause it to collapse. Not suitable for very fine hair.

Some styling, dressing and finishing products

Correct equipment and tools for blow-drying

When you blow-dry, the length of hair dictates the size of the brush that you choose. This is why stylists have a wide and varied range of brushes. To start with, you will only need a basic range of brushes. As you gain experience and master different techniques, you may wish to add to your equipment.

Tool		Effect	Suitability
Denman brush		Use for a smooth finish, e.g. a 'bob' style.	Hair only requiring a slight curve or straight finish; curl cannot be achieved.
Vent brush		Produces a soft, casual 'broken-up' effect.	Good for a quick casual result; not very suitable for curling.
Circular brushes		Good for producing a curled effect. The smaller the brush, the tighter the curl.	Large round brushes are ideal for long hair; smaller brushes for shorter hair. Any round brush can tangle in hair.
Setting rollers for wet setting		Various sizes for different degrees of curl.	Suitable for all hair types to produce soft to firm curls.
Diffuser		Encourages curl into hair by scrunching the hair into the diffuser.	Ideal for permed or naturally curly hair.

Style and finish hair

Tool		Effect	Suitability
Dressing-out combs		Use for backcombing and teasing style into hair.	Use for all dressing-out techniques.
African Caribbean and wide-toothed combs		Use to detangle hair.	Suitable for straight and curly hair.
Velcro rollers for dry setting		Good for body and bounce.	Normally only suitable for dry setting; produce a very soft curl.
Hand dryer		Use to remove moisture from the hair and to produce a variety of blow-dried looks.	High temperature settings should not be used on very fine, fragile or dry hair. Creates body and lift, straight and smooth looks.
Hand dryer with nozzle		Use to remove moisture from the hair and to produce a variety of blow-dried looks.	The nozzle helps to direct the airflow more specifically. Care must be taken not to burn the scalp!

Styling tools and techniques

Following health and safety measures at work

When working in the salon, you are responsible for the health and safety of yourself and your client (see G20). You need to make sure your client is gowned correctly for the service and use the correct PPE to ensure that you don't develop contact **dermatitis** while carrying out styling and finishing services.

Task 2

Using G20 as your reference, complete the table provided on the website to identify the most suitable methods of sterilisation for the styling tools and equipment listed.

A worksheet for this task is provided on the website for you to complete and add to your portfolio.

Information from manufacturers

All manufacturers of hair services and products must, by law, supply manufacturers' data sheets to comply with the Control of Substances Hazardous to Health (COSHH) Regulations 2003. These sheets provide you with everything you need to know about the product you are using – the ingredients, the handling and storage of the product, and any disposal considerations.

The sheets will also tell you the first aid measures to follow if the product comes into contact with the eyes or skin, or if it is swallowed.

What would you do if some of the styling products that you were using accidentally ended up in the client's eye? Ideally, you should call a first aider, but if one is not available immediately then you need to take action. By following the first aid measures stated on the manufacturer's data sheet, you will be able to deal with the problem until a first aider is available.

Your responsibilities relating to legislation

As a stylist, you must be aware of your own responsibilities under the COSHH Regulations (see G20, pages 56–57). All products used in hairdressing are covered by these regulations as they relate to:

- handling chemicals
- storing chemicals
- disposing of chemicals.

Dermatitis

Inflammation or allergy of the skin, sometimes called contact dermatitis. Usually affecting the hands of hairdressers, it causes the hands and fingers to crack and bleed due to constantly being wet and coming into contact with chemicals. Drying hands thoroughly after shampooing, using a good barrier cream and always wearing gloves when using chemicals will help avoid this condition.

COSHH information for: Hydrogen peroxide

General Description

Stabilised acidic aqueous solutions or emulsions containing Hydrogen Peroxide of various strengths for use with:

- Permanent tints
- Bleach powder
- Permanent waves as neutralisers
- Hair lighteners
- Straighteners
- Dye remover

Hazardous Ingredients

- Hydrogen Peroxide up to 60 vol or 10%

Hazard

- Irritant to eyes and skin

Precautions when in use

- Always wear protective gloves
- Avoid contact with eyes and face
- Do not use on abraded or sensitive skin
- Always use non-metallic utensils, to avoid rapid decomposition of the product

Storage Precautions

- Store in a cool, dry place away from sunlight and other sources of heat
- Always store Hydrogen Peroxide in the container supplied
- It is particularly important that no contamination enters the container as this could lead to decomposition resulting in the liberation of heat and oxygen
- Replace cap immediately after use

Manufacturer's data sheet for hydrogen peroxide

Task 3

1. In your salon or college/training establishment, find out where the manufacturers' data sheets and risk assessment sheets are located. Select six products you frequently use and obtain copies of their sheets for your portfolio.
2. Hairspray contains many chemicals, some of which are flammable (easily catch fire). Find out and make a note of the following information for your portfolio:
   - the safety considerations to be taken into account when using hairspray
   - the correct procedure for storing a can of hairspray
   - the correct procedure for disposing of an empty can of hairspray.

A worksheet for this task is provided on the website for you to complete and add to your portfolio.

Salon life

Cutting corners

Joe's story

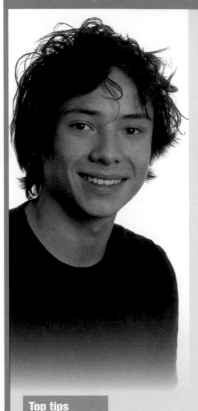

It was a really busy day and the basins were filling up fast so I took my client to be shampooed before checking my consultation sheet with my tutor as I'm supposed to. After shampooing and conditioning, I took my client back to my workstation before asking my tutor to come over so I could talk through what I was going to do. When she finally got to me, she told me off for shampooing prior to discussing the client's needs with her, but as the client wanted a straightforward one-length cut, she was happy for me to begin.

I'd been cutting my client's hair for about 5 minutes when I noticed whitish, brownish 'bits' attached to her hair. I asked her if she had dry skin or had used a product that might have left a residue, but she hadn't. On closer inspection I realised that my client had nits!

I told my tutor straightaway and she confirmed it before explaining the best course of action to my client. Then my tutor told me that because I was halfway through the cut I had to finish it. Afterwards I had to sterilise all the tools and equipment that I had used. I even had to sterilise the work surfaces and the chair and trolley. This took so much time that I lost half my lunch hour.

My tutor praised me on the professional way I handled the situation, but pointed out that had I not gone over to the basin to save time, the infestation would have been spotted at the consultation and I wouldn't have lost half my lunch break! I now know the importance of not cutting corners – if it had been anything worse than nits, I could have unknowingly infected other clients, students or even myself!

Top tips

If you are unsure of anything you see on the hair or scalp and suspect it may be a disease or disorder, always ask for a second opinion. You may not have come across it before, but someone else may have done.

Ask the expert

Q *I have been told that if a client has psoriasis you can still carry out a hairdressing service. Is this true?*

A Yes – as long as the skin is not broken (from scratching the area), most physical (non-chemical services) can be carried out. You would need to make the client aware (if they didn't already know) that they have this skin condition. You can reassure them it isn't contagious but that they may like to consult a pharmacist for a specialised shampoo. In extreme cases, the client should consult their doctor. If you are going to be using any products on the hair you need to be careful with your application, as they may 'sting' the affected areas.

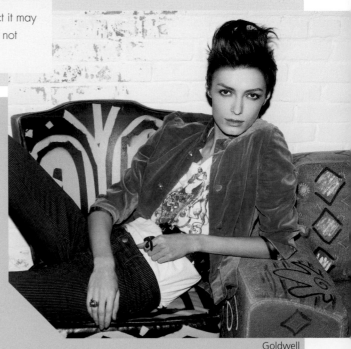

Goldwell

Organising your working area and time effectively

Organising yourself and your time at work is an important part of your role as a stylist. Every salon allows a set amount of time for every process that is carried out, from shampooing to colouring.

Organisation for blow-drying

You must have:

- a hairdryer and other electrical equipment such as electric tongs and straighteners
- a good selection of brushes and combs for blow-drying and finishing
- a selection of styling and finishing products.

A good trolley layout with all the necessary equipment will allow you to spend more time with the client on the service. Generally salons allocate the following timings to each service:

- shampoo and conditioning: 5–10 minutes depending on the length of the hair
- blow-drying: 30–40 minutes, again depending on the length of the hair.

Safe working for you, your clients and colleagues

Personal hygiene

If you have overslept and not had time for a shower in the morning, not only are you going to feel uncomfortable but your work colleagues and clients might as well! Personal hygiene is as important as keeping your tools and equipment clean and sterilised, and you should have the same standards for yourself.

You should:

- make sure you wash your hands before each client, especially if you are a smoker
- use mints or a breath freshener if you have had strong-smelling food the previous night, for example a curry
- wear a minimal amount of jewellery
- ensure your uniform is freshly laundered and ironed
- wear your hair tied back if that is a salon requirement
- wear a small amount of make-up to portray a professional appearance
- wear shoes that are comfortable and that you can stand in for long periods of time
- use your common sense and think about the image you would like to see when you walk into a professional salon
- conduct yourself in a manner when using tools and equipment that will not put yourself or others at risk
- make regular checks of your equipment
- keep your work area clean, tidy and free of trailing wires, products or anything else that could cause harm or injury.

Consultation

For every hairdressing service, an in-depth consultation is the key to success. Without gathering the right kind of information from your client, you will not be able to fulfil her wishes.

Style books

Style books will also help you and your client agree together what kind of look is going to be achieved. Using style books as a basis of discussion also helps you to

251

Unit
GH10

Style and finish hair

Fact or fiction?

Is this statement fact or fiction?

If you do not identify infestations before you shampoo, then you are obliged to complete the service.

To check your answer see page 497.

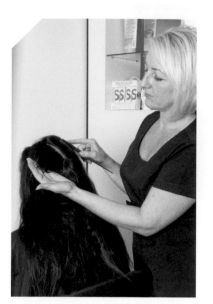

An in-depth consultation is key to success

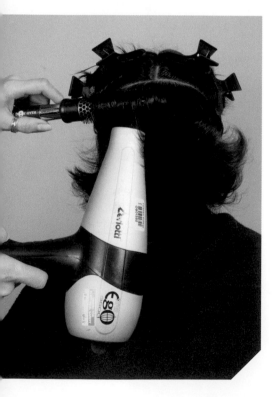

252

Unit
GH10

Style and finish hair

identify to the client what type of products have been used and what kind of aftercare will be needed at home.

Task 4

In pairs and using style books, carry out a consultation on each other. Identify what size brushes and the type of products you will need to achieve the desired end result. Write a short statement giving the appropriate aftercare advice.

Completing the service within a commercially viable time

A salon will work out the timings of its services so that all time is used to its best advantage and that it sees enough clients to make a profit. As a stylist, you need to be aware of the timescale that you have to carry out various services.

Until you gain experience you will not be expected to work to these time constraints, but you need to aware of the times that you have to work towards to be financially viable for your salon.

Blow-dry and finger-dry hair into shape

Most hairstyles have been blow-dried or finished in some way. For daily wear, most people want styles that are easy to manage. In this section you will learn how to use current drying and finishing techniques to be able to produce these styles, taking into account different hair types and critical influencing factors. You will also be looking at the effect blow-drying has on the hair's structure and the effect that moisture in the atmosphere has on the hair.

In this section you will learn about:

- consulting and preparing before styling
- blow-drying hair using correct products and tools
- critical styling techniques that ensure client comfort
- blow-drying and finger-drying techniques.

Consulting and preparing before styling

Consulting the client

During the consultation, check:

- for anything that may prevent you from carrying out the service such as infections and infestations
- the type of hair you are working on – look at the texture and density of hair as this will influence the choice of styling products
- any critical influencing factors that may influence the blow-dry, such as head and face shape and double crowns
- how the client is currently wearing her hair – if the client wants the same style, you have an advantage by seeing her hair before it is shampooed
- how much natural movement there is in the hair – this will affect your product choice and the choice of brush size
- whether there are any natural partings – it is always better to allow the hair to fall into its natural partings as the style will last longer.

Types of questions to ask during the consultation

- Is the curl in your hair a perm or is it naturally curly (if relevant)?
- Would you like a styling product on your hair?
- How would you like your hair blow-dried? (Use style books to help.)
- Is it a daytime or an evening look?
- Do you get any problems with particular parts of the hair? (Let the client identify what she considers to be awkward areas.)

Questions to ask during the service

- Is the heat of the hairdryer comfortable for you?
- Is that enough body and height for you?
- Are you happy with the finished result?

It is important to check during the service that the client is happy with the way her hair is taking shape. This is the time to make any changes that either of you may feel are appropriate or necessary.

Blow-drying hair using correct products and tools

When you have completed your client consultation using the checklist on page 252, you should have gathered enough information to help you decide on your choice of products, equipment and techniques that you are going to use. If you are unable to make all of these choices, then you have not completed a thorough consultation!

Controlling your styling tools

You need to be able to control your equipment and the hair as you blow-dry it. The way in which you manage the hair is very important, as this will affect the finished result. Here are some tips to help you.

- Rough-dry excess moisture from the hair before you begin to style it.
- Take small sections to allow the heat of the hairdryer, electric tongs and heated brush to dry/penetrate the mesh of hair.
- The airflow from the hairdryer should flow over the cuticle in the direction of the hairstyle, not against it – to do so would roughen the cuticle scales, making the hair look fluffy and dull.
- Try not to direct the heat from the hairdryer directly onto the scalp, as this will cause great discomfort to the client.
- When using electric tongs or other electrical equipment, do not allow the tongs to come into contact with the scalp – see the photo, right.
- Do not over-dry the hair. When a mesh of hair is dry you will not be able to alter its shape.
- Adjust the height that the client is sitting at to enable you to work around her effectively.
- Always warn the client if you are going to adjust the position of the seat.
- When blow-drying the nape of the hair, position the client's head downwards so that you can work freely in that area.
- Remember to change hands (with the dryer and brush) so that you can work effectively around the head.
- Section off the bulk of the hair that you are not working with so that you work in a controlled manner.

Top tips

The consultation is the first communication that you have with the client. It is important to spend time questioning the client on her requirements and expectations. It is also the time when you need to complete a blow-drying analysis. It may be useful to prepare a checklist to help you.

253

Unit

GH10

Style and finish hair

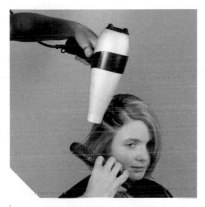

Air should flow from the hair roots down over the hair to the ends

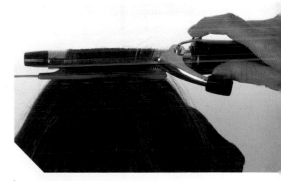

Hold the electric tongs in the correct position so as to avoid contact with the scalp

Top tips

- When blow-drying, always work from roots to points, keeping the cuticle scales flat.
- Keep the dryer moving to avoid burning the hair or scalp.
- Keep an even tension on the hair but do not overstretch it by pulling too hard.

Step-by-step blow-drying technique

1 Section the hair evenly into four equal sections.

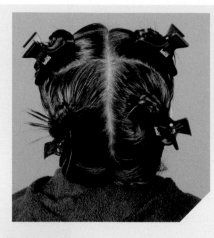

2 Beginning at the nape and working up towards the crown area, style the hair ensuring the direction of airflow from the dryer flows over the hair from root to point.

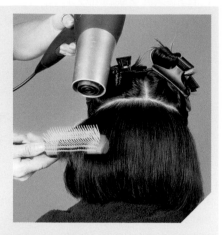

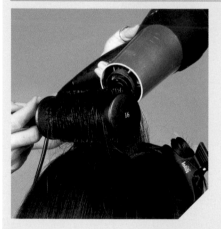

3 Work to the crown area and direct the hair backwards — this helps to achieve root lift and height at the crown area. You may like to change your choice of brush to achieve more root lift at this point.

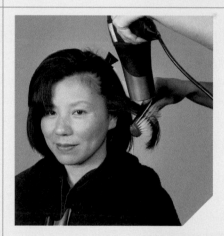

4 Moving to the sides, take a small section and continue to blow-dry the hair under. Be careful not to brush the ear or burn it with the dryer.

5 At the fringe area you may wish to use a different brush depending on the amount of root lift you want to achieve. Remember to change your body position, so the heat of the dryer is flowing over the hair shaft in the correct way.

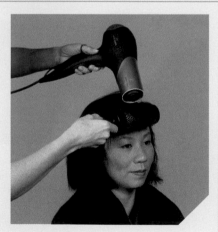

6 Confirm your client is happy and you have achieved a balanced end result. Apply finishing products as required and provide the appropriate aftercare advice.

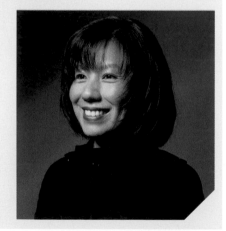

Using the correct tension and meshes of hair to suit the styling tools and process

When blow-drying, it is important that you use the correct size of meshes. This is so that:

- the heat from the hairdryer can penetrate the hair mesh evenly, enabling you to dry the hair evenly
- the mesh of hair suits the length and width of the brush you have chosen, so that hair does not get caught and tangled around the sides
- heat from electrical appliances can penetrate the mesh of hair to achieve the result required
- you work in a methodical manner covering the whole of the head, ensuring all of the hair is dry.

It is equally important that you keep tension even along the mesh of hair when you work so that:

- the curl you may be putting into the hair from either a brush, tongs or hot brush gives you an even result along the section of hair
- if you are straightening the hair, you will ensure an even result.

Task 5

Practise holding the hairdryer in your left hand and using the brush with your right hand, and then change over. You must be able to work with both hands when blow-drying. Ask your tutor to check that the size of the meshes you have taken are correct for the size of the brush.

Applying styling products to control the hair, taking into account critical influencing factors

You have looked at the use of styling products (see page 246), at what they do and their suitability for different types of hair. Styling products can also be used to help you overcome or control some of the critical influencing factors that you may experience.

Styling aids

Because the hair has the ability to absorb water (allowing you to shampoo it), it can also absorb **atmospheric moisture**. By using styling products you are putting a slight barrier on the hair, which will protect the hair from atmospheric moisture and help prevent your finished look from collapsing. Styling products also help to protect the hair from the effects of added heat when styling.

Blow-dries may not last long, because as soon as the hair comes into contact with atmospheric moisture it will start to drop.

The use of setting or styling products will help to produce a longer-lasting blow-dry. There are several types of products but all modern products work in the same way. They coat the outside of the hair shaft in a plastic film. This prevents atmospheric moisture penetrating the cuticle layer.

Top tips

Correct use of heat will allow the hair to be dried into its new shape, leaving it manageable with bounce and shine. Incorrect use of heat will dry out the hair by roughening the cuticle scale and leaving the hair in poor condition.

255

Unit

GH10

Style and finish hair

Atmospheric moisture

Humidity (water) in the air (atmosphere) from, for example, rain, a shower or a bath.

Unit

GH10

Style and finish hair

Factors to consider when styling hair

These modern products are made of plasticisers, e.g. Polyvinyl Pyrolidone, which is a clear film that dissolves in hot water and shampoo. It is therefore removed easily from the hair. The products soften the hair shaft, allowing shapes to be formed readily, and prevent the hair from becoming 'fly-away', which makes it more manageable when it is styled and finished. They also protect the hair from added heat.

Influencing factors

When choosing products, equipment and blow-drying techniques, you should consider the following factors.

Factor	What to consider
Hair texture	Very fine hair will need a product that gives it lift and volume, and some styling brushes would not be suitable.
Haircut	The length of the layers and style will determine what size brush you will use and what type of product. If it is a very textured cut, you may need to use more than one product on the hair.
Head and face shape	These influence the choice of drying technique and how you style the hair.
Hair growth patterns	You may need a 'firm hold' product to help you to style the hair to disguise a double crown or to hold down a fringe with a cowlick.
Hair elasticity	This will influence your product choice and choice of equipment; for example you would not use electric tongs or a heated brush on hair that had poor elasticity because you would be adding heat to already 'stressed' hair. You may choose to use a product that will help to improve the condition of the hair, such as serum or a gloss.
Hair length	If you are working on very long hair, you may need to use a product that is not too heavy, to avoid weighing the hair down. You may want to opt for a light blow-drying lotion.
Hair density	This will have an influence on your product choice. If the client has very thick hair, you will not want to use a product that will increase the volume in the hair.

As well as using styling products to help you control critical influencing factors, you also need to be aware of what equipment and styling techniques can be used to help you with potential problems.

Dealing with critical influencing factors

Problem	Solution
Strong cowlick movement in the fringe area on straight hair	Use a firm hold product at the roots. Blow-dry the hair in the opposite direction to the way it wants to sit. Finish with a firm hold spray.
Flat spot at the back of the head	Use a root-lift product. Direct the heat of the hairdryer into the roots to achieve maximum lift using a round brush (pick the size of brush suitable for the length of hair you are working on).

Changing the hair's structure

When you shampoo, you are not only removing dirt and grease from the hair but you are also changing the properties of the hair that make it possible to alter its shape temporarily by blow-drying.

The hair has two key properties:

- it is **hygroscopic** — able to absorb water
- it has natural elasticity — it will stretch and return to its original shape.

Hair in its natural state is called **alpha keratin**. Hair in its stretched state is called **beta keratin**.

Hygroscopic

Able to absorb water.

Alpha keratin

Hair in its natural state.

Beta keratin

Hair in its stretched state.

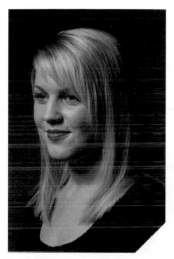 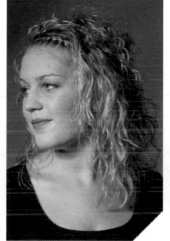 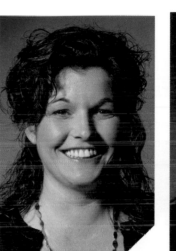 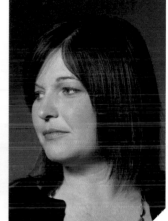

Straight hair becomes curly, changing alpha to beta keratin

Naturally curly hair becomes straight, changing alpha to beta keratin

Without the hair's ability to absorb water and stretch and return to its original shape, you would not be able to alter its shape.

When hair is shampooed, water is absorbed into the cortex. The water breaks down the hydrogen bonds (which are the weaker bonds in the hair) and allows the hair to be stretched. By applying heat to the hair in this stretched state, you can re-form the bonds into a new shape around either a brush or a roller (the hair is now in its beta keratin state). This is called a physical change because it is only temporary and the hair can be blow-dried or set as often as required.

Blow-drying and finger-drying techniques

There are a number of different looks that you can achieve when blow-drying, from a very soft, casual look, to a firmer, more set-looking style. The tools and techniques that you use will help you to produce these looks (look back at pages 247–48 to remind yourself of the equipment available).

257

Unit
GH10

Style and finish hair

Blow-dry on straight, long, one-length hair

The bob is a classic style that when dried correctly will look smooth and sleek. What you will need:

- client with one-length hair
- Denman or medium to large round brush
- selection of styling and finishing products
- sectioning clips
- hairdryer (possibly straightening irons)
- dressing-out combs.

Blow-dry of one-length hair

1 Firstly, hair would be sectioned into four then a section dropped at the nape of the neck and blow-dried under. Sections would then be taken down and blow-dried in this way up to the crown area. Next a section is brought down at the sides and blow-dried.

2 Either a round brush or a Denman brush can be used to smooth the hair at the sides as you continue to work your way up the sides of the head to the parting.

3 Allow the hair to cool before applying finishing products. Check your balance and the client's satisfaction. Provide the appropriate aftercare advice.

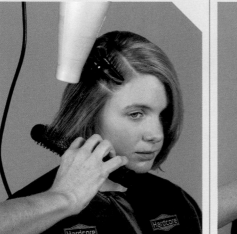 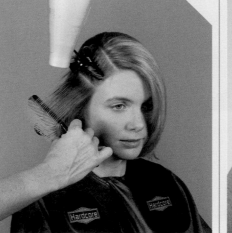 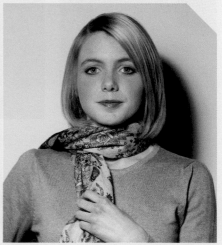

Blow-dry on short, straight or curly layered hair

These are often referred to as 'back and bubbly' styles because they follow a specific design and require a small round brush for a firm hold. When you blow-dry the hair, it will look like little sausages all over the head! What you will need:

- client with short, layered hair
- hairdryer (possibly electric tongs or hot brush)
- selection of round brushes
- sectioning clips
- selection of styling and finishing products
- dressing-out combs.

Step-by-step blow-dry on short, straight or curly layered hair

1 Divide the hair into four and bring down a sub-section of hair at the nape. Blow-dry this section in the direction required.

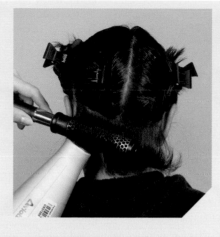

2 Release one of the main back sections and continue to blow-dry the hair in the desired manner.

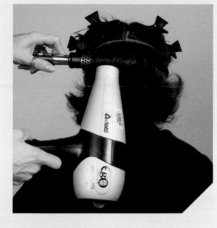

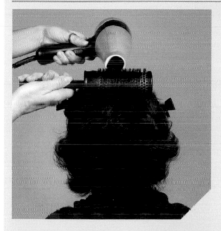

3 At the crown area, blow-dry the hair down creating body and root lift. A larger brush is used to create more volume and less curl.

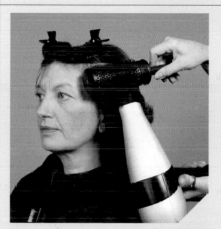

4 Release a section at the side and blow-dry in the desired direction. Maintain good control of your hairdryer to avoid disturbing the hair that you have already blow dried.

5 From the top sections, continue to join the side sections to achieve a balanced shape.

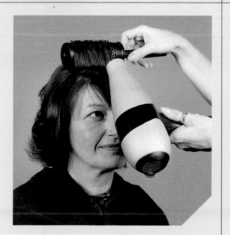

6 The finished result. Run your fingers through the hair to soften the look, while using the cool setting on your hairdryer to close the cuticle and fix the curl. Apply appropriate finishing products to suit the hair type, and provide aftercare advice.

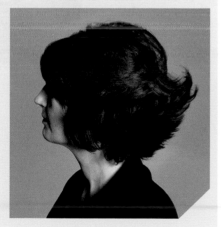

259

Unit
GH10

Style and finish hair

Scrunch-drying on permed or naturally curly hair

Using this technique will encourage the curl into the hair. You want to control the hair so that the curl is well formed and does not appear frizzy. What you will need:

- client with naturally curly or permed hair
- hairdryer with diffuser
- selection of styling and finishing products
- sectioning clips.

Style and finish hair

Scrunch-drying hair

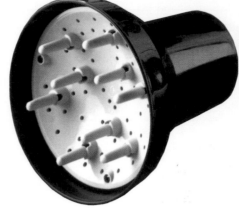

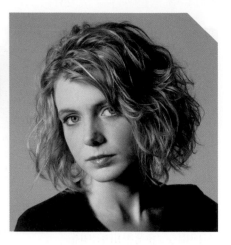

When using a diffuser, the hair should be sectioned to allow you to work in manageable sections. The hair can 'sit' into the diffuser, while you use your hand to scrunch the curl into the hair. The diffuser takes away the force of the airflow and leaves the heat, allowing the hair to dry into its curl.

Finger-drying short hair

1 Apply a small amount of styling product – dispense into your hands and spread evenly through the hair.

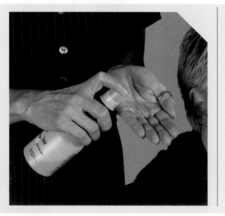

2 Using your fingers, mould the hair and lift the roots to achieve the desired result.

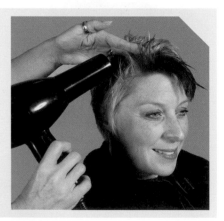

Keeping the hair moist throughout the service

When styling the hair, it is important that the hair does not dry out before you have blow-dried it into the shape required. Use a water spray to dampen the hair slightly; you may find that this will be required more often on fine hair, as it has a tendency to dry out more quickly than thick hair.

If the hair does dry out and you do not moisten it, you will not achieve a smooth finish and the style will not last as long. This is because the hydrogen bonds will have re-formed into the hair's natural state and not taken on the shape of the roller or brush that you are using to style the hair (refer back to page 257).

Ensuring you achieve the volume, balance and curl required

Throughout any of the blow-drying services, always check with your client that:

- you are working towards the style desired by the client – check that the parting is in the right place
- you are achieving the correct amount of width and height that the client requires
- she is happy with the finished result.

Dress and finish hair

In this section you will be looking at how to use heated styling equipment, taking into account health and safety issues. You will also be looking at how to use backcombing and backbrushing techniques and applying finishing products to complete the look required by the client.

Other considerations

- Keep even tension without pulling the hair from the scalp.
- Do not use electrical equipment with wet hands.

Using heated styling equipment

Additional equipment

Other equipment you can use to help give extra support or to smooth and straighten the hair as you blow-dry includes:

- electric (heated) tongs
- hot brushes
- straightening irons
- crimping irons
- heated rollers.

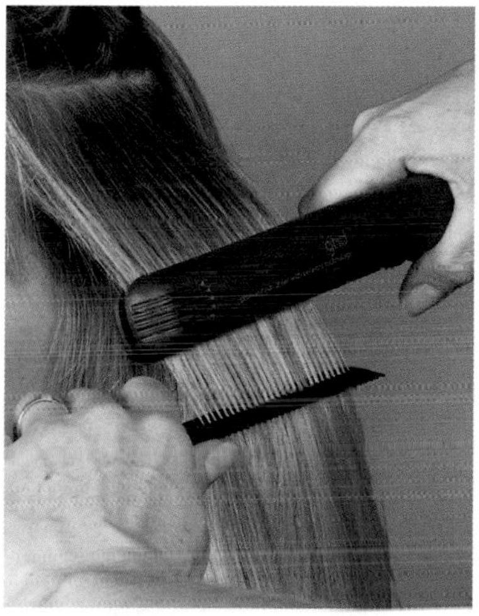

These are very useful pieces of equipment, but they should only be used to add support to the blow-dry that you have already completed. It is not appropriate to rough-dry a client's hair and then go back through with a set of tongs or hot brush to put curl into the hair. The chart below outlines the uses of each of these pieces of equipment.

Straightening irons

Tool	Effect	Suitability	Comments
Electric (heated) tongs 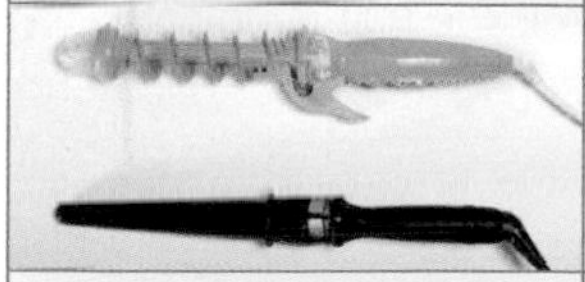	Produces curls, waves and ringlets.	Only to be used on dry hair; useful for all hair types but not very porous or damaged hair.	Hair ends must be wound smoothly around barrel to prevent buckled ends. Make sure that you place a comb between the tongs and scalp to prevent them from touching.
Hot air brushes 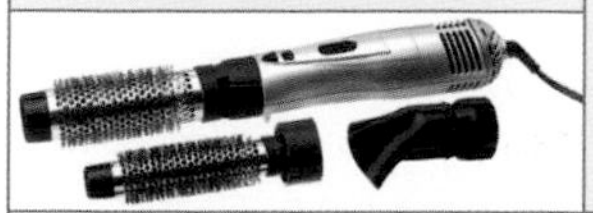	Produces a softer curl.	Only to be used on dry hair; finer sections need to be taken on thick hair.	Easier to work with than electric tongs, but can become tangled in hair. Make sure that you place a comb between the brush and scalp to prevent the brush from touching the scalp.
Crimping irons 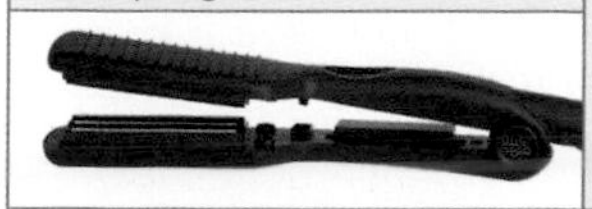	Creates volume in hair, producing a line of crimps.	Only to be used on dry hair; not suitable for very short hair.	The finer the sections of hair, the better the end result.
Straightening irons 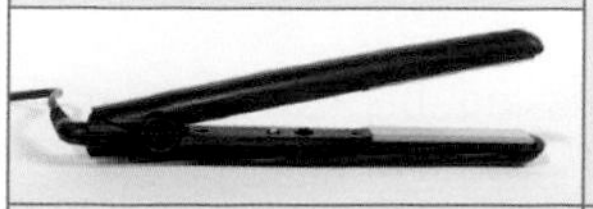	Straightens hair. Curls and waves can also be produced.	Only to be used on dry hair; not suitable for very porous, dry hair.	Overuse dries out hair.
Heated rollers 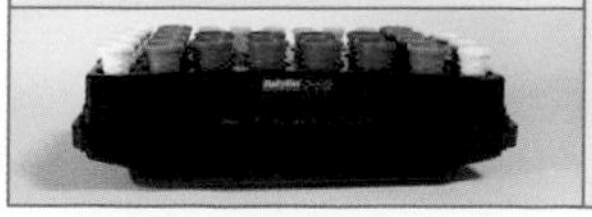	Adds soft curl and body to hair.	Only to be used on dry hair.	If sections taken are too large, the hair can become tangled and the heat won't be able to penetrate the mesh of hair. The rollers need to be allowed to cool while in place to achieve a firm result.

Electrical tools

Unit
GH10

Style and finish hair

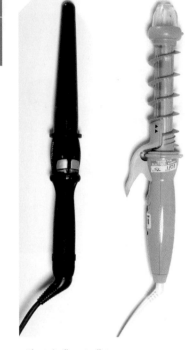

Electric (heated) tongs

Health and safety rules when working with electrical equipment

To minimise the risk of damage to your tools and to work safely you should:

- never place tongs, hot brushes or crimpers directly on the scalp – this will cause serious burns to the client
- make sure the heat is not directed on one spot when using a nozzle attachment on a hairdryer
- always sit tongs and hot brushes on the stand so as not to scorch work surfaces
- always check the heat setting and speed controls before you start blow-drying
- regularly clean the air intake grille at the back of hairdryers to remove dust and fluff to prevent hairdryers from overheating
- put away equipment when not in use
- avoid winding flexes of electrical equipment too tightly when storing
- never store tongs, hot brushes or other electrical equipment until they have cooled down.

You should regularly carry out the following safety checks.

- Make sure all plugs are wired correctly.
- Make sure the dryer cable is safe. (Look for frayed flexes and loose plug tops.)
- Keep your equipment free of product build-up by cleaning frequently with an alcohol-based solution. (Note: only do this when the equipment is cooled and unplugged.)
- Check the heat settings at regular intervals.

By law, all electrical equipment should be checked by a qualified electrician every six months.

Dressing-out techniques

Dressing out a blow-dry

Only dress out a blow-dry if the hair is completely dry. Even if the hair is only slightly damp, it will go back to its original shape, lose its springiness and then you will not achieve the style you want.

To dress out a blow-dry:

- make sure the hair is completely dry
- use heated styling equipment if more movement is required
- loosen the blow-dry by running your fingers through the hair
- apply backcombing if required
- use a dressing-out comb to lift, smooth and shape the hair
- check the balance of the style by using your mirror and turning the client's head to view the style from different angles.

Backcombing, teasing and backbrushing

If you want to add height and width to a blow-dry when dressing, backcomb the hair. If you do not want to add too much height, but want to remove blow-drying marks from the hair, tease the hair into shape using the prongs on a dressing-out comb.

Backbrushing is carried out using the same method as backcombing, but the comb is exchanged for a flat bristle brush. Backbrushing provides a slightly softer effect, and allows you to cover a greater area of hair.

For a fuller account of backcombing, backbrushing and teasing methods, refer to page 286.

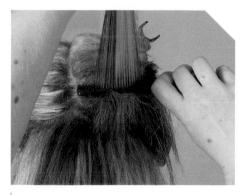

Backcombing

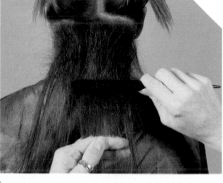

Backbrushing

Applying finishing products, taking into account critical influencing factors

You have looked at the different types of styling products that are available to you (refer to page 246). What you need to consider at this stage is what products you will use to help you to achieve the finished result. Most products can be used on wet or dry hair and will give very different effects on both.

Finishing products are:

- dressing creams
- oils
- sprays
- waxes
- gels.

Finishing products can also be used to help hide any critical influencing factors (see page 256).

If a client has very fine hair, use a product to give the appearance of thickness and bulk to the hair. If the client has dry, fluffy or coarse hair, a finishing cream or oil will give the hair shine and lustre.

Some critical influencing factors cannot always be hidden with styling or products. If this is the case, make sure that you adapt your styling (end result) so that you work with the problems. For example, if you have a client who has very fine, straight hair, you would find it difficult to achieve a really textured look.

Top tips

It is important to look at your client's hair both before and after you have shampooed the hair, so that you can identify any potential problems and address them with your products and styling techniques.

Task 6

In groups or pairs, think of as many critical influencing factors as you can.
Look at each of these in turn and identify the relevant product that you think will help overcome the problem.

A worksheet for this task is provided on the website for you to complete and add to your portfolio.

Confirm the finished look with the client, giving the correct aftercare advice

Throughout the service you should be communicating constantly with your client.

- Confirm the style before you begin.
- Check the client is comfortable.
- Check that you have achieved the intended shape, direction and amount of volume required.
- Is there enough hairspray on the hair?

Finally, the most important question – ask your client whether she likes the end result! The client may have a few suggestions and it is important to listen to and respect her wishes. If, however, you strongly disagree, explain why and come to a compromise (a solution that suits you both).

Provide aftercare advice

Giving your client aftercare advice is an important part of the overall service. You do not want to produce something in the salon that the client will never be able to achieve again – that will only dishearten her!

Explain to the client what you are doing throughout the service:

- what tools and equipment you are using and why you are using them
- show the client the correct angle at which to hold the hairdryer and brush
- explain what products you are using, why you are using them and what you hope to achieve by using them
- show the client the amount of product you are using and the benefits of the product.

Products

When you use products on your client in the salon, it is a good time to discuss aftercare products the client can use at home. This doesn't mean you are doing a 'hard sell' on your client; rather, you are giving advice on how she can achieve the same results that you have produced while maintaining and caring for her hair. As well as recommending products she can use, you can also offer advice on the products she should avoid or perhaps use less of. If a client has a build-up of hairspray (white flakes on the hair shaft) you could suggest she change to a spray gel, which will also give a firm hold.

Heated equipment

Most clients will have used some form of heated styling equipment in the shape of a hairdryer, tongs, hot brush or straighteners. Overuse of any of these pieces of equipment can have a drying effect on the hair and extreme overuse will have a permanent damaging effect on the hair's structure. You should offer advice backed up with a demonstration of the correct use of the heated appliances and recommend heat protector products to help prevent any further damage. You can also introduce the client to conditioning treatments that are carried out in the salon or recommend a product the client can use at home.

Lifestyle

You should always consider your client's lifestyle when discussing suitable style choices for her. If she has a young family, a busy career or is active in sports, she won't have a lot of time to spend on blow-drying and straightening her hair every morning. You will need to work with the natural movement (if any) in the hair and perhaps suggest colour to add further interest. You will need to explain carefully to your client the work involved in the upkeep of her chosen style to ensure suitability.

If you give good aftercare advice, your client is more likely to purchase the products that you have recommended from your salon and to believe in you and the advice given.

Evaluate the result of the treatment with the client

On most consultation sheets there will be a box for the client to say if they were happy with the service and end result. It is good practice to evaluate your own work and performance regularly, so that you can track your progression.

The following questions will help to provide a framework for your self-evaluation.

- Did you select the correct tools, products and equipment?
- Did you achieve an end result pleasing to both yourself and the client?
- Did you complete the work within the set time constraints?
- Are there any areas that you need to improve on?

Check your knowledge

The following questions will help you to check your understanding of this unit.
The answers can be found on pages 497–8.

1   What is the best way to gown your client for a blow-drying process?
  a) Gown and towel
  b) Gown only
  c) Gown and disposable plastic cape
  d) Gown, towel and disposable plastic cape

2   The styling product gel is suitable for which hair type?
  a) Very thick straight hair
  b) Fine hair that requires support at the root
  c) Short textured styles
  d) African-type hair

3   A Denman brush is used to:
  a) produce a small tight curl in the hair
  b) give a smooth finish, for example to a 'bob' style
  c) backcomb and tease hair into style
  d) produce a soft, casual broken-up effect.

4   The purpose of glosses and serums on the hair is to:
  a) reduce frizz and add shine
  b) detangle the hair
  c) give the hair a softer look and feel
  d) maintain curl and replace lost moisture.

5   A manufacturer's data sheet is:
  a) instructions telling you how to use styling products
  b) information on the ingredients, handling and storage of a product
  c) information on what hair types the product is suitable for
  d) the same as a risk assessment sheet.

6   If you discover an infestation when halfway through a service, you should:
  a) stop the service and ask the client to come back when she has treated the hair
  b) refuse to carry on with the service and report to your tutor or manager
  c) continue with the service and give the client advice on whether they should visit their GP
  d) inform all clients and staff in the salon so they can go home and treat their hair.

7   When blow-drying the hair the airflow of the hairdryer should go:
  a) from root to point
  b) from point to root
  c) it doesn't matter because you want to dry all of the hair
  d) up and down the hair shaft.

8 When blow-drying in the nape area you should position the client:
   a) with head upside down for maximum volume
   b) with head upright – you should be the one bending and uncomfortable, not the client
   c) with head tilted forward so you can work freely in this area
   d) standing up so the client is at the right height for you.

9 When blow-dried hair comes into contact with atmospheric moisture it will:
   a) become dry and brittle
   b) become oily and lank
   c) start to drop and return to its natural state
   d) not be affected.

10 Styling products coat the hair with:
   a) water
   b) plasticisers
   c) oil
   d) moisture.

11 Hair in its natural state is called:
   a) beta keratin
   b) dry hair
   c) hygroscopic hair
   d) alpha keratin.

12 Hair is hygroscopic. This means that it has the ability to:
   a) take a curl easily
   b) be extra bouncy after a blow-dry
   c) absorb moisture
   d) hold a blow-dry for 14 days.

13 Styling products will protect the hair against:
   a) heat and moisture
   b) diseases
   c) oil and grease
   d) infestations.

14 Heated styling equipment should be checked by a qualified electrician every:
   a) week
   b) 3 months
   c) 6 months
   d 9 months.

15 The bonds that are re-formed during a blow-drying process are:
  a) the hygroscopic bonds
  b) the disulphide bonds
  c) the peptide bonds
  d) the hydrogen bonds.

16 What effect will humidity have on the hair structure?
  a) It will help to give the style more hold
  b) It will break down the disulphide bonds causing the style to collapse
  c) It will break down the hydrogen bonds causing the style to collapse
  d) It will make styling products feel sticky on the hair

17 How will overuse of heat affect the hair and scalp?
  a) You will flatten the cuticle and not achieve root lift or body
  b) Hair condition will deteriorate; severe damage may include yellowing of the hair, split ends or breakage, and burns to the scalp
  c) You will take longer to complete your blow-drying service
  d) You will dry the hair too quickly and not be able to form the curl or lift you require

Getting ready for assessment

You will be assessed using a combination of assessment methods, as described below. Remember that within each of the services you carry out with a client, you will cover different units. For example, when styling and finishing hair (GH10), you will also have to be aware of health and safety (G20) and advise and consult with clients (G7). You may also have shampooed and conditioned hair (GH8). If you are not sure what you have covered in your service, always ask your assessor or supervisor for advice.

	NVQ	VRQ
Credit value	6	5
Guided Learning Hours	50	30

	NVQ	VRQ
Practical demonstrations, to be observed by assessor	Your assessor will need to observe you on at least three occasions on three separate clients. You must prove that you can: • blow-dry with a brush to create volume • blow-dry with a round brush to create curl • carry out straightening and smoothing techniques with a brush • use a range of heated styling equipment • use four out of the seven products listed • carry out all the remaining ranges in full. Simulation is not allowed for any performance within this unit.	Your assessor will need to observe you on at least three occasions on three separate clients. You must prove that you can: • consider all of the eleven factors listed • use ten out of the twelve tools and equipment listed • carry out finger-drying techniques • carry out straightening and smoothing techniques with a brush • complete either an above or below shoulder length blow-dry • use a minimum of four styling products • use a minimum of four finishing products • give the appropriate aftercare advice. Simulation should be avoided where possible.
Service timings	Blow dry and finish, maximum (above shoulder) – 35 minutes Blow dry and finish, maximum (below shoulder) – 45 minutes	Blow dry and finish, maximum (above shoulder) – 35 minutes Blow dry and finish, maximum (below shoulder) – 45 minutes
Additional evidence	You will be required to complete an independent written paper to support the underpinning knowledge required for this unit. The majority of evidence will be gathered from the observations carried out by your assessor.	You will be required to complete a mandatory written question paper. You will also be assessed through oral questioning.

Task mapping

When you have completed the tasks in this unit, check the table below to see which Performance Criteria (purple), Range (red), Knowledge (green) and Key Skills (blue) you have covered within GH10 to use as additional evidence for your portfolio. Information about which Functional Skills you have covered is available on the website.

Task and page reference	Mapping to Performance Criteria, Range, Knowledge and Key Skills
1 (page 245)	Performance Criteria: 1a, 1b, 1f, 1g, VRQ 1a Range: N/A Knowledge: 1, 5, 6, 7, 8, VRQ 1d Key Skills: C1.2, C1.3, C2.3
2 (page 249)	Performance Criteria: 1e, 1f, 1g, 1k, VRQ 1a, 2c, 2j Range: N/A Knowledge: 3, 12, 13, 16, 18, VRQ 1d, 2l, 2r Key Skills: C1.2, C1.3, C2.3
3 (page 249)	Performance Criteria: N/A, VRQ 2c, 2j Range: N/A Knowledge: 3, 26, VRQ 2r Key Skills: C1.2, C1.3, C2.3
4 (page 252)	Performance Criteria: 1h, 2a, 2b, 3a, 3b, 5a, 5b, VRQ 1b, 1c, 1e, 1f, 2a, 2d, 2f, 2g, 2h, 2i Range: VRQ R1a–k, R2a–L, R5a–e, R7a–c Knowledge: 25, 27, 37–41, VRQ 1e, 1f, 1i, 2l, 2m, 2p, 2q Key Skills: C1.1, C1.3
5 (page 255)	Performance Criteria: 2d, 2e, 2g, 2h, VRQ 1i, 2a Range: 5a, 5e Knowledge: 28–34, VRQ 2l Key Skills: C1.1
6 (page 263)	Performance Criteria: 2g, 3d, 4d, VRQ 1c, 2a, 2d, 2g Range: 4a–g, VRQ R1a–k Knowledge: VRQ 1f, 2m, 2p Key Skills: C1.1, C1.2, C1.3, C2.1A, C2.2B, C2.3

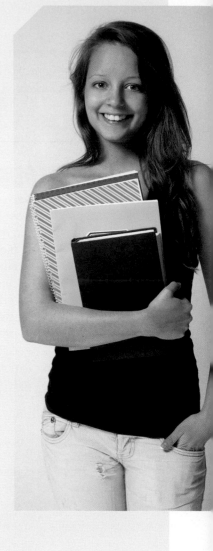

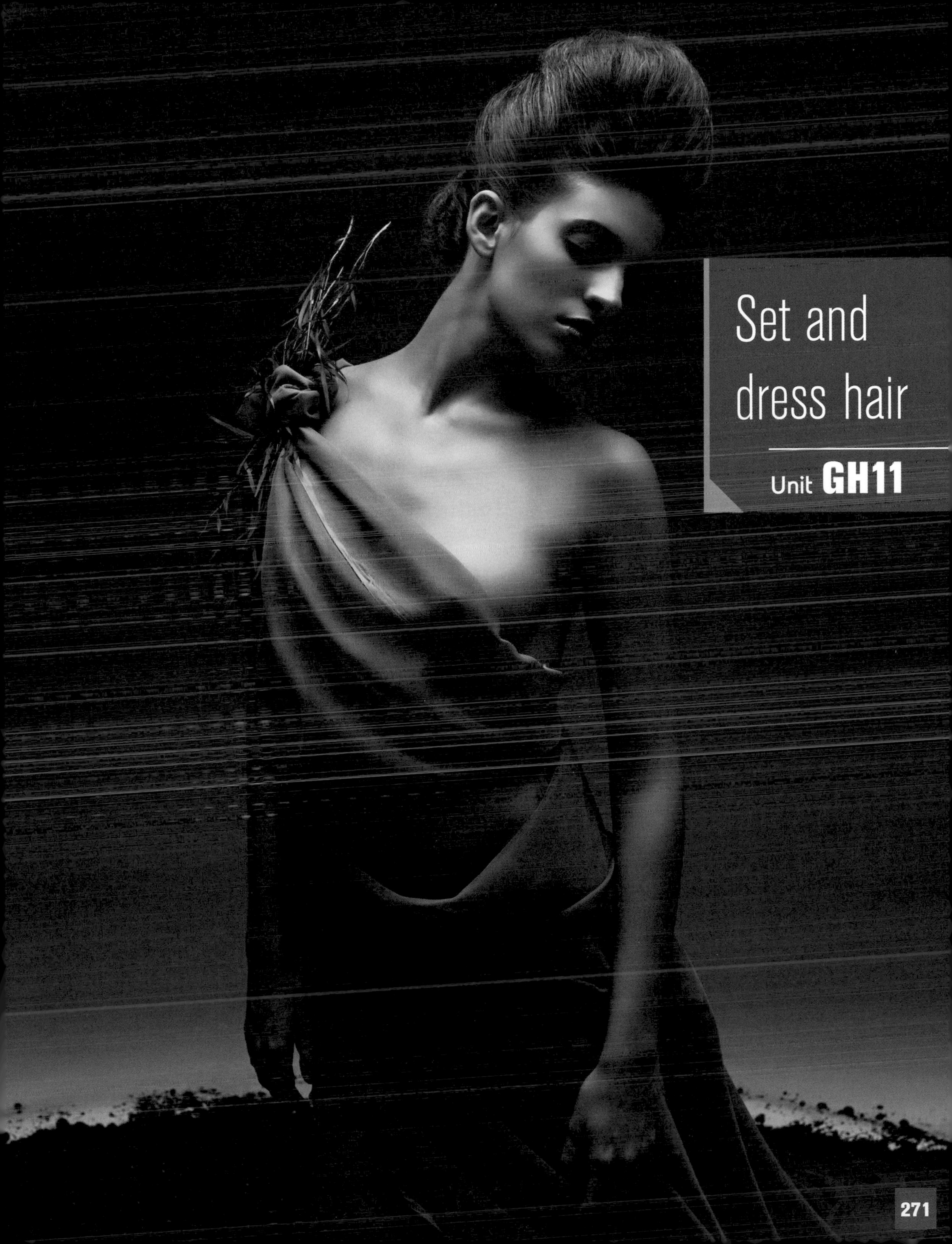

Set and
dress hair

Unit **GH11**

What you will learn:

- **How to maintain effective and safe methods of working when setting and dressing hair**
- **How to set hair**
- **How to dress hair**
- **How to provide aftercare advice**

Introduction

This unit is important because setting and dressing techniques can be used to produce a wide range of looks, and this will help you to progress onto perm-winding techniques. You will be required to work with a wide range of tools and equipment and demonstrate dexterity skills (working with your hands).

You will learn about using rollers; straightening and smoothing; finger-drying and finger-waving; and spiral curling and pin curling techniques on long and short hair. You will also find out about the wide range of styling tools, equipment and products that will enable you to achieve the best results while taking into account critical influencing factors and maintaining a high standard of health and safety as you work.

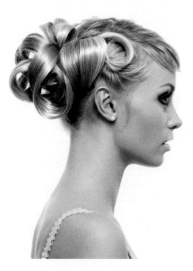

How to maintain effective and safe methods of working

Preparing your client for setting and dressing long hair

Gowning and positioning

Client comfort is always important. You must take care of your client when gowning and positioning her for a service.

When gowning the client for a setting process, you will follow the same procedure as for shampooing (see page 178). If the client is having a dry set (using heated or velcro rollers), or simply having her hair put up, you will only need to use a gown with a towel on top to protect your client from styling and finishing products and natural hair fall.

When you seat your client in the chair at your workstation, it is important that the client is sitting squarely in front of the mirror with both feet flat on the floor or footrest. This is to enable you to move freely around your client and also to ensure that you get an even balance to the hairstyle.

It is important to make sure that you position yourself correctly alongside your client as you are working. All your working positions should feel natural. The more comfortable you are, the less tired you will become.

Your work area

Your work area must be clean and tidy before you receive your client.

Fact or fiction?

Is this statement fact or fiction?

If your client sits with crossed legs, this may affect the dressing-out process and produce an unbalanced end result.

To check your answer see page 498.

Task 1

Using the information in GH10 (page 245), write a brief statement on how you would prepare your work area to receive a client, taking into account all health and safety responsibilities.

Choosing suitable products, equipment and tools

Minimising wastage of products

To work efficiently and effectively with a wide range of products, you need to know how, when and why you are using the products and the amount you should be using. If you use too much of a product then you may not achieve the desired result for your client, and you will also be 'eating into' your salon's profits.

The correct equipment and tools for setting

When you set the hair, the length of hair dictates the size of the roller you use. This is why stylists have a wide and varied range of rollers. To start with, you will need only a basic range of rollers. As you gain experience and master different techniques, you may wish to add to your equipment.

Top tips

It is always better to use a small amount and then apply a little more, rather than squeezing too much out of the bottle or tube and having to throw it away.

273

Unit
GH11

Set and dress hair

Tools for setting hair

Tool		Effect	Suitability
Setting rollers for wet setting		Various sizes for different degrees of curl.	Suitable for all hair types to produce soft to firm curls.
Velcro rollers for dry setting		Various sizes for different lengths of hair and degrees of curl.	Suitable for most hair types. Very straight hair may drop quickly with this form of setting technique.
Heated setting rollers (to be used on dry hair)		Various sizes for different degrees of curl. Produces tumbling curls, body and root lift.	Not suitable for very dry or over-processed hair because of the added heat. Very straight hair may drop quickly with this form of setting technique.
Super flex bendy rollers (Molton Browners)		Hair is wound from one end to the other to produce a waved, spiral effect.	Suitable for most hair types. Care must be taken with very fine, fragile hair as this is a firm winding technique.
Skelox		Various sizes for different degrees of curl on long hair.	Ideal for long hair as the teeth and holes in the roller prevent the hair from becoming tangled.
Conical rollers		Produces a curl that is narrow at the hairline, becoming wider at the top, which makes the curl look like a natural wave.	Can be used on wet or dry hair to produce a natural wave.

Following health and safety measures at work

Your responsibilities relating to legislation

As a stylist, you must be aware of your own responsibilities under the COSHH Regulations 2003 (see G20). All products used in hairdressing are covered by these regulations as they relate to:

- handling chemicals
- storing chemicals
- disposal of chemicals.

Hazard warnings found on products and chemicals

Chemicals and products are considered hazardous if they can be:

- inhaled
- ingested (swallowed)
- in contact with the skin
- absorbed through the skin
- introduced into the body via cuts.

To alert everyone to a hazard, all chemicals that have some type of risk carry a safety symbol.

Sterilising

Sterilisation means the killing of all organisms such as bacteria, fungus and parasites.

There are various methods for sterilising tools and equipment (see page 63). Some methods of sterilisation are more effective than others, and not all equipment can be sterilised in the same way. Your tools should be sterilised after every client so that you minimise the risk of cross-infection and infestation.

Clean equipment

As well as making sure that all of your equipment is sterilised, you need to make sure that it is clean of hair and products. This is especially important with heated styling equipment. If you allow products to build up on the barrel of the equipment, you will find that you have hot and cold spots where the heat cannot penetrate because of the build-up of product. To remove the build-up you need to allow the equipment to cool, then use a soft cloth with a spirit-based cleaner (this will be able to break down the residue) and gently wipe the surface of the piece of equipment. You need to make sure it is completely dry before you switch the equipment back on.

Safe working for you, your clients and colleagues

In this unit you will be working with a wide and varied range of heated styling equipment. It is important to make sure the equipment is fit and safe for purpose (see also page 57, Electricity at Work Regulations 1989). You therefore need to be making constant checks throughout the service. This can be done by visually checking cables and plugs for any frayed or loose wires, and checking the temperature of your equipment.

- If you are using a hood dryer, you can check the equipment is working by simply putting your hand near the airflow and asking the client if she is comfortable.

Fact or fiction?

Is this statement fact or fiction?

All hairdressing equipment can be sterilised using Barbicide®.

To check your answer see page 498.

- When you are using heated rollers, they should not be too hot for you to handle, though take care not to touch the metal rod they sit on to heat up.
- Most professional straighteners indicate when they have reached the correct temperature by a light flashing or a light going off.

You may find the hair is a little hot to the touch after the straighteners or tongs have been used. In this case you will need to develop a technique whereby you use your comb to pick up or move the heated sections of hair that you have been working on. You will also need to make sure that you use your comb to protect the client's scalp when working with both of these pieces of equipment.

Personal, learning and thinking skills – Teamwork

We are all aware that teamwork is an important part of our role as a hairdresser. It aids the smooth running of the salon and promotes a professional atmosphere, which in turn encourages a profitable salon. Have a look at the staffing structure within your salon. Is there anything that you could suggest to enhance the teamwork that is already taking place? Could you introduce a 'buddy' system, whereby if a member of staff was absent their designated 'buddy' would set aside time to bring them up to date? Record your findings and feed back to your manager.

Organising your work area and time effectively

Every salon allows a set amount of time for every process that is carried out, from shampooing to colouring.

Task 2

In your training establishment or college, find out the times allocated to the following services:

- channel, directional and brickwork setting
- full head set with Velcro rollers on hair below shoulder length
- half head directional set with half head pin curls
- full head of pin curls.

A worksheet for this task is provided on the website for you to complete and add to your portfolio.

Organisation for setting and dressing long hair

You must have:

- a hood dryer and other electrical equipment such as heated rollers
- a good selection of brushes and combs for setting and dressing out
- a wide range of setting rollers and a hair net
- pin curl clips, hairgrips and fine hairpins for long hair
- a selection of styling and finishing products.

A good trolley layout with all the necessary equipment will allow you to spend more time with the client on the service.

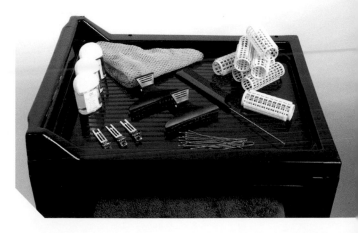

It is important to consider how the trolley is laid out prior to setting and dressing long hair

Unit
GH11

Set and dress hair

Consulting and preparing before styling

Consulting the client

For every hairdressing service, an in-depth consultation is the key to success. Without gathering the right kind of information from your client, you will not be able to fulfil her wishes.

Task 3

In pairs, gather some style books and each choose a style which has clearly been set, tonged or straightened in some way.

- If you are allowed to, cut out the picture from the style book and make brief notes alongside the image. Alternatively, photocopy the image or scan it and then print out a copy.
- Identify which techniques and methods you think have been used.
- State what products you think are the most suitable for that style.
- What aftercare advice would you give to a client with this style?

During the consultation, check:

- for anything that may not allow you to carry out the service, such as infections and infestations
- the type of hair you are working on – look at the texture and density of the hair as this will influence the choice of styling products and the type and size of rollers to be used
- any critical influencing factors that may influence the set, such as head and face shape, and double crowns
- how much natural movement there is in the hair – this will affect your product choice and the type and size of rollers to be used.

Sample questions to ask during the consultation

- How firm would you like the curl to be?
- How long does the set need to last for?
- Would you like any styling and/or finishing products on your hair?
- Is it a daytime or an evening look?
- Do you get any problems with particular parts of the hair? (Let the client identify what she considers to be awkward areas.)

Sample questions to ask during the service

- Is the heat of the hood dryer, tongs etc. comfortable for you?
- Is that enough body and height for you?
- Are you happy with the finished result?
- Do you require any more backcombing or backbrushing?

It is important to check during the service that the client is happy with the way the hair is taking shape. This is the time to make any changes that either of you may feel are appropriate or necessary.

Using the correct tension and meshes of hair to suit the styling tools and process

It is important when setting or dressing out the hair that you use the correct size of meshes. This is so that:

- when placing your rollers they will sit correctly on their own base without **root drag**
- the mesh of hair suits the length and width of the roller you have chosen so that hair does not get caught and tangled around the sides
- heat from electrical appliances can penetrate the mesh of hair to achieve the result required
- you work in a methodical manner, covering the whole of the head and ensuring that all of the hair is dry.

It is also important that you keep tension even along the mesh of hair when you work so that:

- the curl you may be putting into the hair from either a roller, tongs or hot brush gives you an even result along the section of hair
- if you are straightening the hair, you will ensure an even result
- when winding the hair around a roller, tongs or hot brush, you will not get 'baggy' sides.

How to set hair

Setting techniques

There are three key points that apply to both wet and dry setting techniques.

1 *Sectioning* – the section of hair that you take when placing rollers is very important. If the section of hair is too big, you will have 'baggy' ends that will produce an uneven curl result. If the section is too small, you will have 'overcrowding' of rollers and will run out of headspace! The section that you take should be slightly narrower than the length of the roller and no deeper than the width of the roller.
2 *Tension* – good even tension will distribute the hair evenly around the roller, ensuring a uniform curl result.
3 *Angle* – the angle at which you hold the hair when winding will determine the amount of root lift created. For good root lift, the hair needs to be held at 90 degrees from the head. This position should be maintained while the roller is wound to the base. For fashion setting techniques you can drag the roots of the hair if little or no root lift is required.

Root drag

Root drag occurs when the hair is not pulled up at a 90-degree angle, and therefore root lift is not achieved. Instead, the roots would lie flat.

277

Unit
GH11

Set and dress hair

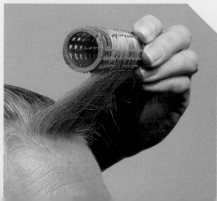

1 Take a section that is slightly narrower than the length of the roller and no deeper than the width of the roller.

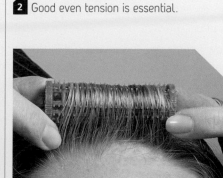

2 Good even tension is essential.

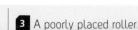

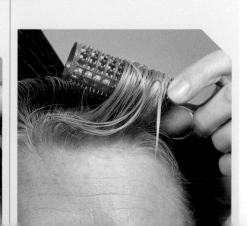

3 A poorly placed roller.

Applying styling products to control the hair, taking into account critical influencing factors

You have looked at the use of styling products (refer back to page 246), at what they do and their suitability for different types of hair. Styling products can also be used to help you overcome or control some of the critical influencing factors that you may come across.

Task 4

Using the information in GH10 (page 246), complete the paragraph about styling and setting aids provided on the website by filling in the missing words. This is important information that you need to understand so you should recap it frequently.

A worksheet for this task is provided on the website for you to complete and add to your portfolio.

Critical influencing factors

When choosing products, equipment and setting techniques, you should consider a wide range of factors, including hair texture, haircut, head and face shape, hair growth patterns, hair length and density.

Task 5

Look back at GH10, page 256, and discuss in groups why critical influencing factors need to be considered when dressing and styling the hair. Make a note of your findings and keep this for reference in your portfolio.

A worksheet for this task is provided on the website for you to complete and add to your portfolio.

As well as using styling products to help you control critical influencing factors, you also need to be aware of what equipment and styling techniques can be used to help you with potential problems.

Influencing factors for setting wet and dry hair

An influencing factor, although it sounds similar to 'critical influencing factor', is not the same thing. When you are considering an influencing factor you are looking more at client requirements and preferences.

When deciding whether to set hair wet or dry, you should consider the following questions:

- How firm do you require the curl in the hair to be? Wet setting produces a firmer curl.
- How much time does your client have for the service? Dry setting or using heated rollers does not take as long as wet setting.
- What type of setting method would suit your client's hair type? Straight hair requires a firmer set; naturally curly or permed hair will hold a curl better.
- How long does the client require the set to last? If it is for one evening, you can use fashion setting techniques. If it is to last a week, you may need to choose a more traditional method of setting that will last longer.

- What is the condition of the hair? If the hair is very dry and damaged, for example, you would not use heated styling tools such as hair straighteners or heated rollers.

Using styling techniques that ensure client comfort

When you shampoo, you are not only removing dirt and grease from the hair, you are also changing the properties of the hair that make it possible to alter its shape temporarily by blow-drying or setting.

Task 6

Look back at GH10, page 257, to recap on the properties of hair and what happens to hair during shampooing and blow-drying, then complete the worksheet provided on the website and add it to your portfolio.

Wet and dry setting

Carrying out wet and dry setting techniques safely

Wet setting the hair involves shampooing, and you need to remember to gown your client correctly for this part of the service. After shampooing, towel-dry the hair to remove any excess moisture, comb the hair through, then apply the product you have chosen.

With dry setting you will not be shampooing the hair, but you still have to prepare the client and the hair for the service (for example gowning). You should brush the hair through to remove any tangles and then apply a setting aid (product) if one is required.

The different effects of wet and dry setting

Wetting the hair causes the hydrogen bonds in the hair to break down. This allows you to change the shape of the hair by blow-drying or setting. When you wind wet hair around a roller and add heat to the hair, the bonds re-form into their new shape around the roller — this is how you are able to style the hair time and time again.

Dry setting the hair does not break down the hydrogen bonds (except a few from your application of styling product). It involves 'baking' the hair into its new shape around the roller. Care has to be taken when doing this — you do not want to over-dry the hair, causing damage.

Dry setting is very useful for fashion setting techniques — it will produce a softer curl, ideal for preparing the hair for hair-up techniques.

Products for setting

Styling products coat the hair with a protective barrier that will help to prevent moisture getting through and causing the set to collapse. Look back at the chart on page 246 to remind yourself of the products available.

Coloured mousse and coloured setting lotions clearly state in the manufacturers' instructions that they should be used on wet hair. You will not achieve an even distribution or colour result if applied to dry hair.

Fact or fiction?

Is this statement fact or fiction?

It is up to the client to inform you of any critical influencing factors.

To check your answer see page 498.

279

Unit

GH11

Set and dress hair

Fact or fiction?

Is this statement fact or fiction?

Hair should only be dry set when it is clean.

To check your answer see page 498.

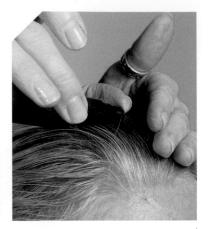

Applying setting lotion

Wet setting

- *Mousse* – towel-dry the hair, comb through and section. Use a large-toothed comb and evenly comb the mousse from the roots to the ends of the hair.
- *Coloured mousse* – make sure that you have gowned your client correctly and you are wearing the correct protective clothing (gloves and apron). Coloured mousse will stain the client's skin so great care must be taken with application. Repeat the procedure above.
- *Setting lotion* – can come in spray form or individual bottles. When using setting lotion from a bottle, place your forefinger slightly over the top of the bottle and sprinkle onto the hair, keeping the client's head back to avoid accidents.
- *Coloured setting lotion* – make sure that your client is correctly gowned and you are wearing protective clothing. Coloured setting lotions will stain the client's skin and, as this is a runny product, great care must be taken when applying.

Dry setting

- *Thermal setting lotions* – these are sprayed onto dry hair and activated by applying heat.
- *Setting lotions (not coloured)* – use the same application method as for wet hair.

Tools and equipment for setting

What you will need:

- a pintail comb – this is used to section and comb through the mesh of hair
- a selection of rollers – the length of the hair and degree of curl required determines the size of the roller used
- setting pins – these are used to secure the rollers
- pin curl clips – these may be required for shorter hair that will not wind around a curler
- styling products – these will make the hair more pliable, add body and protect it from atmospheric moisture
- water spray – the hair must not be allowed to dry out when wet setting
- hair net – this covers the rollers when placing the client under the dryer and stops any small hairs escaping from the rollers
- hood dryer – this supplies an even distribution of heat all around the head.

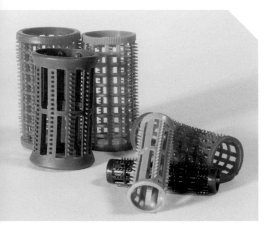

A selection of wet setting rollers

Setting techniques

There are various techniques that can be used to set the hair.

Channel

This type of setting technique is uniform in its layout. Begin at the front hairline, directing the hair backwards, and place a row of rollers in a channel down the centre of the head. Then move to the crown area and, still directing the hair downwards, place a section of rollers each side of the middle channel. Finish by placing another set of rollers at the sides of the head. All of the rollers should be seated in channels down the head.

Brickwork

Think of bricks in a wall; this is how you will be placing the rollers in the hair. Begin at the front hairline and place one roller, then move behind this roller and take another section of hair, starting in line with the middle of the first roller. Continue in this way working down the head, remembering that some alterations in the position of the rollers may be required due to the shape of the head.

Directional

As the name suggests, place the rollers in the direction that you want the hair to be dressed. Incorporate all of the setting techniques when completing a directional wind, as long as the rollers are wound in the direction you wish the hair to sit.

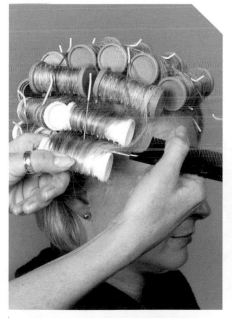

Channel setting using heated rollers

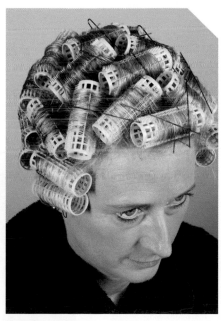

Brickwork setting on wet hair

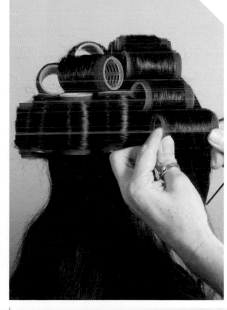

Directional winding

Salon life

Putting a smile on the face

David's story

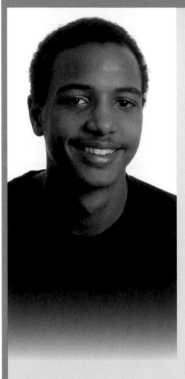

I had real difficulty when positioning rollers so that I didn't have bits of hair left in tiny sections that I couldn't get a roller into. I found this especially frustrating with brickwork setting. When I first joined the college and watched the demonstrations, it all looked so easy. But after weeks of practising, and very sore fingers, I realised that this was because the tutors had been doing it for years! I knew that I had to take my sections a fraction smaller than the roller size, hold the hair at 90 degrees to the head for the correct root lift, and follow a pattern with the rollers the same as a brick wall. But despite this, I still couldn't produce the same result as the demonstration block.

I went to my tutor for help. She pointed out that when I reached the area just below the crown, I wasn't taking the head shape into account – I was placing my rollers in an upside down U-shape and the sides were gradually coming into the middle to meet each other, so I had overcrowding. My tutor explained that I was creating a sad face and what she wanted was a smiley face!

My tutor showed me how to open up the rollers to create the smiley face. By not placing the last two rollers at each end when I was working just below the crown area, this meant that the next row underneath started to angle up into a smile. I did this for two or three sections until I could place the rollers across the whole of the head again. I don't think I am ever going to forget how to place the rollers for a brickwork set!

Top tips

Always make sure that the hair is kept damp throughout the entire setting process. This will help to ensure even tension over the whole head.

Ask the expert

Q *I always seem to get some buckled ends when I set hair. Do you have any suggestions on how I can avoid them?*

A Try to get your sections as neat as you can. The tension needs to be the same for the whole mesh of hair, and you need to use your thumbs to hold the ends of the hair around the roller as you start winding down. If the ends of the hair are uneven and difficult to hold together, you can use the prong of your pintail comb to help you wrap the ends around.

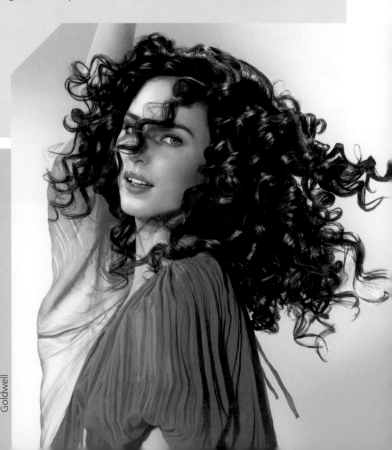

Goldwell

Pin curling techniques

Pin curling techniques are also used in setting, and are very useful for shorter hair that may not wind around a roller easily. You can achieve tight, medium or loose curls.

a) *Flat barrel* – this will sit flat on the head with an open middle and produce a curl that is even from roots to points; this will produce flat movement. Also used for reverse pin curling to create a soft 's' formation.

b) *Barrel* – this creates lift from the root, producing soft curls or waves, and can be used in place of a roller; this will produce volume.

c) *Clockspring* – this will also sit flat on the head with a closed middle. It produces a curl that is looser at the root and gradually tighter towards the ends. Usually used at the nape of the neck.

Spiral curling

This technique is generally used on hair that is below shoulder length. The hair is wound around the roller (or bendy roller) from points to roots along the length of the roller. This will produce a spiral effect similar to how naturally curly hair would fall.

Keeping the hair moist throughout the service

When styling the hair, it is important that the hair does not dry out before you have placed your roller in the correct position. Use a water spray to dampen the hair slightly; you may find that this will be required more often on fine hair as it has a tendency to dry out more quickly than thick hair.

If the hair does dry out and you do not moisten it, you will not achieve a smooth finish and the style will not last as long. This is because the hydrogen bonds will have re-formed into the hair's natural state and not taken on the shape of the roller that you are using to style the hair.

Ensuring you achieve the volume, balance and curl required

Throughout any of the setting and finishing services, always check with your client that:

* you are working towards the style desired by the client – check that the parting is in the right place
* you are achieving the correct amount of width and height that the client requires
* she is happy with the finished result; for example, have you used enough backcombing?

How to dress hair

Dressing long hair is all about controlling the hair, sectioning off the hair not required at various stages and secure pinning. Dressing hair can be as easy or as complicated as you wish to make it! The techniques may look complicated, but if you break them into simple step-by-step stages and work in a methodical manner, you will be able to reproduce all of the styles shown in this section.

You will be looking at how to use heated styling equipment, taking into account health and safety issues. You will learn how to use backcombing and backbrushing techniques, how to apply finishing products, and how the use of added hair ornamentation can enhance the finished result.

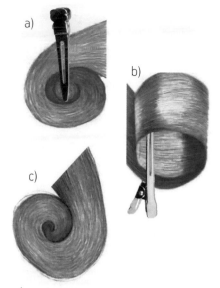

a)

b)

c)

a) Flat barrel, b) barrel and c) clockspring pin curls

283

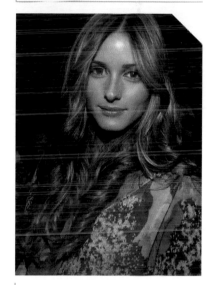

Spiral winding

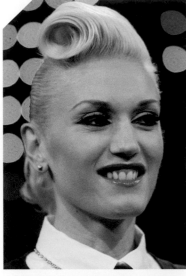

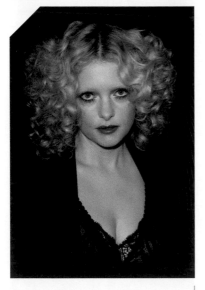

Looks created using curling techniques

Preparing your client

When consulting with your client prior to the service, follow the consultation checklist shown on page 276. Other questions that you need to consider are:

- Does the hair need to be set to achieve the desired result?
- Can I achieve the amount of curl needed by dry setting the hair?
- How much time does the client have?
- How long is the style expected to last?
- Is there enough hair (length and thickness) to enable me to achieve the end result?
- Will the chosen style suit the client's face and personality?

If your client has straight hair and would like it up with some curls on the top, you would need to set the hair. If a client wanted a straight, sleek style, then you would not need to set the hair prior to dressing.

It is always useful to have a style book showing long hairstyles so that you can confirm the required look with your client.

It is also important to check with the client while you are dressing the hair that she is happy with what you are doing and it is how she expected the hair to look. It is no good waiting until the end and then discovering that, for example, the style is not going to suit the dress she is wearing or is not going to be appropriate for the occasion that she is going to.

Leaving your client's hair free from sectioning marks

To avoid creating sectioning marks in the hair, when you carry out setting or hair-up looks you need to pay particular attention to the spaces between the rollers and sections taken for long hair work. You may need to run your fingers gently through the hair to soften the channels created by the rollers or sections and use backcombing, backbrushing or teasing techniques to leave the hair free of sectioning marks. (See pages 262–63 for backbrushing and backcombing techniques.)

Using heated styling equipment

Additional equipment

Other equipment you can use to help give extra support when you set the hair includes:

- electric (heated) tongs
- hot brushes
- crimping irons
- straightening irons
- heated rollers.

See the chart on page 261 for details of these tools.

In addition, hot air brushes can be used to produce a natural, soft curl effect. They should only be used on wet hair; the hair is rolled around the brush and the curl formed as the heat dries the hair. They are ideal for clients who have difficulty using both a brush and a hairdryer.

A hot brush is ideal for a client who has difficulty using both a brush and a hairdryer

Health and safety rules when working with electrical equipment

To minimise the risk of damage to your tools and to work safely you should:

- always check that the client is comfortable and not too hot when under a hood dryer
- never place tongs, hot brushes or straighteners directly on the scalp — this will cause serious burns to the client
- always sit tongs and hot brushes on the stand so as not to scorch work surfaces
- always check the heat and speed controls before you start setting
- put away equipment when not in use
- avoid winding flexes of electrical equipment too tightly when storing
- never store tongs, hot brushes or other electrical equipment until they have cooled down.

By law, all electrical equipment should be checked by a qualified electrician every six months.

Choosing products and equipment suitable for dressing hair

What you will need:

- a wide, flat bristle brush (Isinis or paddle brush) for smoothing over the hair
- hairgrips for securing the hair
- fine pins — useful for creating a smooth finish and tucking in ends
- covered bands — for securing plaits without damaging the hair
- tail comb and dressing comb for creating the final finish
- mousse or gel — can be used if the hair is wet and then dried to give a firm hold
- dressing cream — will help produce a sleek appearance on dry hair
- shine spray — for evening hair-up looks it puts a soft shine on the hair
- hairspray — a light hold hairspray will aid in the dressing out of the style
- gel spray — for a firmer hold when the style is completed; also good for producing spiky finishes.

Critical influencing factors

When deciding on which style to dress the client's hair, take into account the following factors.

- *Density or thickness of the hair* — very fine hair may look 'gappy' if the wrong style is chosen; very thick hair may look too bulky if put up into a vertical roll.
- *Hair texture* — if the hair is very coarse in texture, depending on the style required, the hair might have to be straightened to smooth it or set to form soft curls.
- *Hair length* — if the client has long hair which is layered, you may find that short pieces of hair will fall out from a plait, for example.
- *Head and face shape* — if the client has a high forehead, don't scrape the hair back too severely from the face. If the client has a long face shape, do not give her a style with too much height which makes the face look even longer.

When considering head and face shapes, your aim is to achieve balance. The idea is to draw the eye away from the least flattering point and towards the balance of the style.

Top tips

When you place your client under the dryer, either use a timer or check the time on your watch or a clock to make sure that the client is not left under the dryer unnecessarily. Check the temperature control of the dryer and remove any setting pins or pin curl clips that may cause discomfort. If there are any rollers seated on the client's ears, place cotton wool underneath.

285

Unit

GH11

Set and dress hair

Fact or fiction?

Is this statement fact or fiction?

You can rough-dry the hair and then use heated styling equipment to add curl, volume and movement.

To check your answer see page 498.

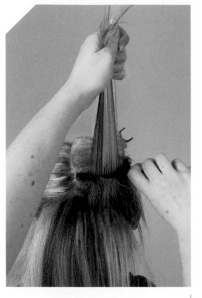

Backcombing

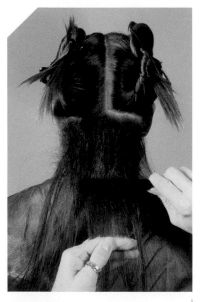

Backbrushing

Dressing-out techniques

Backcombing and teasing

If you want to add height and width to a set when dressing, backcomb the hair. If you do not want to add too much height but want to remove roller marks from the hair, tease the hair into shape.

If the hair is very thick, section off the hair so that you begin at the nape area. Take a section of hair and hold between the first two fingers and thumb. Place your dressing comb into the hair about halfway up and push the hair back towards the roots. The number of times you do this on a mesh of hair will determine how much backcombing you put into the hair.

When teasing the hair, use the prongs on a dressing-out comb. Since these prongs are far apart they will allow some of the hair to fall through without being affected. Again, if the hair is very thick, section the hair off and begin at the nape area working upwards towards the crown.

Always consult with your client about how firm they require the end result and confirm the finished look by using the back mirror to show them all angles of the style.

Backbrushing

Backbrushing is carried out in the same way as backcombing, only you swap the comb for a brush. It is best to use a flat bristle brush as this will not tear or damage the hair. Again, if the hair is very thick, divide the hair off and work in sections. By choosing to backbrush instead of backcomb, you can cover a greater area of hair and produce a slightly softer effect.

Applying finishing products, taking into account critical influencing factors

You have looked at the different types of styling products that are available to you (refer to page 246). What you need to consider at this stage is what products you will use to help you achieve the finished result. Most products can be used on wet or dry hair and will give very different effects on both.

Finishing products are:

- dressing creams
- waxes
- oils
- gels
- sprays.

Finishing products can also be used to help hide any critical influencing factors (see page 256). If a client has very fine hair, use a product which gives the appearance of thickness and bulk to the hair. If the client has dry, fluffy or coarse hair, a finishing cream or oil will give the hair shine and lustre.

Some critical influencing factors cannot always be hidden with styling or products. When this is the case, make sure that you adapt your dressing out (end result) so that you work with the problems. For example, if you have a client who has very fine, straight hair, you would find it difficult to achieve a really textured look.

Controlling and securing long hair

Dressing long hair requires secure pinning of the hair in such a way that the grips are not visible to anyone looking at the hair. The grips should not be so firm as to cause discomfort to your client, but should be firm enough for the style to hold.

The secret to dressing long hair is not to be afraid of the amount of hair that you are working with and using the right tools and equipment for the job. It is a good idea to practise your long hair techniques on a block first, so that you get used to handling long hair, working with your equipment and learning to secure the hair firmly without causing discomfort to the client.

With most long hair work it is a good idea to secure all the hair that you are not working on out of the way. This will allow you to see where you are working and you will not be trying to hold fistfuls of hair in one go.

You will need to make sure that you have all of your equipment to hand so that you don't discover you have run out of grips or other equipment when you are halfway through pinning up your client's hair.

You will need to check with the client that the hair feels secure but that none of the grips or pins are uncomfortable.

Vertical roll (French pleat)

The vertical roll is a versatile way in which to dress the hair. When you have secured the roll, the ends of the hair may be protruding from the top of the head. You can tuck these ends in, producing a very formal roll, or curl or straighten them to produce a more fashionable, casual look. The hair may require a lot of backbrushing (done with a bristle brush) for volume, which is then smoothed over to produce a sleek finish.

287

Unit

GH11

Set and dress hair

Set and dress hair

Step-by-step French pleat (vertical roll)

1 Consult with your client on the type of look she wants to achieve. This could be a classic roll or a more modern version.

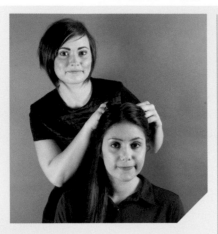

2 To add body to fine hair you may need to backbrush the hair. This will provide you with a firm base to work from. Section the hair and push the hair back into itself to create a slightly matted look at the root area.

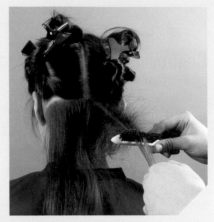

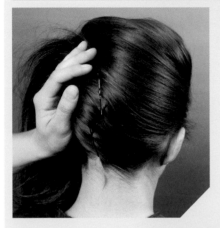

3 Lightly brush over the top section taking care not to remove all of the back-brushing. You should be lifting the hair up from the nape area. Begin your pinning slightly off centre so that your roll will sit in the middle. Criss-cross your grips for added secureness.

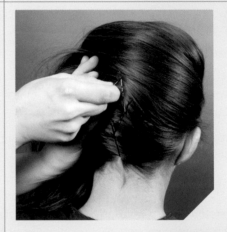

4 If the hair is very thick you can double-grip by placing another line of grips over the grips already placed in the hair. The last grip at the top needs to be turned upside down to prevent the hair from sliding out.

5 Gently brush the hair over to form the roll and hide the layer of grips. Secure the roll to the head by slightly opening the grips and placing them as close to the roll as possible.

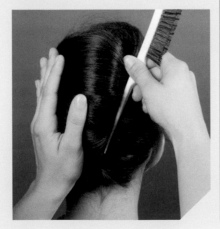

6 The finished result should be checked for balance, then the appropriate finishing products applied and aftercare advice given.

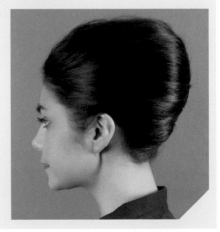

Rolls

1 The hair is evenly wound around the Velcro rollers to suit the direction of the required finished style.

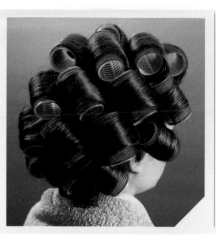

2 The hair is dressed in rolls to produce a classic style suitable for most occasions.

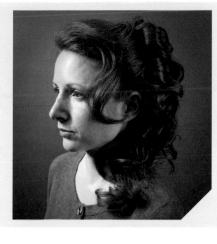

289

Unit
GH11

Instructions for creating rolls

- Consult with the client on her requirements.
- Choose the appropriate size and type of roller and styling products.
- Decide on the type of wind to be used – channel, brickwork or directional.
- Set the client's hair, remembering to check on her comfort throughout.
- Allow the hair to dry or cool, depending on the setting technique used.
- Remove grips and rollers, allowing the hair to cool if necessary.
- Gently run your fingers through the client's hair to remove setting marks.
- The rolls may require a small amount of teasing at the roots for support.
- Secure the roll at either end so the grip is invisible.
- You can build up height by placing one roll on top of another.
- Shine sprays, gel sprays and hairsprays can all be used to finish the look.
- Use a back mirror to check that your client is happy with the look from every angle.

Using accessories

Hair accessories or ornamentation can be used to enhance your finished style. A client might bring in pins, clips or flowers that match her outfit or jewellery. Alternatively, your salon may wish to offer these with an additional charge.

If the use of accessories is discussed at a prior consultation you may need to guide your client on the most suitable accessory for her hair type/texture. If the hair is fine, a large bulky accessory wouldn't be suitable. If the client has thick, dense hair, a small pin or clip would be difficult to see.

Care needs to be taken when 'fixing' the accessory into place so that it is comfortable, secure and doesn't cause damage to either the hair or scalp.

Applying products

When you have dressed the hair into a style, you may need to use finishing products to enhance the style by smoothing or adding texture to the finished look. If you are using sprays, protect your client's face. Either use your hand to stop any of the product coming into contact with the client's face or use a clear plastic face shield if your salon has one.

Checking and confirming the balance of the style to the client's satisfaction

When you have completed your hair-up design, check that you have achieved the intended shape and balance and that the client is happy with the end result. To do this you will need to check the shape and balance of the hair-up design from all angles. It is important to do this as other people and the client will not just be looking at the hair from one direction. Check that you have not left any flat spots or gaps in the hair. You will need to use a back mirror to show the client her hair from all angles.

When showing the client her hair, you should show the profiles (sides), the back and the crown of the style. By doing this you can get the client to confirm that she is happy with the end result. The client will know that her hair looks as good from the back as it does from the front.

How to provide aftercare advice

General aftercare advice

As part of the complete service, you must give your client the correct aftercare advice on her hair. Hair-up styles are usually meant for one night only. However, some clients like to keep their hair up longer if they can, and other clients may have their hair put up once a week and have a comb out to tidy up their hair in between visits.

Aftercare advice for a one-off, hair-up style

If you have put the client's hair up early on in the day and it has to last right through to the evening, give the following advice.

- Re-tong any tendrils that may lose their curl by the end of the day.
- Use a small prong comb to lift, tease or gently backcomb any areas that may require it (demonstrate the techniques to the client).
- Re-apply hairspray in the evening to ensure the style will last.
- Advise the client to avoid humid areas (such as a steamy bathroom or kitchen), as the moisture in the air will make the hair drop.
- You might like to give the client a few extra grips, just in case! The client should not need them if the hair is secured correctly, but it will give the client peace of mind and show thoughtfulness on your part.

Aftercare advice for regular weekly clients

Some clients (usually older) may only have their hair washed and set once a week and have a comb out in between each visit.

- If they use hairspray, advise clients to spray the hair from a good distance so that there is no build-up of hairspray on their hair.
- Advise clients to use a prong comb to lift, tease or gently backcomb any flat spots.
- They shouldn't have very hot baths and should protect their hair when in the shower as the moisture will make the style collapse.
- When they do have their hair taken down for shampooing, it will require a thorough brush through to remove all of the loose natural hair fall that cannot escape when the hair is up.

- Explain to the client about the amount of hair a person loses on average per day, so they will not worry that they are losing too much hair. Explain that the hair gets caught up and cannot fall away because of the way they wear their hair. This means that when it is taken down there will be a lot of natural hair fall in one go.
- Offer advice on the best types of products for them to use during the week to keep the shine and lustre of their hair.
- You can offer advice about the best brushes and combs to use for their hair.
- You can suggest the types of clips, pins and grips that are best to secure their hair with and that will not cause any damage.

All of this advice and any other top tips that you might have are all part of offering a complete service to your client.

Unit

GH11

Set and dress hair

Check your knowledge

The following questions will help you to check your understanding of this unit.
The answers can be found on pages 498–99.

1 Coloured mousses and setting lotions should be applied to:
a) dry hair
b) wet hair
c) towel-dried hair
d) either wet or dry hair; it doesn't matter.

2 The purpose of a hair net used in setting the hair is to:
a) prevent any small hairs escaping from the rollers
b) hold the rollers in place
c) protect the client from the heat of the hairdryer
d) just use as a finishing touch to the set.

3 What effect does a 'dry' setting process have on the hair's structure?
a) It will break down the hydrogen bonds and re-form them around the new shape.
b) It will break down the disulphide bonds and re-form them into the new shape.
c) It will break down the keratin in the hair and re-form it into its new shape.
d) It will 'bake' the hair into its new shape.

4 When you carry out a directional set, you will place the rollers:
a) in a channel beginning at the front hairline
b) in the direction you want the hair to be dressed
c) like bricks in a wall
d) randomly to see what effect you can achieve.

5 A flat barrel pin curl will produce:
a) an open middle, with a curl that is even from roots to points
b) root lift, producing soft curls
c) a closed middle with a curl that is looser at the root and gradually tighter towards the ends
d) a closed middle, with a curl that is even from points to roots.

6 Pin curling techniques are used in setting:
a) when you want to be quick and take bigger sections of hair
b) when you want to create a 'messier' look
c) when the hair is freshly permed
d) for shorter hair that may not wind around a roller easily.

7 The purpose of hot brushes is to:
a) temporarily straighten wavy or curly hair
b) produce a soft, casual look
c) produce ringlets in the hair
d) produce a line of crimps.

8 The angle at which the hair is held during setting will determine:
   a) the distribution of hair around the roller
   b) a uniform curl result
   c) the amount of root lift created
   d) how many rollers you can fit onto the head.

9 'Baggy' ends are created by:
   a) the hair being too thick
   b) the section of hair taken being too large
   c) the section of hair taken being too small
   d) the client moving while under the hairdryer.

10 Good, even tension will:
   a) prevent the set from dropping when coming into contact with atmospheric moisture
   b) create root drag for fashion setting techniques
   c) stop the hair becoming tangled in the roller
   d) distribute the hair evenly around the roller, ensuring a uniform curl result.

11 Why is it important to give aftercare to the client after the service?
   a) So you don't receive any complaints
   b) To ensure the client understands how to maintain the look at home
   c) So you can sell retail products
   d) So you can demonstrate your knowledge

12 Why is it important to allow the hair to cool before removing rollers?
   a) So you don't burn your fingers
   b) To give you time to fill in the client record card
   c) To allow the curl to set
   d) To allow the cuticle scales to close

293

Unit
GH11

Set and dress hair

Unit
GH11

Set and dress hair

Getting ready for assessment

You will be assessed using a combination of assessment methods, as described below. Remember that within each of the services you carry out with a client you will cover different units. For example, when setting and dressing hair (GH11), you will also have to be aware of health and safety (G20) and advise and consult with clients (G7). If you are not sure what you have covered in your service, always ask your assessor or supervisor for advice.

	NVQ	VRQ
Credit value	6	5
Guided Learning Hours	50	30

	NVQ	VRQ
Practical demonstrations, to be observed by assessor	You are required to complete three performances, which must include: • one curled effect • one smooth effect • one rolled effect. One of these performances must be of a set using rollers secured with pins. You are required to use four out of the seven types of products listed, but you must show your knowledge and understanding of the remaining products in order to prove competency. All other ranges must be completed. These performances will be observed by your assessor. Simulation is not allowed for any evidence requirements within this unit.	You are required to complete three performances, which must include: • one curled effect • one smooth effect • one rolled effect. One of these performances must be of a set using rollers secured with pins. You are required to use four out of the seven types of products listed, but you must show your knowledge and understanding of the remaining products in order to prove competency. All other ranges must be completed. These performances will be observed by your assessor. Simulation is not allowed for any evidence requirements within this unit.
Service timings	Set and dress above shoulder length hair (excluding drying) – 35 minutes Set and dress below shoulder length hair (excluding drying) – 45 minutes	Brick wind, maximum (above shoulder) – 35 minutes Brick wind, maximum (below shoulder) – 45 minutes Directional wind, maximum (above shoulder) – 35 minutes Directional wind, maximum (below shoulder) – 45 minutes
Additional evidence	You will need to complete an independent written paper to show your understanding of the knowledge requirements.	You will need to complete an independent written paper to show your understanding of the knowledge requirements.

Task mapping

When you have completed the tasks in this unit, check the table below to see which Performance Criteria (purple), Range (red), Knowledge (green) and Key Skills (blue) you have covered within GH11 to use as additional evidence within your portfolio. Information about which Functional Skills you have covered is available on the website.

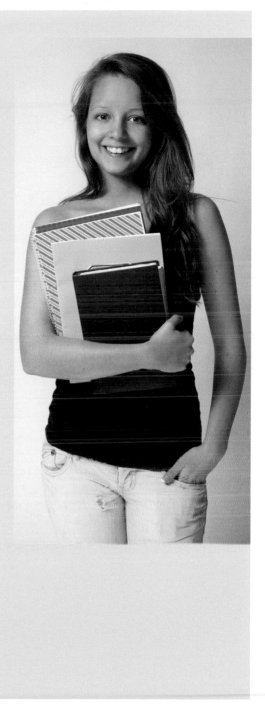

295

Unit

GH11

Set and dress hair

Task and page reference	Mapping to Performance Criteria, Range, Knowledge and Key Skills
1 (page 272)	Performance Criteria: 1a, 1b, 1c, 1g, VRQ 1a, 2a, 2c, 2j Range: N/A Knowledge: VRQ 1d, 2r, 2t Key Skills: C1.2, C1.3, C2.3
2 (page 275)	Performance Criteria: 1l Range: VRQ R3a, R3b Knowledge: 2 Key Skills: C1.2, C1.3, C2.3, N1.1, N1.2, N1.3, N2.1, N2.2, N2.3
3 (page 276)	Performance Criteria: 1h, 2h, 2k, 3e–h, 4a, 4b, VRQ 2a, 2d, 2g, 2h, 2i Range: VRQ R3a, R3b, R3c, R5a–e, R6a–f, R7a–c Knowledge: VRQ 1e, 1f, 2l, 2m, 2p, 2q Key Skills: C1.2, C1.2
4 (page 278)	Performance Criteria: 2g Range: N/A Knowledge: 19, 20, VRQ 1g, 1h Key Skills: C1.2
5 (page 278)	Performance Criteria: 2i, VRQ 1c, 2d Range: 6a–h, VRQ R1a–k Knowledge: 30, VRQ 1f Key Skills: C1.1, C1.2, C1.3, C2.1A, C2.2B, C2.3
6 (page 279)	Performance Criteria: N/A Range: N/A Knowledge: 19, 20, 23, VRQ 1g, 1h Key Skills: C1.2

Cut hair using basic techniques

Unit **GH12**

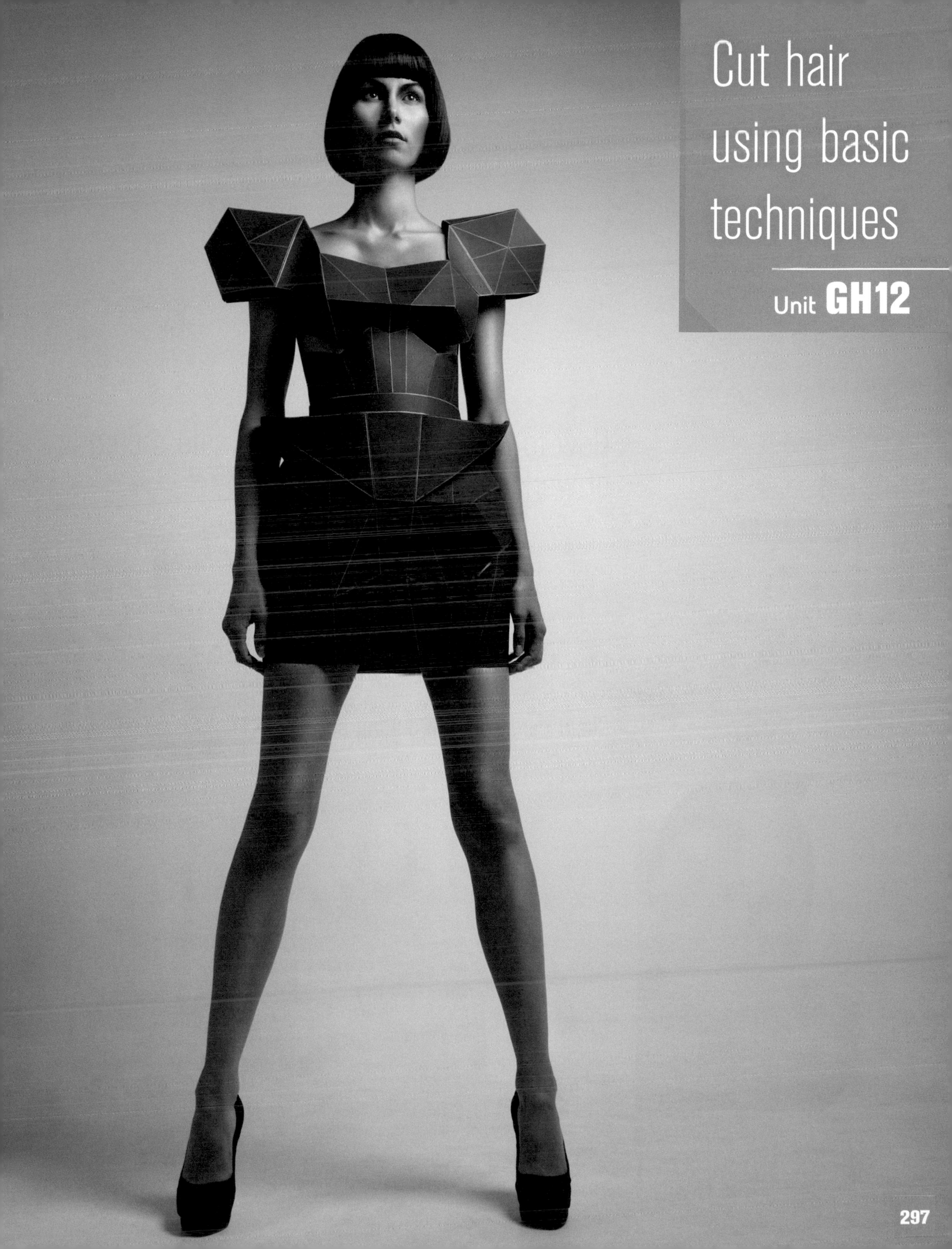

Cut hair using basic techniques

What you will learn:

- **How to maintain effective and safe methods of working when cutting hair**
- **How to cut hair to achieve a variety of looks**
- **How to provide aftercare advice**

Introduction

This unit is the core of your hairdressing qualification. It will guide you through the skills you will need to learn to be able to cut hair. You must master these skills before you can become a professional hairdresser.

The unit looks at the different cutting tools, their uses and their effects. It also covers safety, hair-cutting techniques and the cutting of wet and dry hair. You will also consider critical influencing factors — hair textures, hair growth patterns, head and face shapes and how to give appropriate aftercare advice.

How to maintain effective and safe methods of working

It is essential that you work safely and effectively when cutting hair. One of the requirements of this section is that you ensure your work standards meet health and safety laws and regulations for both the client and yourself. By following these laws and regulations you will help to minimise the risk of **cross-infection** and **infestation**.

You should be able to organise yourself and your equipment so that your tools are suitable to achieve the desired look and your work methods minimise the risk of damage to tools and equipment. Time spent on the preparation of the client and the duration of the service must be within the timescale required by the salon.

Client care during a cutting service

Gowning

Throughout the hairdressing service, it is your responsibility to make sure that your client remains comfortable — having hair cut and styled is a pleasurable experience. As part of this service, you must make sure that you gown your client correctly so that hair cuttings do not go onto the client's clothing or cause her any irritation.

Some stylists prefer to gown the client after the consultation so that they can see how the client dresses, which gives the stylist an idea of style suitability. When you are ready to begin the service, you are then ready to gown the client.

For a cut on wet hair, first use a normal cutting gown. Over this place a towel, then a plastic disposable cape on top (this double protection will ensure the client does not get wet). When you have completed the shampoo, towel-dry the client's hair and replace the plastic cape with a cutting collar.

When cutting dry hair, you should use a cutting gown and then place a cutting collar around the client's neck. Using a neck brush, gently brush in sideways strokes to remove the hair cuttings from the client's face and neck. You must make sure that you clean your neck brush on a regular basis to prevent any cross-infection or infestation between clients.

Cross-infection

The transfer of a disease or infection from one person to another.

Infestation

A term applied to parasites which live in or on another living creature in large numbers.

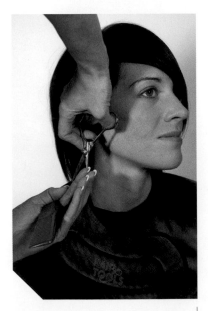

Plastic cape and towel replaced by a cutting collar

Positioning the client

The positioning of the client is very important as it can affect the line and balance of the haircut.

Once the client is seated and you are ready to cut, check that she is comfortable and is sitting correctly. If the client has her legs crossed, this will encourage her to lean to one side, with one shoulder up and one shoulder down, and this will throw you off line when cutting, resulting in an uneven finish.

The client should be sitting with the small of her back against the back of the chair and with both feet on the floor or on a footrest. This will ensure that she is sitting squarely in the chair and not lopsided.

Positioning – you the stylist

You also need to consider your own posture and position when you are working at your workstation.

Some salons may have their workstations situated close together. You then have a trolley alongside you, which will take up space. If you work on a client without bending your knees, you may find that you will be bumping into your work colleague. It will also put a strain on your back if you are not standing in the correct position and could result in spinal problems and fatigue.

Health and safety issues

Every client must be treated with care and attention from the beginning to the end of the service. Good health and safety practices must apply to all clients.

It is essential to keep your work area clean, tidy and free of waste. Hair cuttings should be swept away and disposed of in a bin, not piled up in the corner of the room. Tea, coffee and magazines should be removed from your workstation in preparation to receive your next client. Remove any used product packaging and dispose of it in the relevant place. Make sure equipment is allowed to cool and is correctly stored.

Spillages

All spillages should be mopped up immediately and not left for others. It is your responsibility under the Health and Safety at Work Act to ensure the environment is safe for colleagues and clients.

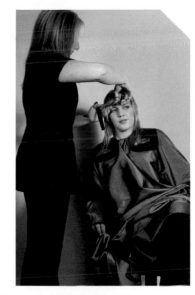

Incorrect sitting position

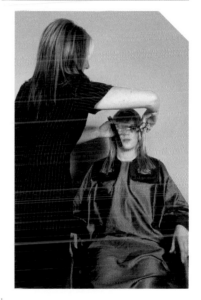

Correct sitting position

Potential hazards in the salon

Hazard	Ways to avoid	When referral may be necessary
Spillages	Take care when using products. Mop up any excess water after shampooing.	If the spillage is corrosive or an irritant.
Slippery floors	Sweep up hair immediately after cutting. Mop up any spillage from products.	When grease, wax or polish is spilt.
Tools or equipment	Store equipment correctly. Allow electrical equipment to cool before storing, making sure there are no trailing wires.	When a piece of equipment is broken or defective.
Bags, coats or stock left on the floor	Hang coats on a coat rack and ask clients if they can tuck their bags underneath their seat.	If an object is too heavy to move and is blocking an exit.

299

Unit
GH12

Cut hair using basic techniques

Task 1

Look back at unit G20, pages 46–47, on risk assessment. Using the blank risk assessment form provided on the website, identify as many risks associated with cutting as you can.

A worksheet for this task is provided on the website for you to complete and add to your portfolio.

Choosing the right tools and using them correctly

You will need a variety of tools and equipment to help you complete a haircut successfully. You need to understand their uses, the methods of sterilisation for them and how to use them safely.

Scissors

Scissors are the most important piece of equipment for a hairdresser. Scissors vary in design, size and price. The best way to find out if a pair of scissors suits you is to pick them up and see if they are comfortable to hold. Hands and fingers vary in size, so holding scissors is the only way to tell if they suit you.

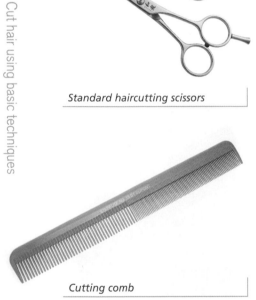

Standard haircutting scissors

Cutting comb

This is an essential piece of equipment. Combs are available in different sizes to suit your needs and the type of hair you are working with. If you are using clippers, you will require a cutting comb that is more flexible than the normal straight, rigid cutting comb. The flexibility of the comb used for clipper work or a scissor-over-comb cut allows you to work closely and follow the client's head shape (see page 306).

Cutting comb

Thinning scissors

The purpose of thinning scissors is to remove bulk from the hair without removing length. There are two main types: those that have two notched (serrated) blades and those that have one ordinary blade and one notched blade. The spaces between the notches vary in size and determine the amount of hair that is removed.

Scissors with two notched blades will take off more hair than thinning scissors with one notched blade and one ordinary blade. Notched scissors with wide spaces between the notches will remove more hair than thinning scissors with smaller spaces between the notches.

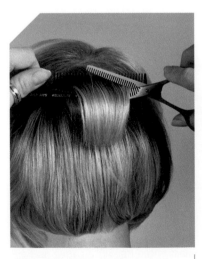

Thinning scissors in use

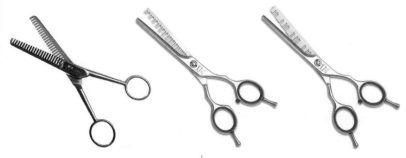

Three types of thinning scissors

Thinning scissors are also called:

- texturising scissors
- serrated scissors
- notched scissors.

They should be looked after in the same way as standard scissors.

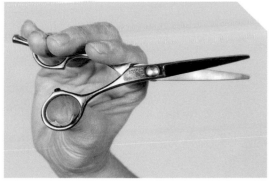

The correct way to hold scissors

Razors

The most commonly used razors are open or cut-throat razors, shapers or safety razors. The more modern razor has a disposable blade and a guard over it so only a small amount of the hair is cut. This also gives added protection and helps prevent cutting the client's skin. The disposable razor is easy to use. Once the blade becomes blunt it can be replaced quickly and easily, ensuring you do not tear the client's hair.

Razoring is usually carried out on wet hair as this reduces the friction on the hair and is less painful for the client. (Razoring dry hair can pull and be uncomfortable!) Look after razors in the same way as scissors, making sure that you dispose of used blades – known as sharps – in a sharps bin (see page 65).

Electric and rechargeable clippers

Clippers are generally used for short, graduated styles. They are used on dry hair only. They can give the effect of a scissor-over-comb cut and are used in both men's and ladies' hairdressing.

Clippers work by the bottom blade remaining fixed while the top blade moves at a very high speed. You can add clipper attachments to vary/alter the length of the cut, depending on the size of the grade that you attach – the higher the number is on the grade, the longer the hair will be; the lower the number on the grade, the shorter the hair will be.

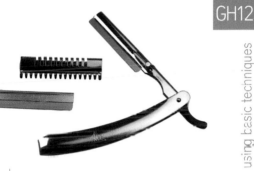

Safety razor

Clipper attachment grades run from 1 to 8

Rechargeable clippers

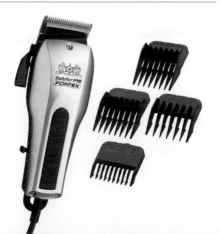

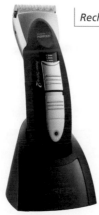

Rechargeable clippers are generally smaller than electric clippers and give a closer haircut. They can be used to trim behind the backs of the ears or other hard-to-reach areas. Different heads are available for these clippers for use in hair sculpting. After use they should be replaced on their stand for recharging.

You should oil both types of clippers after every use to maintain them and to make sure that they run smoothly. This will help to prolong their life.

Neck brush, water spray and sectioning clips

You will require these items when cutting.

- *Neck brush* – removes cuttings from the client. You should use this throughout the haircut. To maintain good health and hygiene standards and care for your equipment, you will need to wash your neck brush in warm soapy water on a regular basis.
- *Water spray* – used to damp down hair that dries too quickly. If the hair is allowed to dry out halfway through the cut, you will not achieve even tension. You should empty the water from your water spray on a regular basis. This will help to prevent the water becoming stagnant or leaking onto other tools and equipment.
- *Sectioning clips* – these divide/section large quantities of hair. These can be sterilised by immersing them in Barbicide® solution for the manufacturer's recommended time.

Using tools that are safe and fit for their purpose

It may help you to have a daily ritual, either when you get your equipment out or when you pack it away; a quick checklist will ensure that you do not overlook any safety issues. Equipment that you are using should not be damaged or broken in any way. You need to make sure that teeth are not missing from combs, hairbrushes should be free of any loose hairs and all equipment should be cleaned and sterilised on a regular basis.

Using equipment safely to minimise the risk of damage to tools

When working with electrical equipment, you need to make sure that you follow good codes of practice. To ensure that you are working safely, use the following list. (This list is not exhaustive.)

- Do not use electrical equipment with wet hands.
- Check plugs and wires are not loose/damaged before use.
- Use the correct piece of equipment for the job you want to do.
- Replace equipment carefully after use, ensuring it is clean and in good working order.
- Switch off electrical items when not in use and unplug to avoid trailing wires.
- When putting away electrical equipment, avoid folding flexes too tightly as this will cause them to short-circuit if they get damaged.

In accordance with the Electricity at Work Regulations 1989, all electrical equipment should be checked every six months by a qualified person, who should then place a sticker on the equipment to show that it is safe to use. The salon should keep a record of the visit for future reference.

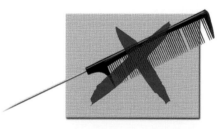

Equipment that you are using should not be damaged or broken in any way

Task 2

What would you do if you accidentally cut a client? Discuss your response in pairs or groups, and record your findings before you read on.

What to do if you accidentally cut a client

- Put on protective gloves.
- Apply a small amount of pressure to stem the blood flow, either with a pad or towel.
- Call for a first aider. (Do you know who your first aider is?)
- Remain calm while the first aider is coming and speak reassuringly to your client.
- Fill in an accident report form – this ensures that you have a record of what happened should this be required for future reference. You should also inform the salon manager or your trainer. (Do you know where your accident report forms are kept?)

Protecting yourself

For your own health and safety, you need to be aware of potential hazards to yourself, for example the possibility of cross-infection of hepatitis and the HIV virus from exposure to blood. Prevention is better than cure. You can have a vaccination for hepatitis A and B if you are in a high-risk group, of which hairdressing could be considered one. You are at risk because of the potential of cuts from scissors and sharps – this increases the risk of exposure to blood. The use of protective gloves may be necessary as a preventative measure.

If you have an open cut, make sure that it is covered with a dressing so that if you accidentally cut a client you will not be at risk from cross-infection of blood.

Good organisation and time management

You need to be prepared for every client, which means you must have the right tools available to cover every aspect of the hairdressing services that your salon offers.

Good organisation means:

- a full trolley layout
- all equipment is clean and sterilised
- record cards and style books are at hand ready for the consultation
- a tidy working area that is free of excess waste (cut hair), and that has no slippery surfaces or potential hazards. Remove any equipment not needed, for example free-standing climazones.

Using your time effectively

You should always be organised and ready for the client's arrival. Each salon has its own time allocation for services offered. For example, most experienced stylists will allow only 20 minutes for a dry cut and a maximum of 45 minutes for a cut and blow-dry. As a trainee, you should be aware of the time it takes you to cut a client's hair. It is expected that you will take longer than an experienced stylist for your first cuts.

It is important to have all of the relevant equipment ready to hand before you receive your client. This will also help you to use your time effectively. Before you receive your client, you will need to get out the relevant record card and look at the appointment page to see what service the client is having. By doing this you will then be able to set yourself up to receive the client with all of the equipment that you are going to need.

Top tips

When cutting children's hair, you need to be aware that they may not be able to sit as still as you would like. Their attention span is shorter and their movements can be sudden. Try to give them something to occupy them, such as a book or toy. This will help them to sit a little longer and prevent any cuts or injuries to yourself or the child.

303

Unit

GH12

Cut hair using basic techniques

Task 3

Find out how long your salon allows for each of the following services:

- wet cut and rough dry
- dry cut
- cut and blow-dry on hair above shoulder length
- cut and blow-dry on hair below shoulder length.

Compare this with your group and discuss any differences.

Working within a commercially viable time

You will have researched how long your salon or training establishment allows for the services that it offers and this will be the timeframe that you will be trying to work within.

By breaking the service down into stages, it should show you how much time you will have to spend on each stage and give you a timescale to work towards. What you do not want to do is watch the clock. This will not only get you flustered but it will also make the client feel uncomfortable. All you need to do is be aware that you are on track and not running over on one part of the service as this will have a knock-on effect on the rest of the day's services.

Health, hygiene and sterilisation

You should prevent cross-infection of blood by covering any open cuts when working. Tools must be sterilised to ensure that you minimise any risk of cross-infection or infestation that can be passed on by your equipment. Refer to the table in G20 (page 63) for the best methods of sterilisation for cutting tools.

Disposal of used sharps

'Sharps' is the term used in hairdressing to describe the blades used in safety razors.

Salons should supply a yellow sharps bin for the disposal of blades. It is a hard plastic bin that cannot be pierced and is collected by the local health authority to be incinerated (burned). If you put a disposable blade from your razor/hair shaper in an ordinary black bin liner, the person emptying the bin may be cut.

Fact or fiction?

Is the following statement fact or fiction?

Washing tools and equipment will ensure you won't pass on any infections.

To check your answer see page 499.

Task 4

Investigate the sharps bin in your training establishment.

- Where is it kept?
- What else can be disposed of in the sharps bin?
- Who collects it for emptying, and how often?

Personal hygiene

As well as looking after your tools and equipment, you must also make sure that you take your own personal hygiene into account to minimise the risk of cross-infection and infestation. (Please refer to G20, page 73.)

You may be required to wear a uniform in many establishments. This may be so that you comply with the college's or salon's health and safety policies, which will have taken hygiene points into account.

How to cut hair to achieve a variety of looks

In this section you will be looking at how to complete a thorough consultation, and the different cutting techniques and factors that you have to take into consideration to complete a successful haircut.

Consultation

Before cutting the client's hair, you should carry out a thorough consultation with her. There are a number of important factors to consider before the service can take place and these can be addressed by completing a consultation cutting checklist before you begin. A suggested checklist is given here (right).

You will be checking the hair and scalp for any infections or infestations (see table on pages 145–48 in G7) that may not allow you to carry out the service. You will also be looking at the hair growth patterns, hair texture, density, head and face shape and the elasticity of the hair, as these are critical influencing factors that you will need to identify. These will be described below.

When you carry out the consultation, it is a good idea not to gown up your client straightaway. Seeing the way she dresses will help you to determine the personality and the type of lifestyle she may lead. For example, a client who is conservatively (soberly) dressed may not appreciate an emerging cut. The use of style books will help to give both you and the client a clear picture of the end result that you hope to achieve.

Consultation checklist

Client's name: _____ Tel. no: _____
Address: _____
Date: _____ Stylist: _____

Factors to consider

Client requirements:
What are your client's wishes? _____
What are your client's expectations of the haircut? _____
Face shape: Square Round Oval Oblong Heart Diamond
Body proportions: (tall/petite) _____
Hair type/movement: European Asian African Caribbean
Has the hair got a wave/curl in it? _____
Hair texture: Very fine? Very coarse?
Density of hair: (How much hair do you have to work with?)

_____

Natural growth patterns: Double crown Widow's peak Cowlick Nape whorl
Hair condition: _____
Porosity and elasticity: _____
Client personality/dress/lifestyle: _____
Client limitations: _____
Check whether the client will be able to maintain the style at home: ☐
Suggested style: _____
[Use the information gathered above to suggest or guide your client towards a style that you both feel suits her needs.]
Cutting techniques and reasons: _____

_____

[List the techniques you are going to use and your reasons for using them. Make sure that the chosen cutting techniques, for example, razoring, suit the hair's condition. (This will also act as a record card of your consultation and the cut for future reference.)]
Aftercare advice given: _____

_____

Task 5

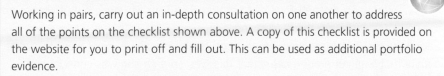

Working in pairs, carry out an in-depth consultation on one another to address all of the points on the checklist shown above. A copy of this checklist is provided on the website for you to print off and fill out. This can be used as additional portfolio evidence.

Task 6

Find as many different formats of consultation card as you can. Some should be in electronic form. What are the particular features that occur each time? Compare and discuss in your groups and record your findings for evidence in your portfolio.

Critical influencing factors

A critical influencing factor is anything that you may have to take into account that will have an effect on the end result that you hope to achieve.

Hair density

When you talk about the hair's density, you are referring to the amount of hair that an individual client has per square inch on her head. On some heads of hair you can see the scalp through the hair, which means that the client does not have very dense hair. On other heads there may be a lot of hair per square inch, meaning the client has very dense hair.

It is sometimes easy to get density and texture of hair confused. You will need to remember that density refers to the amount of hair on the head and texture refers to the diameter of an individual hair, not the amount of hair the client has.

Hair texture

You should examine the hair's texture very carefully during your consultation with the client because this may affect the cutting technique that you choose to use. If you decide on a particular cutting technique because of the hair's texture, you will have identified a 'critical influencing factor'. For example, if the client has very fine hair, you may choose the club cutting method to increase bulk in the hair. On the other hand, you would not want to increase bulk in thick hair (also a critical influencing factor), so you might choose a thinning technique for this hair texture.

You can identify the texture of the hair by separating a few strands of hair and placing them across the palm of your hand. The texture of the hair usually falls into three categories: fine, medium and thick. You will need to look at the hair closely and decide which one of these categories the hair falls into to determine the hair's texture.

Head and face shapes

When consulting with the client, before deciding on the length of the cut, you should take into consideration the client's head and face shape because these can become critical influencing factors in your choice of style and length for the cut.

You should be able to see that careful consideration needs to be taken when choosing a style to suit a particular face shape. If you make the wrong choice, you could end up enhancing a feature that the client wants to detract from and not emphasise. Some of the potential factors to consider are:

- *Foreheads* – a high forehead can be disguised by cutting in a fringe; a fringe may not be suitable for a small forehead because it will quickly grow out of shape, and may look too heavy for the face shape.
- *Ears* – are the ears large, very small or do they protrude? A client wouldn't want a style that was cut around her ears if this was an area she was conscious of.
- *Flat occipital bone* – this is the protruding bone at the back of head and helps to give shape to many hair styles. If the client's head is flat in this area, you will need to leave length or bulk in your design to compensate for this.

Hair growth patterns

This refers to the way in which the hair grows from the roots. On some heads of hair, growth patterns are very apparent. For example, if the client has a cowlick in the middle of her fringe and the fringe has 'jumped up', this will be obvious to you. In another case, the client may have blow-dried her hair so well that she has disguised a double crown or strong hair growth movement.

To identify hair growth patterns, you will need to take fine meshes of hair down around the hairline and secure the rest of the hair out of the way, then look closely at the direction in which the hair is growing. Some hairlines may sit perfectly in the direction that you want them to; others may push in the opposite direction, making it difficult for you to carry out a particular haircut.

You need to look very closely at potential problem areas when the hair is dry and take a second look as a safeguard if you wet the hair. By deciding to leave length because of the client's hair growth patterns, you will be identifying a critical influencing factor.

Elasticity

We test the elasticity of the hair to see how good the internal strength of the hair is. Remember, porosity testing is to determine the condition of the outside of the hair shaft. (Refer to G7, pages 138–44, for hair tests.) If the hair is in bad condition, you may choose not to use razoring techniques on the hair. This is because if the hair is very fragile, it may not be able to withstand this method of cutting as it can put extra stress on the hair.

Preparing for cutting

Before you receive clients, check that:

- your work area is clean and tidy
- all equipment is to hand and sterile
- client record cards, style books and consultation checklists are ready.

When you receive clients:

- carry out a consultation — complete a cutting checklist to help you to achieve the desired result (see page 305)
- gown them up (see page 298)
- prepare their hair for cutting.

Hair preparation

During the consultation, it is important to consider whether you are going to complete the cut on wet or dry hair. There are a number of factors you need to take into account when deciding this.

- *Cost* – in most salons it is usually more expensive for a client to have a wet cut. This is to cover the cost of water, shampoo, conditioners and the extra time taken by the stylist.
- *Time* – if the client has come in during her lunch hour, she may not have the time to have a cut and blow-dry.

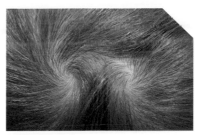

This is a double crown – the parting may have to be changed to distribute the hair more evenly either side of the head to disguise the double crown

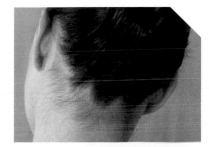

The nape hairline grows unevenly – the hair should not be cut above the hairline

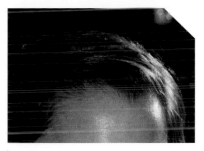

A widow's peak – you would leave a heavier fringe to disguise a widow's peak

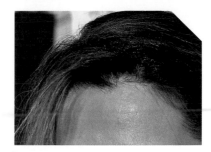

This is a cowlick in the fringe area – the fringe needs to be made heavier to help the hair stay down

Cut hair using basic techniques

- *Influencing factors* – some heads of hair may have very awkward hairlines or growth patterns. By wetting the client's hair, it becomes more difficult to identify these growth patterns, as wet hair can be manipulated in any direction. When the hair is dry, the growth patterns are more apparent and you can adapt the cut as necessary.
- *Techniques* – some cutting techniques require you to cut the hair when wet, for example razoring, while others such as clippering must be carried out on dry hair.

Advantages and disadvantages of cutting wet and dry hair

| Wet hair | | Dry hair | |
Advantages	Disadvantages	Advantages	Disadvantages
• More precise lines. • Hair is easier to manage and control. • Hair can be manipulated into style during cutting.	• Client may be uncomfortable if salon temperature is too cool. • Unable to see bulk/ weight lines in hair (especially permed/ naturally curly hair).	• Hair will be the same length when finished. • Easier to see the bulk to be removed from hair. • Easier to identify and remove split ends.	• Hair flies everywhere (client uncomfortable). • Cut can be uneven. • Hair can be hard to control; hard to keep even tension. • Client may have greasy/ dirty hair.

Accurately establishing and following cutting guidelines

When you are ready to begin your cut on the client, you need to make sure that you work in a methodical manner. You will be working through the haircut by dividing the hair into small workable sections.

Firstly, you will need to decide where you are going to begin your haircut. If you are beginning in the nape area, you will need to comb down a fine mesh of hair; this is classed as a section of hair. As you work through the haircut, you will continue to bring down new sections of hair, making sure they are neat and level.

Hair that you are not working on will need to be secured out of the way. The sections of hair should be no more than 1.25 cm deep; this will enable you to see your previous guideline through each section of hair.

By following these guidelines, you will be able to work around the head, using your time to the maximum benefit and ensuring you achieve the desired result.

Correct sectioning – the hair is divided into four parts and secured

Incorrect sectioning – uneven sectioning, hair taken from either side with no precise lines and no methodical working method

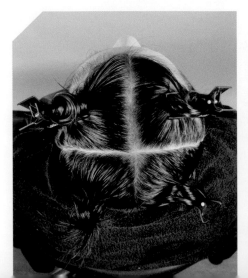

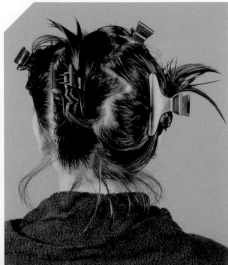

Cutting techniques

Club cutting

This method leaves the ends of the hair blunt and level. It is sometimes called the blunt cut. The technique is the most commonly used one for removing length from the hair and is ideal for fine hair, as it gives the appearance of increasing bulk. It can also help to reduce the tendency of the hair to curl.

Club cutting is very suitable for both straight and curly hair. Sections are combed through and held with tension, ensuring that the ends of the hair are blunt and level. This technique can be used on hair that is either above or below the shoulders and on wet or dry hair.

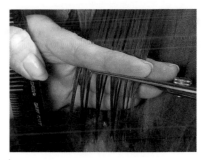

Club cutting

309

Top tips

When club cutting, the section taken must be combed through so that the hair is smooth and held with even tension to ensure an even result.

Unit
GH12

Cut hair using basic techniques

Freehand cutting

This technique is mainly used on straight hair when cutting a one-length look. As the name of the technique suggests, you do not hold the hair with tension — the hair is combed into place and cut freehand.

The freehand technique gives you a truer indication of where the hair will sit when dried because you will not have used tension by pulling the hair down. The technique is therefore often used to cut fringes as they have a tendency to 'jump up' after they have been cut. It is also better suited to one-length looks that are cut above the collar. Cutting hair above the collar length requires a very blunt, even line — by combing the hair down flat onto the neck and cutting freehand, you will be able to achieve this precise line. The freehand cutting technique is rarely used for cutting curly hair as the hair does not sit in one place; the curl in the hair means it will lift and not remain stationary to allow it to be cut freehand.

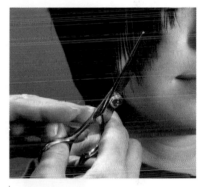

Freehand cutting

Step-by-step freehand cutting

1 Hair may be cut freehand around or over the ear to achieve an even blunt line without any graduation.

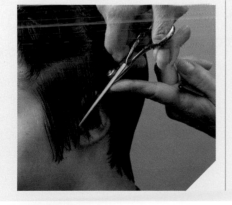

2 The hair is combed down flat into the nape of the neck, and then cut freehand without picking up the section or using tension on the mesh of hair.

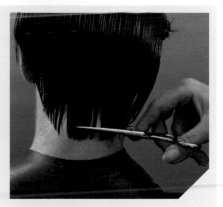

Fact or fiction?

Is this statement fact or fiction?

Clippers can be used on wet and dry hair.

To check your answer see page 499.

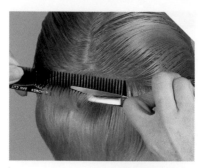

Scissor-over-comb technique

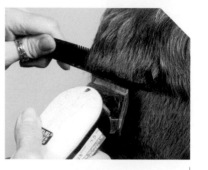

Clipper-over-comb technique

Scissor-over-comb

This technique is used to cut hair very short following the natural contours of the head. It is most frequently used in the nape area or around the ears and is often used in barbering to taper the hair into the hairline.

The technique can be used on wet or dry hair, although you will achieve a better result on dry hair, as the cutting line is clearer.

Clipper-over-comb

With clipper-over-comb, clippers are used instead of scissors to give a similar effect to scissor-over-comb. Both techniques allow you to cut the hair shorter than if you were holding the hair between your fingers.

Thinning

There are various cutting techniques that can be used to thin the hair as well as using thinning scissors and razoring techniques (for information on tools, see pages 300–1).

Some of the thinning techniques that you will be using are also referred to as texturising techniques. The thinning method of cutting removes bulk from the hair without removing the overall length. Thinning can be carried out on wet or dry hair. On dry hair, it is more obvious where the bulk/weight is in a haircut (the only exception is when using a razor).

Technique		Suitability	Benefit
Weave cutting		This technique is best suited to medium, straight or wavy hair and can be carried out on wet and dry hair. (It can be used on short or curly hair but other methods would be more suitable.) It is not suitable for partings, hairlines and the crown area.	Creates different lengths of hair. The shorter pieces will stand up, supporting the remaining hair, and can create lift on 'flat spots' on the head.
Pointing/ chipping		Ideal for straight and wavy hair on most hair lengths.	This technique will break up hard lines in the hair. It is often used to soften the edges of a haircut around the face. It will subtly remove bulk from the ends of the hair.
Castle cutting		Can be carried out on wet or dry hair, straight and wavy. The best results are achieved on short hair.	Gives a shattered edge look to the style. Removes bulk from the ends. If used 'deep' into the hair it will create a very textured look.

Technique		Suitability	Benefit
Razoring		Ideally to be carried out on wet hair to prevent any tearing or discomfort to the client. Not recommended on very fine, fragile hair.	Will encourage the hair to curl if a wave is present. Can be used to remove length and bulk from the hair, leaving the ends soft and feathered.
Thinning		Not recommended for very fine hair. Can be used on large areas on either straight or curly hair.	Removes bulk without removing length. Overuse will result in the ends becoming very wispy.
Slicing		Ideal for medium length to long hair, straight, wavy or curly. Not suitable for fine hair.	Mainly used to remove bulk and texturise the hair. Can also remove length. Will produce a soft finish to cuts.

Avoid using thinning techniques on front hairlines, natural partings or the crown area. This may produce unwanted spiky effects.

Thinning techniques

Step-by step guides to the one-length look

When asked to describe a one-length cut, most people would point to a bob cut on straight hair. However, a one-length cut can be carried out on curly hair (either permed or naturally curly), which would look totally different although it is the same cut. You need to remember that different factors have to be taken into account for every head of hair that you cut. Each client and head of hair is unique. The main purpose of a one-length cut is to keep maximum weight in the hair.

Cutting techniques for a one-length look

There are two main types of technique to achieve a one-length cut:

- club cutting (see page 309)
- freehand cutting (see page 309).

Both types of cut can be used on either wet or dry hair.

312

Unit
GH12

Cut hair using basic techniques

Step-by-step cutting of straight one-length hair

1 Section the hair into four equal sections and drop a fine mesh of hair at the nape. This is referred to as the base line. Note that the head is tilted forwards to prevent unwanted graduation.

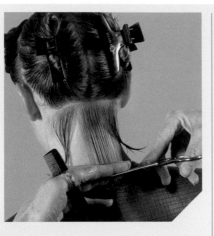

2 Continue to bring even sections down. Always begin cutting the new section in the middle of the head, working out to either side. Work your way up to the crown area in this manner.

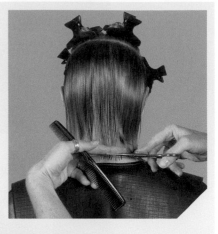

3 Check the length and balance of the haircut by taking hair from the same place on each side of the head. Run your fingers down to check the length is even.

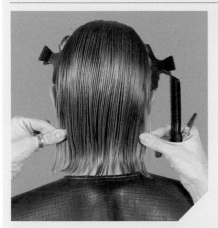

4 Connect the sides to the back by dropping a fine mesh of hair and cut from the back sections working towards the front.

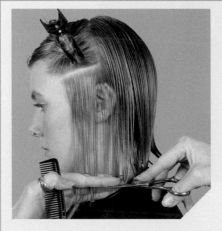

5 Continue to bring all of the sections down, working towards the client's parting.

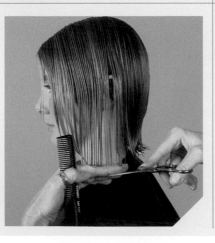

6 Confirm with your client that they are happy with the finished result, and provide the correct aftercare advice.

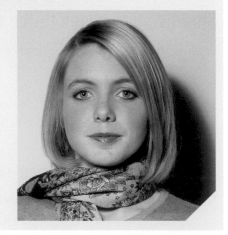

Important factors to consider when cutting one-length hair

- Tilt the head forward when cutting the back sections — to prevent unwanted graduation.
- Section evenly — for an accurate cut.
- Keep tension even — for an accurate cut.
- The hairline at the sides is finer than the nape hairline — allow for this hair to 'jump up'.
- Make sure there is no hair caught behind the ear when cutting the sides.

Important factors to consider when cutting curly one-length hair

- Allow for the hair to get shorter as the curls dry.
- Apply more tension to your sections to achieve an accurate cut.

Step-by-step guides to layered looks

Uniform layer cut

This technique involves putting layers into the hair following the natural shape of the head. Imagine a client with a crash helmet on – think about how the shape of the helmet follows the shape of the head. In a uniform layer cut, the layers are cut to the same length all over the head, hence its name.

Step-by-step uniform layer cut

1 Drop a fine mesh of hair in the nape and cut the baseline to the desired length.

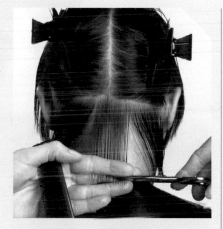

2 Take a panel of hair from the crown down the middle of the head to the nape baseline. Cut the hair, beginning at the crown at an angle of 90 degrees to the head.

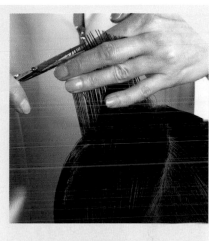

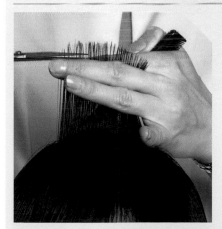

3 After working in 'orange segments' through the back, go back to the top crown hair and pull up a section of hair at 90 degrees to the head. Continue to remove the appropriate length.

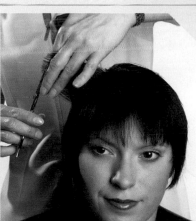

4 Following the head shape round, continue to cut the hair either side of the section, working towards the front hairline.

5 When all inner layers have been cut 90 degrees to the head, go back to the perimeter length and remove any unwanted hair to ensure a clean, even shape.

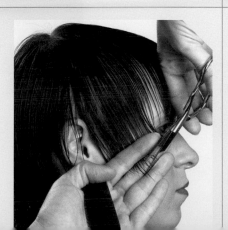

6 Confirm the finished look meets the client's expectations and offer the correct aftercare advice.

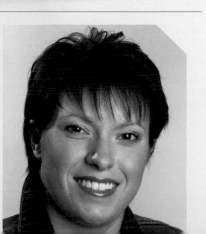

313

Unit
GH12

Cut hair using basic techniques

Unit
GH12

Cut hair using basic techniques

Graduated layer cut

This technique involves changing the angle of the layers that you are cutting. The angles can be anywhere between 45 and 180 degrees. Increasing or decreasing the angle of the layers will determine the amount of weight left in the hair.

Step-by-step graduated layer cut

1 Working from the bottom baseline, decide on the angle you will be cutting to achieve the weight that is to be left in the haircut. Hold the hair at a 45-degree angle with the hand turned out towards you to ensure you can achieve your angle.

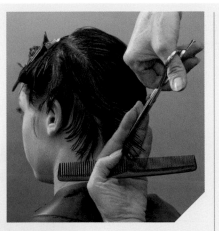

2 Having achieved the desired length and angle in the first section, use as a guideline and proceed to work out on either side of the middle section to behind the ears.

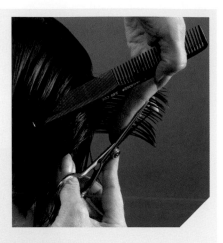

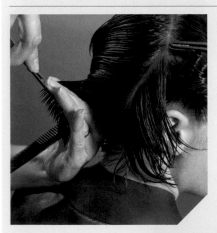

3 As you work closer to behind the ear, begin to slightly over-direct the sections, reducing elevation; this will enable you to maintain the length and angle required.

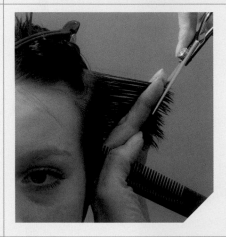

4 If you are completing an asymmetric graduated layer, one of your side sections will be cut shorter, either above or on the ear. Decide where you want your perimeter baseline to sit and then use this to continue angling the hair at 45 degrees to maintain weight and length in top sections.

5 On the opposite side, which is going to be longer, use the last back section behind the ear as a guide and continue to decrease the elevation and increase the over-direction.

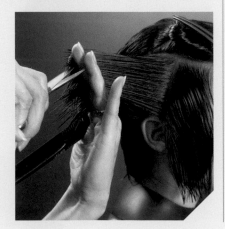

6 The finished result. Check for balance and provide aftercare advice.

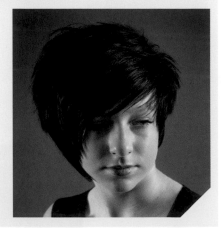

Step-by-step long graduated cut

1 A panel of hair is taken from the crown and cut following the head shape at 90 degrees.

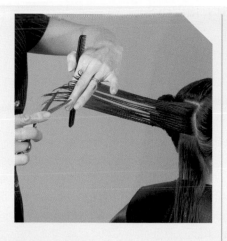

2 Working down towards the base line, continue to pull the hair out following the head shape.

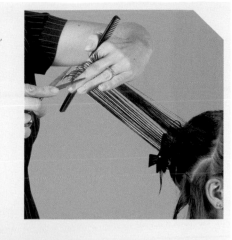

Cut hair using basic techniques

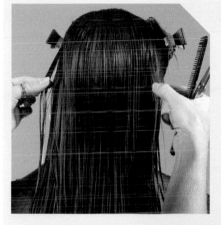

3 Continue to work in 'orange segments' around the head using a piece of the old section with a piece of the new section to ensure a balanced result. Check the balance by running your fingers down the hair lengths.

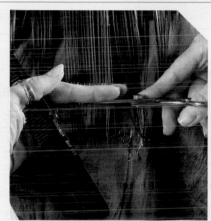

4 When the layers have been completed, the baseline/perimeter will need to be tidied up to achieve an even, clean, blunt line.

5 To shape the hair at the sides, determine where the shortest length is going to sit and work downwards to connect to the base line. Pull the hair forward if you wish to maintain length.

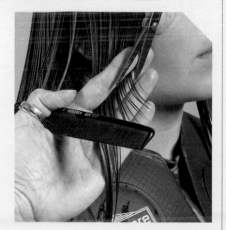

6 Comb through and check the length and end result with the client, making sure you have an evenly balanced haircut.

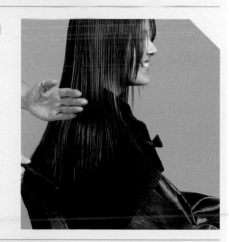

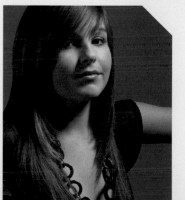

7 Apply styling products, blow-dry the client's hair in the desired style and provide the appropriate aftercare advice.

Adapting your cutting techniques to take into account critical influencing factors

You have looked at cutting methods/techniques and critical influencing factors. Now you need to put the two together.

When you are going to carry out a hair cutting service on a client, you will need to establish during your consultation what critical influencing factors (if any) you have to consider.

It is important to check through the client's hair before and after you shampoo the hair. This is because not all critical influencing factors are apparent on either wet or dry hair. If a client has straightened her hair and you have carried out your consultation on straight hair, when you take her to the basin and wash the hair, you may discover that she has a very strong natural wave in her hair which means that you may need to use a different cutting method from the one you had discussed.

It is important to carry out your consultation on dry hair and then re-check the hair when it is shampooed to make sure you have identified all the potential critical influencing factors.

Client satisfaction

Consulting, checking and confirming the client's satisfaction with the finished cut

As you are progressing through your cut, you will need to adjust the position in which you work around the head.

If you think about tennis players, they do not stand in one position on the court and stretch to reach the ball; they move around the court and adjust their positioning so that they achieve their end result to win the game.

Although heads come in different shapes and sizes, they are all round. If you stand 'square on' to a head of hair and try to cut the hair in this position, you will not achieve a balanced shape. You will need to move around the head as you work so that you are covering all angles of the haircut. This will help you to achieve an accurate cut, ensuring that you have even distribution of weight and balance throughout the style.

Cross-checking your haircut as you work is another factor that will help you to achieve even distribution and weight throughout the style. To cross-check a haircut, you will need to take sections/meshes of hair in the opposite direction to the way in which you have carried out your haircut. You should still hold them at the same angle as you did for the original haircut and continue to work in small methodical sections so that you are covering the whole of the haircut.

A mirror is another good tool to use to check the shape, weight and balance of a haircut. If you stand directly behind your client and lift sections of hair, you will be able to use the mirror to confirm that they are of the same length, that you have used the same angle on both sides and have achieved a balanced result.

When you have gained experience, you can also carry out this process without using your mirror. You will be able to check sections through feel, looking to see if the hair is 'sitting' in the style you have cut, seeing if the weight left in the hair is working, giving you the effect both you and the client wanted to achieve.

By cross-checking and using your mirror to check the weight and angles of your cut, you are giving yourself and your client the opportunity to make any changes to the haircut before you get to the drying stage. It is important to check with your client that she is happy with what you have done and is ready for you to dry her hair into the finished result.

> *Cross-checking a uniform layer haircut*

317

Unit

GH12

Cut hair using basic techniques

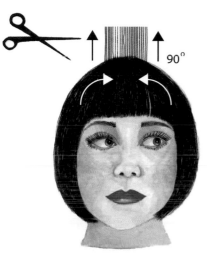

Hair is held up and cut at 90 degrees for the main haircut. To cross-check, the hair is combed and a section taken in the opposite direction, still held at 90 degrees and checked.

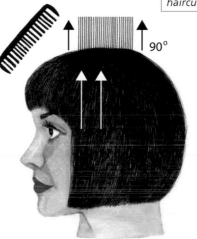

Section taken along the head to cross-check the cut.

How to provide aftercare advice

Giving aftercare advice is important as part of the whole service. You would not expect to go to a hi-fi shop and purchase a stereo system and not receive information or instructions on how to use the equipment that you have bought. The same applies to providing your client with information following any service given in the salon.

The types of information on aftercare that you should be giving your client include:

- how often she should come back into the salon for a trim to maintain the look (remember that on average, hair grows 1.25 cm (½ inch) per month; some hair may grow more quickly or slowly but this gives you a good indication of how frequently the style will need to be trimmed)
- which products are best suited to your client's hair type and will help to recreate the look you have achieved
- which tools (for example, correct size of brush) and equipment are best for achieving the look.

Basically, you are trying to give information that will help the client to maintain her hair and achieve the desired effect.

You can talk to your client about the use of products and drying techniques during the service and give her information on how much the average head of hair grows each month, so that she will have a better understanding of why it is important to come into the salon for regular trims.

Salon life

Confidence with cutting

Hannah's story

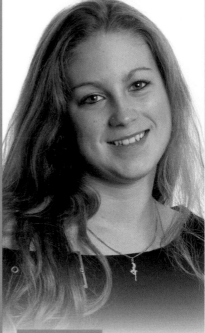

I am in the last few months of my hairdressing qualification and have been working in the industry for the last year, gradually building up my client base. I am really pleased with how things have been going, but was slightly concerned because the main bulk of my work has been colouring. I felt OK with the basic cuts but was a little uncertain with more angled styles.

After chatting with my tutor at college about the problem, I went through my hair magazines and cut out several pictures of cuts that I felt I would struggle to recreate. I took them into college and sat down with my tutor. She got me to draw all over the pictures to show where I thought the cutting angles were and write what angle the hair was held at. When I broke a cut down into areas rather than looking at the whole look in one go, it became much more obvious how the hair had been sectioned and what cutting angles had been used. I have done this quite a lot now and am finding that I can break a picture up in my mind and look at it in segments to help me work out the cutting methods and techniques used to create the style. I was so surprised to see that most haircuts are based on the basic cuts we have been taught, with sometimes only a slight variation on a few angles.

Top tips

If you are going to cut out magazine pictures, get them laminated so they can be reused over and over again.

Ask the expert

Q *I have watched several of the stylists in my salon carry out cuts in completely different ways, but they want to reach the same end result. Does this mean that one of them is cutting incorrectly?*

A No, if you lined a group of stylists up and asked them all to carry out the same cut, they would (most likely) all do something different. We advise our students to watch different people's techniques and try them all to see which one works for them. As long as they achieve the finished result without any health and safety issues, that is all that matters. We are all individuals, so our cutting will be different.

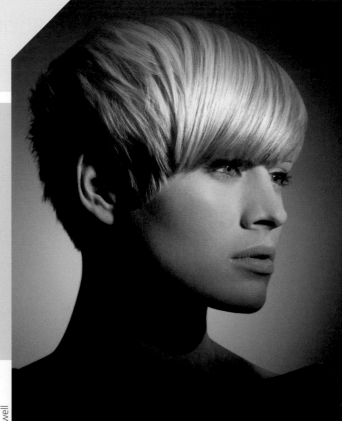

Goldwell

Check your knowledge

The following questions will help you to check your understanding of this unit.
The answers can be found on page 499.

1 Thinning scissors are also known as:
 a) bulk removing scissors
 b) serrated scissors
 c) curl enhancing scissors
 d) razoring scissors.

2 It is important to sterilise equipment after every client to:
 a) make your tools and equipment look and smell nice
 b) keep yourself busy between clients
 c) minimise the risk of cross-infection and infestation
 d) make sure they work properly.

3 'Sharps' is the term given to:
 a) the prong on pintail combs
 b) scissors
 c) a blunt haircut
 d) the blades in safety razors.

4 When the hair's 'texture' is referred to, this means:
 a) the amount of hair a client has on her head
 b) how much the hair can stretch and return to its original shape
 c) how damaged the cuticle may be
 d) whether a single strand of hair is fine, medium or thick in diameter.

5 Critical influencing factor means:
 a) any factor that you have to take into account when adapting your haircut
 b) any disease or disorder present on the hair or scalp
 c) how much money the client wishes to spend on a haircut
 d) how much time you have to carry out a service.

6 A freehand cutting technique involves:
 a) not using a comb on the hair
 b) not using tension on the hair
 c) not using sectioning clips on the hair
 d) not wetting the hair.

7 The purpose of club cutting the hair is to:
 a) create a 'shattered' edge
 b) make the ends of the hair blunt and level
 c) remove bulk but not length from the ends of the hair
 d) allow the hair to curl up into its natural position.

8 The scissor-over-comb technique is used when:

   a) you need to be quick and haven't got time to section all of the hair

   b) thinning the ends of the hair out

   c) you need to get in close to the head, where the hair is too short to pick up

   d) you need to create hard lines.

9 Clippers are sterilised using:

   a) Barbicide®

   b) an autoclave

   c) boiling water

   d) sterilising wipes and sprays.

10 During a one-length cut the head is tilted forward to prevent:

   a) unwanted graduation

   b) the sides from 'jumping' up

   c) the stylist getting backache

   d) the hair from 'bouncing' up.

11 It is important to cross-check your haircut because:

   a) this makes you look professional

   b) you can check you have achieved a balanced shape

   c) it gives you the chance to work body into the hair

   d) you can talk the client through the haircut.

12 Tension is important when cutting hair because:

   a) all haircuts have to be cut the same way

   b) it allows you to determine how much the hair will 'jump up' for the finished result

   c) it ensures you achieve a balanced result

   d) it makes the hair easier to cut.

13 Using a scissor-over-comb technique will allow you to:

   a) cut hair that is too dense for you to hold

   b) cut very fine hair to give a thicker appearance

   c) cut curly hair without using too much tension

   d) cut the hair shorter in the nape of the neck.

14 If you cut the hair using a 90-degree angle all over the head you will achieve a:

   a) long graduation

   b) uniform layer

   c) short graduation

   d) one-length cut.

15 A hair growth pattern is:
   a) how fast the hair grows
   b) how long the hair will grow
   c) the movement of the hair at the root area
   d) the movement of the hair at the mid-lengths and ends.

16 A short graduated haircut is cut at a:
   a) 45-degree angle
   b) 90-degree angle
   c) 180-degree angle
   d) 110-degree angle.

Getting ready for assessment

The assessment for the cutting hair unit is similar whether you are doing the NVQ or VRQ. You will be assessed using a combination of assessment methods, as described below. Remember that within each of the services you carry out with a client, you will cover different units. For example, when carrying out a cutting hair service (GH12 or GB3), you will also have to be aware of health and safety (G20) and giving clients a positive impression (G17) at all times. You may also shampoo and condition hair (GH8) and set or dress hair (GH11). If you are not sure what you have covered in your service, always ask your assessor or supervisor for advice.

	NVQ	VRQ
Credit value	8	8
Guided Learning Hours	80	75

	NVQ	VRQ
Practical demonstrations, to be observed by assessor	You are required to complete eight cutting performances, two for each of the four cutting looks (fringes can be incorporated into any of the cutting looks). These looks must include a: • one-length cut that is above the shoulder • short graduation incorporating the use of scissor-over-comb. Simulation is not allowed for any evidence requirements within this unit. You must complete all of the ranges listed.	You are required to complete eight cutting performances, two for each of the four cutting looks listed in the ranges (fringes can be incorporated into any of the cutting looks). These four looks must include a: • one-length cut that is above the shoulder • short graduation incorporating the use of scissor-over-comb. Simulation should be avoided where possible.
Service timings	Cut hair – all techniques 45 minutes	Cut hair – all techniques 45 minutes
Additional evidence	Knowledge and understanding will be assessed by an independent written paper.	Knowledge and understanding will be assessed by an independent written paper.

Task mapping

When you have completed the tasks in this unit, check the table below to see which Performance Criteria (purple), Range (red), Knowledge (green) and Key Skills (blue) you have covered within GH12 to use as additional evidence within your portfolio. Information about which Functional Skills you have covered is available on the website.

Task and page reference	Mapping to Performance Criteria, Range, Knowledge and Key Skills
1 (page 300)	Performance Criteria: 1g, 1i, VRQ 2i Range: N/A Knowledge: 3, 4, 5, 7, 11, 12, 13, 14, VRQ 1d, 2j, 2p Key Skills: C1.2, C1.3
2 (page 302)	Performance Criteria: 1e, 1f, 1g, 1k Range: N/A Knowledge: 8, 12, 14, VRQ 1d, 2p Key Skills: C1.1, C1.2, C1.3
3 (page 304)	Performance Criteria: 1j Range: VRQ R2a–e Knowledge: 2 Key Skills: C1.1, C2.1, N1.1, N1.2, N1.3, N2.1, N2.2, N2.3

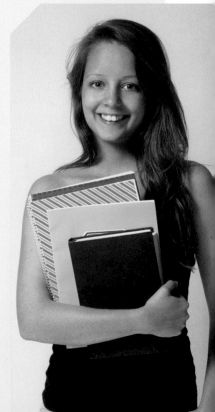

4 (page 304)	Performance Criteria: VRQ 2i Range: N/A Knowledge: 3, VRQ 1d, 2p Key Skills: C1.2, C1.3, C2.3
5 (page 305)	Performance Criteria: 2a, 2b, VRQ 1b, 2a, Range: N/A Knowledge: 15, 18, 19, 20, VRQ 1c, 1f, 1g Key Skills: C1.1, C1.2, C1.3, C2.3
6 (page 305)	Performance Criteria: VRQ 1b, 2a Range: N/A Knowledge: VRQ 1c, 1f, 1g Key Skills: C1.1, C1.2, C1.3, C2.3

323

Unit
GH12

Cut hair using basic techniques

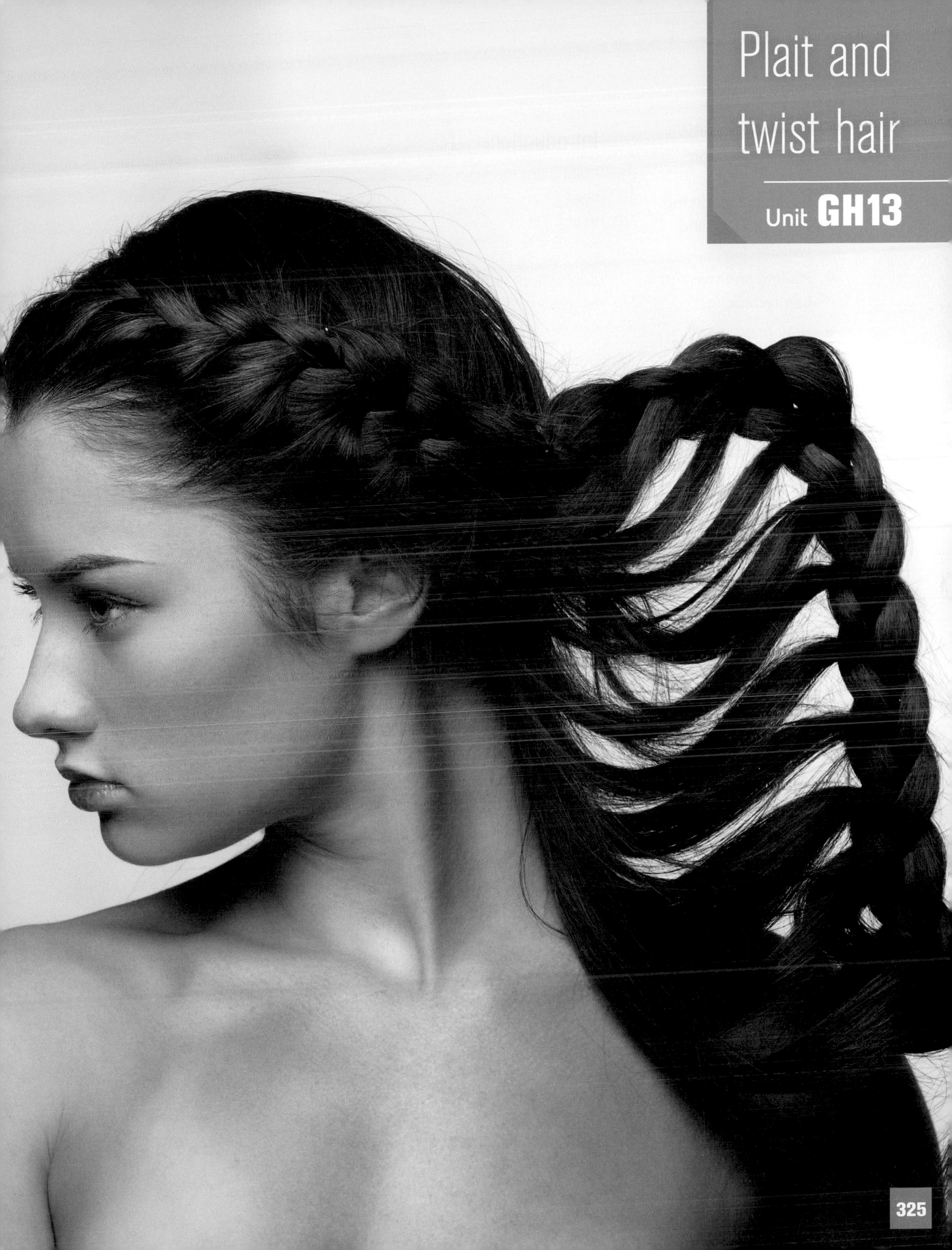

Plait and twist hair

Unit **GH13**

Unit

GH13

Plait and twist hair

What you will learn:

- **How to maintain effective and safe methods of working when plaiting and twisting hair**
- **Plaiting and twisting hair techniques**
- **How to provide aftercare advice**

Introduction

Plaiting and twisting hair is an art and can take a long time to perfect. You will need a huge amount of practice in creating the five different looks necessary to gain this unit of your Level 2 qualification. This unit consists of using plaiting and twisting techniques to achieve a variety of different looks: multiple cornrows, French plait, fishtail plait, two-strand twists and flat twists. You will need to have a high level of manual dexterity to become competent at these techniques as many require the use of very small sections of hair being worked in a very intricate, methodical sequence.

At one time plaits were only seen on small children and were personified by the character Heidi in the 1970s TV series. Plaits and twists have become more fashionable lately due to high-profile stars such as Kylie and Fergie (from the Black Eyed Peas) wearing a combination of plaits and twists within their hairstyles for their music videos and for major events like red carpet award ceremonies. The trend has also been widely used on catwalks during the unveiling of the new season's fashion ranges and has made its way down to the high street. The great advantage of plaits and twists is that they keep the hair away from the face so a plait around the front hairline is practical as well as providing a funky focal point to the hairstyle.

Fact or fiction?

Is this statement fact or fiction?

Cornrow plaiting originated in India.

To check your answer see page 499.

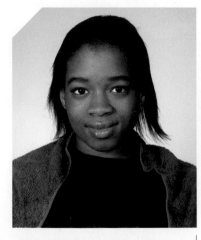

Gown client correctly for plaiting and twisting

How to maintain effective and safe methods of working

Preparing and protecting your client

It is vital to the well-being of your client that you follow your salon's rules for preparing and protecting your client during plaiting and twisting services. You must always consider the effects of the products you are using and their potential for harming your client. This will help you evaluate any risks and prevent accidents happening.

Firstly, you will need to gown your client and use a towel to protect their clothing from products and natural hairfall.

Task 1

Write down your salon's requirements for client preparation for plaiting and twisting hair and keep in your portfolio for evidence.

Posture

You must make sure your posture is good while plaiting and twisting hair, as these services require you to bend in awkward positions so that you can get in the correct position to plait and twist the hair closely into the scalp. As hairdressers we stand for long periods of time and poor posture can lead to fatigue and more permanent risks of bodily injury, especially back and shoulder problems.

Clients should be seated comfortably and squarely in the salon chair with both feet on the floor or footrest for even posture. If your client has her legs crossed, ask her politely to uncross them, or her plaits or twists may be unevenly positioned.

Health and safety issues

It is also very important to protect yourself from the occupational hazard of the skin complaint **dermatitis**, which has caused such severe skin problems for some hairdressers that they have had to change careers. If you always wear gloves when necessary, this will help prevent dermatitis. (Refer to G20, page 55.)

Effective working methods

As a salon employee or college trainee, you will be expected to use all products carefully and effectively. Safe and effective working methods will include the following:

- *Minimising the wastage of products* – always use the right amount of product for the individual client's hair. Never overload the hair with plaiting and twisting products as the excess will cause the hair to become too oily to work with or excess product could end up on the floor causing potential health and safety risks. Wastage of product is not cost-effective to the salon and will result in the salon's profits declining.
- *Minimising the risk of cross-infection* – during the consultation for plaiting and twisting hair, you will need to evaluate the condition of your client's hair and scalp prior to the service. If you find any risk of cross-infection to yourself, your colleagues and other clients, you must not continue with the service. These would be classed as **contraindications** (see G7, pages 144–48).
- *Making effective use of your working time* – you should always make the best use of your time in the salon. You can do this by making sure you have all tools, equipment and products ready to hand before your client arrives for her appointment. If you were an employer paying an hourly rate, would you pay someone for wasting time? If you do not make the most effective use of your working day, you will not be deemed competent for your Level 2 qualification and a salon owner with a business to run will not want to employ you.
- *Ensuring the use of clean resources* – would you like to sit in a dirty salon or have dirty brushes or towels used on you? All clients have the right to know that the salon tools, equipment and resources used on them are totally clean and sterilised if necessary. A dirty salon will not attract or keep clientele.
Refer to G20, page 63 for the best methods of sterilisation for your tools and equipment.
- *Minimising the risk of harm or injury to yourself and your clients* – you and your salon have an obligation to your clients and visitors to ensure their safety. Your salon also has an obligation to you as an employee to ensure your safety while you are at work. All members of the salon team must make sure they know how to work safely to avoid accidents happening in the salon. This can be done by following all of the salon's health and safety policies, rules and regulations. See G20, pages 49–51.

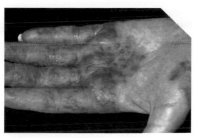

Contact dermatitis

327

Unit

GH13

Plait and twist hair

Dermatitis

An inflammation or allergy of the skin, usually affecting the hands of hairdressers. It causes the hands to crack and bleed due to constantly being wet and coming into contact with certain chemicals. Drying hands thoroughly after shampooing, using a good barrier cream and always wearing gloves when touching chemicals will help to avoid this. Sometimes called contact dermatitis.

Contraindication

In this unit a contraindication could be the presence of traction alopecia (see pages 330 and 331) or **folliculitis**.

Folliculitis

Inflammation of the hair follicles. This can occur when the hair is pulled tight into plaits or twists which open the follicle slightly, allowing bacteria to enter. The follicle will then become infected and yellow pustules will form at the base of the follicle.

Task 2

Write down what dermatitis is and explain how to avoid developing it while carrying out plaiting and twisting services.

Top tips

A clean and tidy working area helps you work efficiently and presents a good professional image to your client.

Working area

Your working area must be kept clean and tidy at all times to prevent hazards and potential accidents. Always wipe up any spillages of water or plaiting and twisting products immediately to avoid slippery patches on the floor. Once you have finished with a piece of equipment, always put it away so you have as much space as possible to work in. Used towels should be placed immediately in a towel bin, so that it is obvious to staff and clients that they are ready for washing.

Task 3

What would you consider to be contraindications to plaiting and twisting hair? List five contraindications and explain why they would prevent you from carrying out a plaiting or twisting service.

A worksheet for this task is provided on the website for you to complete and add to your portfolio.

Task 4

How might wastage happen in your salon? How can you help to minimise wastage? Write down three methods and keep this in your portfolio for evidence.

A worksheet for this task is provided on the website for you to complete and add to your portfolio.

Commercial timing

It takes skill and accuracy to plait and twist hair perfectly, and you will need a great deal of practice before you become competent. As a Level 2 Hairdressing student, you have Performance Criteria (PCs) and range statements (Ranges) for plaiting and twisting to meet before your assessor can be sure you are competent. In addition to these PCs and Ranges, you also need to prove you can plait and twist the hair neatly and precisely in a commercially acceptable time.

- Multiple cornrows: 120 minutes – full head
- French plait: 20 minutes
- Fishtail plait: 20 minutes
- Flat twists: 45 minutes
- Two-strand twists: 30 minutes – single, 120 minutes – full head

Your awarding organisations will also provide this information in their assessment guidance.

Plaiting and twisting hair techniques

Consultation and communication

A vital part of this service, as always, is a thorough consultation. You need to use all the good communication skills you have learned to be as confident as possible when asking your client questions before and during the plaiting and twisting service. The plaiting or twisting style chosen must be completely clear to both you and your client so that the finished style has been agreed. You do not want to spend time and effort completing intricate plaits to be told when finished that the style is not what the client wanted!

A client's lifestyle can influence the choice of style when plaiting and twisting hair. If the client is an active sportsperson, a style which keeps the hair away from the face and that needs little maintenance (e.g. cornrows) may suit the client more than twists which may come loose/out as they are competing in a sports event. However, some plaiting or twisting styles which result in the hair being tightly secured to the scalp may not be considered suitable by certain employers.

Tools for plaiting and twisting

It is important to use the correct tools to achieve good results. When plaiting and twisting you need to have a good-quality pintail or tail comb which will have fine teeth for sectioning and a pointed tail which will not scratch the scalp. Another tool which may help you is a postiche brush, which is a thin brush specifically for use during long hair work. It has narrow bristles and a pointed end (similar to a tail comb) which is good for sectioning. You will also need a wide-toothed comb and sectioning clips to secure hair out of the way while you are working.

Sectioning and securing

Neat and precise (known as clean) sectioning is an important part of both plaiting and twisting services to ensure you work neatly and accurately and produce precise work. Even if your plaits and twists are perfect, if your sectioning is uneven your finished design will not been deemed competent. You must have a plan of the finished plaiting and twisting direction and design so that you can section cleanly and evenly. This is so you have a vision of the pattern and where you want the hair to go.

When securing your plaits and twists you should never use normal elastic bands, as these will rip and tear the cuticle scales. You should only use bands for professional use such as covered elastics or mini silicone bands, which are specially designed to hold the hair securely but will also be kind to it at the same time. There are lots of different kinds of either covered elastic bands or silicone bands which are less abrasive to the cuticle scales when securing hair. Some stylists like to use pipe cleaners as they twist around and secure the ends of the hair without damaging it. Twists can be secured with grips, tiny jaw clips or bands depending on the look you are creating.

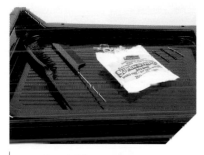

Tools for plaiting and twisting – postiche brush, pintail comb, mini silicone bands and hair grips

329

Unit

GH13

Plait and twist hair

Unit
GH13

Plait and twist hair

Factors affecting plaiting and twisting

Hair density

The amount of hair your client has needs to be taken into account before plaiting or twisting. Sometimes the hair is too sparse for a particular style and this will need to be explained to your client. Also, if the client has lots of hair it will not only increase difficulty in sectioning but will also take longer for you to achieve the finished result.

Hair texture

The thickness or thinness of your client's hair will have an effect on the finished plaiting or twisting style. Some hair textures are deceiving and the hair looks thicker than it actually is. Fine hair left long and loose can look quite normal in texture, but if you plait this type of hair it can look really thin and wispy. Thick hair can cause problems when sectioning, especially if you are doing really small and complex sectioning, as the thickness of the hair can get in your way. Try to be as dominant with the hair as you can (hold the hair with good **tension** and be as firm as you can without causing your client discomfort) and keep the hair you are not working with sectioned out of your way.

Head and face shape

When assessing your client's head and face shape you need to take into account any prominent features or shapes. For example, if a client has an excessively large nose you would not want to give them a full head of multiple cornrows as this will only emphasise the client's nose. The idea is to try to maximise any good features or shapes and minimise the focus on any negative features.

Hair elasticity

Assessing the hair's elasticity is something you have learned about in G7. (Go back to page 141 to refresh your memory if necessary.) The hair's elasticity is important to this unit as any service that puts tension on the hair has the potential to break or snap delicate hair or hair with little elasticity. For this reason you should be wary of plaiting hair with tension or hair that you feel is weak, delicate or lacking in good elasticity. Some children's hair is delicate as the protein of the hair (**keratin**) sometimes doesn't harden fully until children reach their teenage years.

Hair length

The hair needs to be long enough to enable you to plait or twist it into a style. If the hair is not long enough it will be really difficult to create the style and the plaits or twists may fall out during the special occasion! Be honest with your client to avoid disappointment. If the hair is too long it may be too heavy to hold twists and they may also fall out. You would not want this to happen while your client is dancing at a special occasion ball or during the first dance at her wedding! Be honest with your client once you have assessed the viability of the chosen style.

Tension

How firmly a mesh of hair is held during plaiting and twisting the hair. Tension should always be kept even, as uneven tension will produce uneven plaits or twists.

Keratin

Protein found in hair, nails and skin.

Traction alopecia

Hair thinning or hair loss due to excessive tension on the hair follicle. This can be a result of wearing the hair in tight plaits or twists. The source of the tension needs to be removed and the client may need to be referred to a **trichologist**.

Trichologist

A person who is qualified to diagnose and treat hair and scalp disorders and diseases.

Task 5

Write down the meaning of traction alopecia and explain how this condition is caused.

Scalp condition

If your client has any scalp condition that is infectious (for example scabies, head lice, ringworm, impetigo) you must not proceed with the plaiting or twisting service as this will be putting you, your colleagues and the rest of the salon's clients at risk of cross-infection. If your client has a condition that is not infectious but that can be unsightly, for example psoriasis in its dry state, then it may not be advisable to show the scalp by plaiting into multiple cornrows or by sectioning into small twists, which would make the scalp condition visible to all.

Desired look

Magazines and style books are ideal visual aids to show your client before deciding on a chosen style. It also allows you to be confident in knowing the style the client has chosen is the same style you have in your mind to create. Sometimes clients are not aware of the correct names for styles or techniques, so make sure you are both positive about the intended style result.

Controlling the hair when plaiting and twisting

To ensure you produce even plaits and twists, it is important to maintain a comfortable and even tension while working. If your tension is loose, the plaits and twists will be too loose and may fall out. However, if your tension is excessively tight you will cause discomfort to your client and may even cause **traction alopecia**. If a client comes into the salon and you notice broken hair around the hairline where the hair has been plaited, you should advise your client to have a break from plaiting so that the tension in this area is relieved. If you plait hair with this condition you may well contribute to the breakage and a worsening of the condition. The client may need to see her GP for a referral to a **trichologist**.

Products for plaiting and twisting

There are certain products developed especially for helping to control the hair while plaiting and twisting. These products also help to keep the hair in shape once the finished result has been achieved. You need to follow the manufacturer's directions when applying these products so that you do not overload the hair, making it appear greasy or too hard and crispy. This will also ensure you use plaiting and twisting products cost-effectively, which will mean better profits for your salon.

Products for plaiting and twisting are:

- *Sprays* – used before or after plaiting and twisting hair to keep the style in place.
- *Serums* – these are silicone-based products used before plaiting or twisting to smooth the cuticle scales when styling.
- *Gels* – strong liquid-based products used before plaiting or twisting hair which dry hard to keep hair in place.

Plaits and twists

To be deemed competent in this unit you need to practise and create the looks on the following pages. Once you have practised and feel confident you can produce the looks neatly and cleanly, you are ready for assessment.

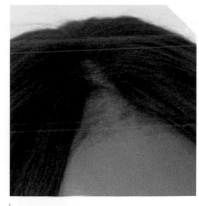
Traction alopecia

331

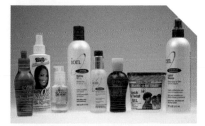
Spray, serum and gel for plaiting and twisting

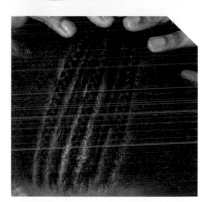
Multiple cornrows, lots of three-strand plaits which sit on top of their base.

Fact or fiction?

Is this statement fact or fiction?

Cornrow plaiting is also known as cane row.

To check your answer see page 499.

Step-by-step French plait

A French plait is a single inverted plait using all the client's hair.

1 Beginning at the front hairline, take a small triangle of hair and split into three equal sections. Ensure this is centred or the plait will look one-sided.

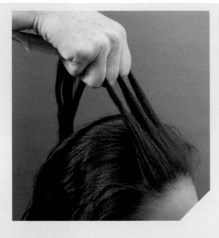

2 The outside section is crossed over the centre section of hair. Ensure the plait stays central while you are progressing. Adjust your hand hold so that you can hold all three sections with even tension. Begin by taking one of the outside sections and cross it over the middle section. Repeat this for the opposite outside section. You should do this twice before adding in extra hair.

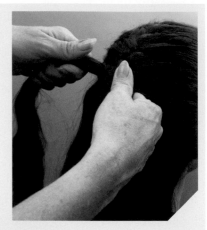

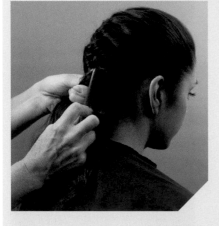

3 Now add new sub-sections of hair to the existing sections you are holding. Start by running a pintail comb or a 'free' finger from the front hairline on one side of the head to the base of the plait. Add this new section of hair to the section you have just crossed over the centre of the plait and hold with even tension.

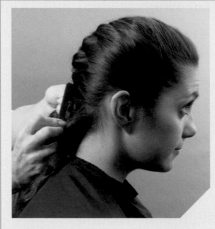

4 This method of adding a new sub-section of hair every time an outside section is crossed over a centre section is repeated on both sides of the head. It helps to use your thumb to anchor the hair in place to keep tension firm throughout.

5 It is important to keep the tension equal on both sides of the head while working so the finished plait will look even. You should be regularly combing the hair through with either your fingers or a pintail comb to keep the sections even, clean and knot free.
It is also a good idea to tilt the client's head as you work, as this will help to maintain tension.

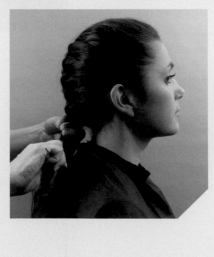

6 Plait the remaining three sections together in a normal plait and secure the ends with a hair band. You may wish to use hairspray to 'tuck' any loose strands into place.

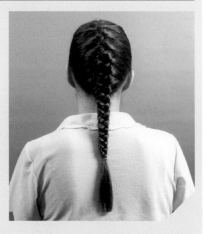

Step-by-step fishtail plait

A fishtail plait is achieved by crossing even sections of hair over each other to create a herringbone look. The fishtail plait can be used to finish off a French/scalp plait or the hair can be put into a ponytail before a fishtail plait is carried out.

Note: on more mature clients this technique is often carried out on hair that has been brought over to one side of the head; younger clients can wear the look centrally at the back.

1 Before starting a fishtail plait the hair must be brushed through and completely tangle free. Start by dividing the hair into two equal sections.

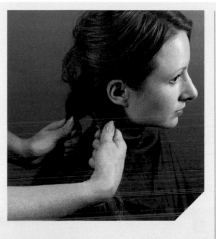

2 Using your forefinger, take a small sub-section from the back of the left-hand section and pass this over to the right-hand section. Combine this with the section you are holding in your right hand. Maintain good tension.

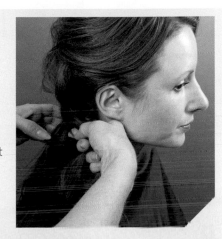

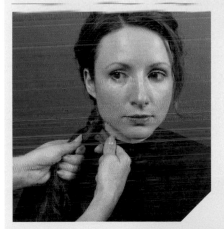

3 Now take a small sub-section from the back of the right-hand section and pass this over to the left-hand section, maintaining good tension throughout.

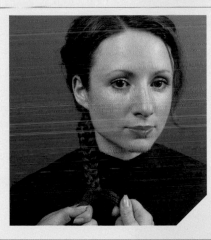

4 Repeat this method, keeping good tension and small, even sub-sections until all of the hair is plaited.

5 Secure the ends with a hair band.

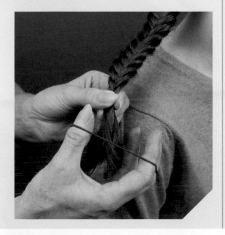

6 The finished fishtail plait.

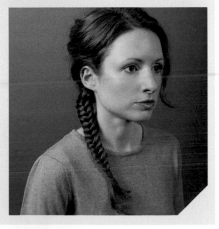

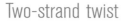

Twist out

A two-strand twist which is untwisted after it has dried.

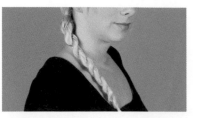

A two-strand twist

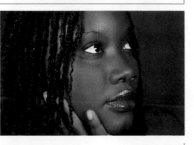

Two-strand twists

Two-strand twist

In this style, the hair is twisted left over right, left over right until the twist is complete. This can be done on wet or dry hair and can be used before a **twist out**.

Task 6

Use the internet or magazines to research plaiting and twisting styles and patterns. Use the images you find to create a visual aid to show clients the plaiting and twisting styles available. Try www.virtualhaircare.com and the *Hairdressers Journal International* as well as hairstyling magazines.

Step-by-step flat twists

In this style, the hair is rolled and twisted by hand flat to the scalp.

1 Take a central, narrow section from the front hairline to just before the crown. Use your pintail comb to ensure even sectioning.

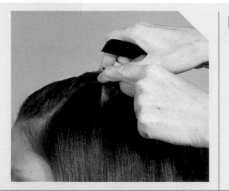

2 Twist and roll the section flat from the front hairline to the back of the section. Maintain firm tension as you are twisting.

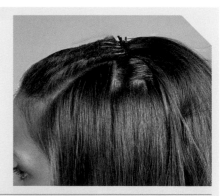

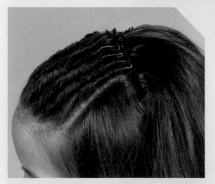

3 Secure firmly with grips. These can be crossed over each other to anchor the hair securely.

4 Repeat this method until all the hair is twisted flat on one side, down to the ear section.

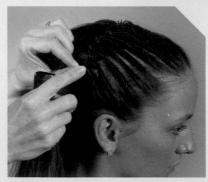

5 Repeat evenly on the opposite side of the head until all the front sections are twisted flat and secured firmly.

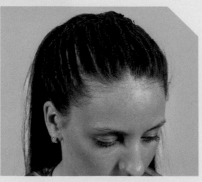

6 Incorporate the rest of the hair into the finished look and provide the appropriate aftercare advice.

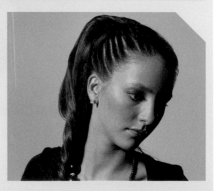

How to provide aftercare advice

In order to maintain the plaits or twists, it is important to give your client clear advice on suitable homecare products and their use. If your client goes home without knowing how to care for her plaits or twists, they are unlikely to last for the time generally expected. Anything rubbing or causing friction on the hair will have a detrimental (harmful) effect on plaits or twists.

To ensure the condition of the hair is maintained, it is important to give guidance on how to remove the plaits and twists. If your client is unaware of the correct procedure and rips out the bands securing the plaits and tries to pull the plait out from the root, this will not only cause knotting but will also be painful and damage the hair.

You should advise your client to be methodical about removing plaits and twists. Using a tail comb, always work from the points of the hair, undoing the plait and working up to the root. Use a wide-toothed comb to comb through the hair once all the plaits have been removed. It is advisable to carry out a deep conditioning treatment once the plaits or twists are removed to replace moisture and strengthen the cortex.

Advise your client that a lot of hair may fall out once the plaits or twists are removed and that this is quite normal. The longer the plaits or twists have been in, the more hair will fall out. Explain that this is only natural hair fall which would have ended up in the client's brush if the hair had not been in plaits or twists. Everyone loses between 80 and 100 hairs a day, and if these hairs are not able to fall out because they are stuck in a plait or twist, then you will see them all fall out once the plait or twist is removed.

Always recommend homecare advice and products to your client so that she can maintain the hard work that you have carried out. For cornrow plaits which may stay in the hair for weeks, it is advisable to recommend a light oil to keep the scalp moisturised. Your client may wish to shampoo the hair while in cornrow plaits, and you should recommend light gentle shampooing movements using a moisturising shampoo to avoid drying the scalp.

Top tips

A satin or silky pillow case may help prolong the life of plaits or twists.

335

Unit

GH13

Plait and twist hair

Task 7

Write down the types of products available in your salon for plaiting and twisting. State when and why you would use these products. Make a note of the manufacturers' instructions on how to use these products economically.

A worksheet for this task is provided on the website for you to complete and add to your portfolio.

Salon life

A fragile client

Joy's story

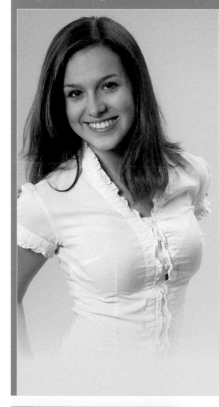

When I was training I was asked by a client to do multiple cornrow plaits. Although I could do cornrows easily, I was a bit concerned because the client's hair looked quite fragile at the hairline. I asked the client if she had had problems with the hairline before and she said no, so I continued with the plaiting service.

A couple of weeks later the client returned to the salon and said her hair had started to break around the hairline. When I looked properly at the client's hairline, I could have cried. The hairline had receded right back and what was there was really wispy. I felt dreadful to have let this happen. I removed the plaits and carried out a deep penetrating conditioning treatment to help restore some protein and moisture to the hair. The client never returned to the salon and I still feel bad about plaiting her hair, as I should have said no to the plaits when I saw the hairline was weak. I will never make this mistake again!

Top tips

Never go against your instincts and always rely on your professionalism. If you don't think you should carry out a service, state this to your client and fully explain the reasons why, including outlining the possible consequences should you carry out the service.

Ask the expert

Q   *Why do some clients' hairlines become weak and break when in plaits?*

A   This is due to excessive tension being placed on the hair shafts at the hairline. It can cause the hair to become weakened at the root, and if the pressure continues the hair will be pulled out and break off. It takes a long time for the hair to regenerate and therefore the hairline can look sparse for a considerable period.

Check your knowledge

The following questions will help you to check your understanding of this unit.
The answers can be found on pages 499–500.

1 State what traction alopecia means.

_____

2 Why is it important to minimise the risk of cross-infection and infestation when plaiting and twisting hair?
   a) So that you look good to the client
   b) To ensure that you do not pass on any infections or infestations to clients and colleagues
   c) So that you do pass on any infections or infestations to clients and colleagues
   d) So that you stay clean yourself

3 What are the potential consequences of excessive tension on the hair when plaiting and twisting?
   a) The client may lose hair through a condition called traction alopecia
   b) The client may moan at you for pulling too tight
   c) The client may not tip you if you pull too hard
   d) The client may lose hair through a condition called alopecia areata

4 Why should you section hair accurately when plaiting and twisting hair?

_____

_____

_____

5 State three methods of securing plaits and twists.

_____

_____

_____

6 Why is it important to use products economically when plaiting and twisting hair?

_____

_____

_____

7 Why is it important to recommend homecare advice to your client after plaiting or twisting services?

_____

_____

_____

8 Why is it important to give good advice to your client regarding removing the plaits or twists?

_____

_____

_____

9 How can your client's lifestyle influence the choice of the style of the plaits or twists?

_____

_____

_____

10 Why might there be lots of hair fall when the plaits or twists are removed?

_____

_____

_____

Unit

GH13

Plait and twist hair

Getting ready for assessment

You will be assessed using a combination of assessment methods, as described below. Remember that within each of the services you carry out with a client, you will cover different units. For example, when plaiting and twisting hair (GH13), you will also have to be aware of health and safety (G20) and advise and consult with clients (G7). You may also shampoo and condition hair (GH8) or set or dress hair (GH11). If you are not sure what you have covered in your service, always ask your assessor or supervisor for advice.

	NVQ	VRQ
Credit value	4	5
Guided Learning Hours	37	30

	NVQ	VRQ
Practical demonstrations, to be observed by assessor	You will be assessed on at least four occasions and each occasion must be for a different look. You have to prove you can create all the plaits and twists in the range: • *Multiple cornrows* – lots of three-strand plaits which sit on top of their base. This is also known as a cane row. • *French plait* – a single inverted plait using all the client's hair. • *Fishtail plait* – a plait achieved by crossing even sections of hair over each other to create a herringbone look. • *Two-strand twists* – the hair is twisted left over right, left over right until the twist is complete. • *Flat twists* – the hair is rolled and twisted by hand flat to the scalp. Simulation is not allowed for any performance evidence within this unit.	You need to take into account all the factors R1a–k. Select the appropriate styling and finishing products and give the correct aftercare advice.
Service timings	Multiple cornrows (over 50 per cent) – 45 minutes French plait – 30 minutes Fishtail plait – 30 minutes Two-strand twists (over 50 per cent) – 45 minutes Flat twists (over 50 per cent) – 45 minutes	Twists (50 per cent of head) – 45 minutes Scalp plait 30 minutes
Additional evidence	It is likely most evidence will be gathered from the observations made by the assessor, but you may be required to produce other evidence to support your performance if the assessor has not been present. This unit requires mandatory written questions.	You will need to complete a written question paper.

Unit

GH13

Plait and twist hair

Task mapping

When you have completed the tasks in this unit, check the table below to see which Performance Criteria (purple), Range (red), Knowledge (green) and Key Skills (blue) you have covered within GH13 to use as additional evidence within your portfolio. Information about which Functional Skills you have covered is available on the website.

Task and page reference	Mapping to Performance Criteria, Range, Knowledge and Key Skills
1 (page 326)	Performance Criteria: 1a, VRQ 1a, 2a, 2c Range: N/A Knowledge: 1, 4, VRQ 1d Key Skills: C1.2, C1.3, C2.3
2 (page 327)	Performance Criteria: 1b, 1f, VRQ 2c, 2j Range: N/A Knowledge: 3, 5, 6, VRQ 2r Key Skills: C1.2, C1.3, C2.3
3 (page 328)	Performance Criteria: 1f, 1g, VRQ 1c, 2d Range: VRQ R1a–k Knowledge: 10, VRQ 1f Key Skills: C1.2, C1.3
4 (page 328)	Performance Criteria: 1f Range: N/A Knowledge: 27 Key Skills: C1.2, C1.3
5 (page 330)	Performance Criteria: N/A Range: N/A Knowledge: 14, 15, 16, 17 Key Skills: C1.2, C1.3, C2.3
6 (page 334)	Performance Criteria: Practising 2a, 3a Range: 2a–e Knowledge: 19, VRQ 1e Key Skills: C1.3
7 (page 335)	Performance Criteria: Practising 2g, 3a, 3b, VRQ 1b, 2a, 2g Range: Practising 4a, VRQ R5a–e, R6a–f Knowledge: 25, 26, 27, 28, VRQ 2m, 2p Key Skills: C1.2, C1.3, C2.3

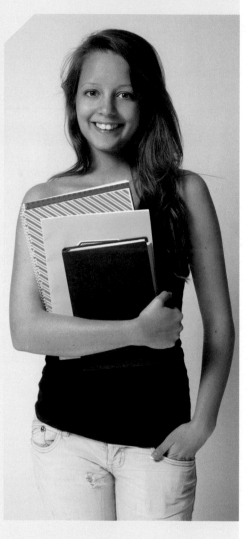

Perm and neutralise hair

Unit GH14

Goldwell

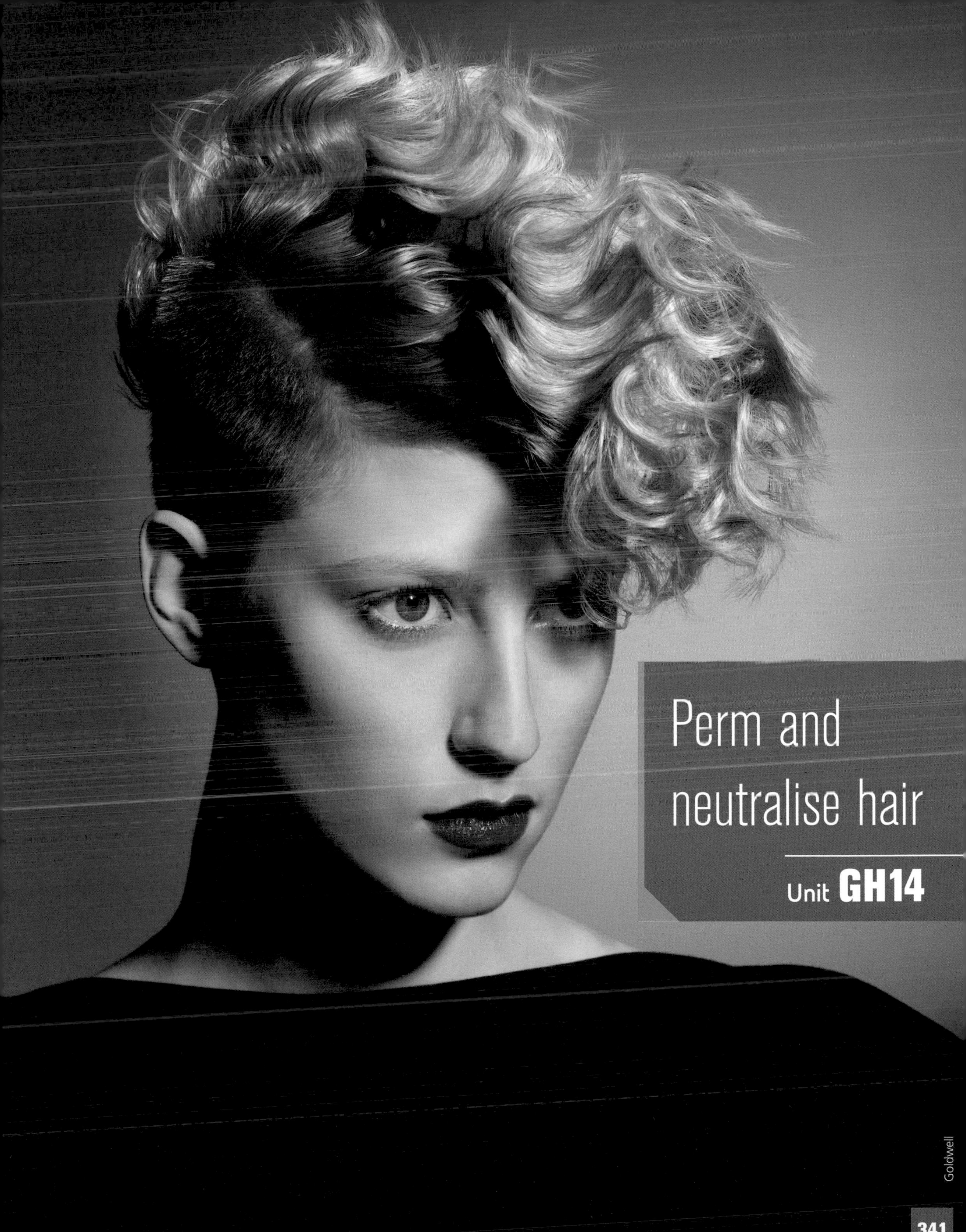

What you will learn:

- **How to maintain effective and safe methods of working when perming and neutralising hair**

- **How to prepare for perming and neutralising**

- **How to perm and neutralise hair**

- **How to provide aftercare advice**

Introduction

Perming and **neutralising** are permanent chemical processes that change the structure of the hair (perming comes from the old-fashioned term 'permanent wave'). They can be damaging to the hair if you do not understand what effect the chemicals have on the hair structure. Anyone can buy a home perm from the chemist, but if you do not know what the chemicals in the perm and neutraliser are capable of doing to the hair and scalp, the results can be disastrous. Therefore, it is very important to understand the hair structure, especially the cortex region where the chemical changes take place during both perming and neutralising, in order to achieve a professional result. The correct use of aftercare products such as restructurants is also extremely important.

This unit contains all the information you will need to know about perming and neutralising. (Before you begin this unit, look back at the section Facts about hair and skin, pages 2–5, for a reminder of the hair's structure.)

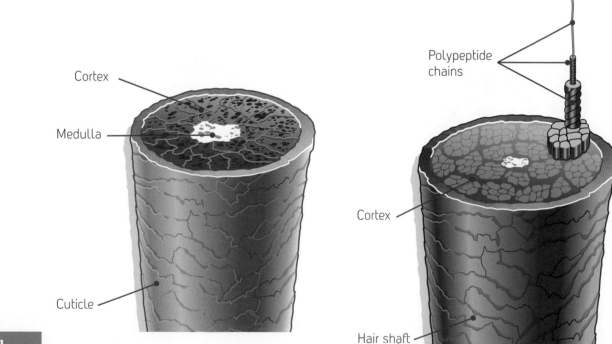

Cortex

Medulla

Cuticle

Polypeptide chains

Cortex

Hair shaft

Perming

The process of curling hair by chemically altering its internal structure (the cortex).

Neutralising

The chemical process that fixes the hair in a new position after it has been altered by the action of perm lotion.

How to maintain effective and safe methods of working

It is vital that you follow all health and safety rules and regulations during the perming and neutralising process to ensure the highest level of client care possible. This will also ensure you reach a high standard of work, as health and safety is an essential part of every process you carry out as a professional stylist.

How perms work

Perming involves three stages.

1 softening
2 moulding
3 fixing

The softening stage

Perm lotion opens and swells the cuticle scales, so that it can enter the cortex. Some acid perm lotions need added heat to help open the cuticle scales – remember the pH scale from Facts about hair and skin (see page 13). Mildly acid products close the cuticle scales. Always read and follow the manufacturer's instructions.

The moulding stage

The perm lotion enters the cortex where it deposits hydrogen. The hydrogen attaches itself to the **disulphide bonds** and breaks them apart into separate individual sulphur bonds. (Not all disulphide bonds are broken during perming.) The hair, which has been softened, is now able to take on the shape of the perm rod. This is known as moulding.

The fixing stage

Neutralising removes the hydrogen from the cortex by adding oxygen (a process of oxidation). The hydrogen attached to each sulphur bond combines with the oxygen molecule, creating H_2O (water). This process joins together the separated, individual sulphur bonds to re-form disulphide bonds in a new position, which permanently fixes the curl.

343

Unit

GH14

Perm and neutralise hair

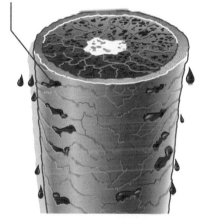

Perm lotion opens and swells cuticle scales

The softening stage

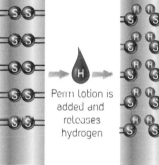

Before perming, disulphide bonds intact

The hydrogen attaches itself to the disulphide bonds and breaks them into single sulphur bonds

Perm lotion is added and releases hydrogen

The moulding stage

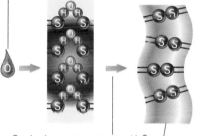

Neutraliser is added and oxygen is released. Oxygen joins with the hydrogen to make H_2O (water)

$2 \times$ hydrogen + oxygen = H_2O, which is rinsed from the hair

Sulphur bonds re-form to make disulphide bonds in a newly curled formation, which permanently fixes curl

The fixing stage

Disulphide bonds

Two sulphur atoms bonded together, found within the cortex region of the hair. Forming part of the protein of the hair (keratin) these bonds help to maintain the hair's elasticity. Being strong, they can only be broken by the addition of perm lotion.

Preparing your client

Gowning

The chemicals used in perm lotion and neutralisers can cause a colour change in some fabrics. It is important to ensure the client's clothes are fully protected with a towel, chemical gown (this is plastic coated and will stop any liquid penetrating it), second towel for extra protection and plastic cape.

Consultation

A thorough consultation is an essential start to a successful perming result. In addition to the normal areas to assess, such as hair texture and porosity, you need to ask the client some specific questions relating to the perm.

- Do you have any perm, colour, bleach or relaxer on your hair?
- Is your skin sensitive to perm lotion?
- What size curl do you require?
- How do you manage your hair at home – do you set, blow-dry or leave to dry naturally?
- Do you have any problem areas that do not perm very well?
- Are you on any long-term medication? (This could have affected the internal quality of the hair, which may lead to the hair becoming too fragile for the perming process. In the worst cases, the hair can break, so this is an important question to ask.)

Once you have the answers to these questions you can decide:

- if any hair tests are necessary
- what size perm rods and winding technique to use
- which perm lotion and application technique to use.

Health and safety issues

Perming and neutralising involves the use of chemicals and you have to know and understand your responsibilities when using these products. You must always read and follow the manufacturer's instructions for the particular product you are using. If you decide, for whatever reason, that you no longer need to read the instructions, you will be showing a complete disregard for the safety and well-being of your client and going against the professional standards of the hairdressing industry.

Task 1

Compare two different manufacturers' instruction leaflets for two different perm lotions. Write down and compare the:

a) ingredients
b) processing times
c) neutralising times
d) rinsing times.

A worksheet for this task is provided on the website for you to complete and add to your portfolio.

Personal protective equipment (PPE)

When applying perm lotion and neutraliser, it is important to protect yourself from the possible effects of the chemicals. You must wear an apron to protect yourself from any splashes of perm lotion or neutraliser. As mentioned earlier, these chemicals can discolour fabrics.

It is also very important to protect yourself from the occupational hazard of the skin complaint **dermatitis**, which has caused such severe skin problems for some hairdressers that they have had to change careers. If you always wear gloves when applying perm lotion and neutraliser to avoid contact with these chemicals, you will minimise the risk of this happening to you.

Under the Personal Protective Equipment at Work Regulations, your employer has a responsibility to provide protective materials and gloves for you to use and you have a responsibility to wear them.

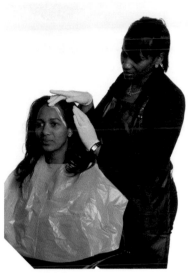

345

Unit
GH14

You and your client must be properly protected before applying perm lotion, relaxer and neutraliser

Task 2

1 Write down what you could do to help prevent yourself getting the skin condition dermatitis.
2 Why do you think it is important to follow these precautions?

Control of Substances Hazardous to Health Regulations (COSHH) 2003

Under the Control of Substances Hazardous to Health Regulations (COSHH) 2003, you must read the data sheets provided by the manufacturer of the perm so that you know how to handle, store and dispose of the chemicals used in the product.

Generally, perms should be stored in a cool, dry place away from bright sunlight. They should be used in a well-ventilated area and the manufacturer's instructions must be followed. When disposing of any leftover perm lotion or neutraliser, you should dilute the chemicals by flushing them down the sink with plenty of water.

Effective working methods

As a salon employee or college trainee, you will be expected to use all products carefully and effectively. Safe and effective working methods will include:

- *Minimising the wastage of products* – always use the right amount of product for the individual client's hair. Never overload the hair with perm lotion or neutraliser as the excess will drip off the hair onto the client and the floor, causing potential health and safety risks. Wastage of product is not cost-effective to the salon and will result in the salon's profits declining.
- *Minimising the risk of cross-infection* – during the consultation for the perm you will need to evaluate the condition of your client's hair and scalp prior to perming. If you find any risk of cross-infection to yourself, your colleagues and other clients, you must not continue with the perm. These would be classed as contraindications (see page 144).
- *Making effective use of your working time* – you should always make the best use of your time in the salon. If you were an employer paying an hourly rate, would you pay someone for wasting time? If you do not make the most effective use of your working day, you will not be deemed competent for your Level 2 qualification and a salon owner with a business to run will not want to employ you.

Dermatitis

An inflammation or allergy of the skin, usually affecting the hands of hairdressers. It causes the hands to crack and bleed due to constantly being wet and coming into contact with certain chemicals. Wearing gloves when shampooing, using a good barrier cream and always wearing gloves when touching chemicals will help to avoid this. Sometimes called contact dermatitis.

Perm and neutralise hair

- *Ensuring the use of clean resources* – would you like to sit in a dirty salon or have dirty brushes or towels used on you? All clients have the right to know that the salon tools, equipment and resources used on them are totally clean and sterilised if necessary. A dirty salon will not attract or keep clientele.
- *Minimising the risk of harm or injury to yourself and your clients* – you and your salon have an obligation to your clients and visitors to ensure their safety. Your salon also has an obligation to you as an employee to ensure your safety while you are at work. All members of the salon team must make sure they know how to work safely to avoid accidents happening in the salon. This can be done by following all of the salon's health and safety rules and regulations.

Task 3

What would you consider to be contraindications to perming? List five and explain why they are contraindications.

A worksheet for this task is provided on the website for you to complete and add to your portfolio.

Task 4

How might wastage happen in your salon? How can you help to minimise wastage? Write down three methods and keep in your portfolio for evidence.

A worksheet for this task is provided on the website for you to complete and add to your portfolio.

Working area

Your working area must be kept clean and tidy at all times to prevent hazards and potential accidents. A clean and tidy working area also helps you work efficiently and presents a good professional image to your client.

Posture

You must also make sure your posture is good while working, as hairdressers stand for long periods of time and poor posture can lead to fatigue and more permanent risks of bodily injury.

Organisation and stock control

It is important to build into your working day time to organise yourself for your client's service before she arrives. When perming, this means organising your perm trolley to include:

- perm rods in different sizes
- end papers
- sectioning clips
- barrier cream
- towels
- gloves and apron
- perm lotion
- pre-perm spray or lotion.

If you do not organise yourself in readiness for the perm, you will be wasting valuable time. Your employer will want you to use all of your time at work effectively and your clients will not want to be kept waiting.

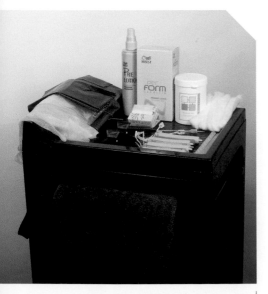

It is important to lay out all the equipment you will need for perming prior to the service

Stock control

In order for the salon to function effectively, you are required to follow stock control procedures. This will ensure that all perming products and equipment such as cotton wool, end papers and gloves are reordered when necessary and are available for use as and when required. A salon may lose business if the perm the client usually has is out of stock. There may not be another perm suitable to use on the client's hair and she may get the impression of a disorganised salon that does not care about its clients.

Commercial timing

It takes skill and accuracy to wind a perm perfectly and you will need a great deal of practice before you can perm a client's hair competently. As a Level 2 Hairdressing student, you have practical outcomes for perming and neutralising to meet before your assessor can be sure you are competent. In addition to these practical outcomes, you also need to prove you can wind a perm accurately in a commercially acceptable time.

Personal, learning and thinking skills – Effective participation

Once you have started to practise perming you will understand that it is not as easy as it looks. It is vital that you learn how to place straight perm rods in the hair at the right angle to ensure you do not cause chemical damage to the hair. A good way to learn this skill is to observe and assist a competent, experienced stylist as they perm hair. You can pick up a huge amount of skills and tips while passing up perm rods and perm papers! Ensure you pay particular attention to the angles being used to place the perm rods in the hair. Afterwards, try to recreate the perm winding techniques yourself, using the skills you have learned while observing.

Timing for perm winding techniques (winding only)

- Post-damping (applying perm lotion after rods are wound) – 45 minutes

The above timing is a target for you to work to and aim for. Remember, you should always follow manufacturers' instructions. Try not to be disappointed if you cannot achieve targets instantly: put all your energy into producing an accurate perm winding result and your timing will improve with practice.

Try perm winding on a practice block head if you have one, or ask someone patient to be your model. Ask your trainer or an experienced stylist to show you the following techniques.

How to section the head into nine sections

This sectioning technique is helpful when learning how to place the perm rods correctly over a whole head of hair.

How to practise winding a section at the nape area first

This is achieved by taking sections of hair as wide and nearly as long as the perm rods you are using. Pull the sections out at a 90-degree angle and try to keep hold with good **tension** so that the hair stays straight and looks tidy. Then put a perming end paper at about the middle of the section of the hair and try not to bunch the hair together in the paper. Once the end paper is in place, you can place the perm rod in

Top tips

Perming sundries such as neck strip cotton wool, end papers and gloves need to be replenished regularly.

Top tips

An uneven, messy perm wind will produce a poor perm result. Perfect your winding skills first and then practise speed winding to become commercially competent.

Tension

How firmly a mesh of hair is held during perm winding. Tension should always be kept even, as uneven tension will produce uneven curl results.

Carry out a thorough consultation and any hair tests necessary

Always read the manufacturers' instructions for the products chosen

Be organised and keep your area tidy as you work to avoid accidents happening

Wear the correct personal protective equipment: gloves and apron

Work efficiently throughout the perm – avoid wastage of products and sundries; minimise cross-infection by checking for any contraindications and by working safely with clean tools

Use your time effectively throughout the perm (time is money in the salon) and make sure all your resources are clean, minimising the risk of harm and injury to yourself and your client (remember the Health and Safety at Work Act)

Make sure you maintain a good level of stock

Always record the perm lotion used, rod size used, processing time and final curl result for future reference

Health and safety for perming services.

the middle of the end paper and, still holding with good tension, slide the perm rod and the end paper up to the ends of the hair. Make sure the ends of the hair go past the perm rod slightly (otherwise they will buckle and look frizzy) and then fold the end paper around the perm rod and keep winding around until all the hair is wound down to the scalp. Ask your tutor or assessor to check.

Completing client records

It is especially important to keep your clients' records up to date when perming. Records should contain all the relevant information such as date of the perm, products used, size of perm rods used, amount of processing time needed, whether heat was used during processing, perm result, price of perm and any other information you feel is necessary to record.

The record needs to be filled in accurately so note down the information while the perm is processing or immediately after your client has left the salon, otherwise you will forget how long the processing time was. Never guess at how long you think the perm took.

How to prepare for perming and neutralising

In this section you will be taken through the steps and information needed to ensure you have the understanding to prepare your client fully for perming and neutralising processes. Once you have prepared a client thoroughly in readiness for perming and neutralising, you will realise that everything you do during preparation has an effect on the subsequent perm and is critical to the service.

Questioning your client about contraindications and recording responses

Remember, a contraindication is something that prevents you carrying out the service. It is vital that you ask your client if she suffers from any contraindications to establish whether it is safe to carry out the perm. Perming lotion can irritate sensitive or allergic skin and can be very painful if applied to skin with disorders such as psoriasis.

It is important to record your client's responses to the questions you ask about contraindications in order to have proof that she was asked before the service in case of any problems which may occur during or after the perm. A good way of making sure that this is standard procedure in your salon is to have some standard contraindication questions printed on your client's record card, which can be ticked when they have been asked. You could also ask your client to sign the record card to validate that the questions were asked and their responses were accurately recorded.

Hair tests for perming and neutralising

You should always explain the importance of tests to your client so she is aware that you are checking to see whether the hair can withstand the chemical process you are going to carry out.

Elasticity test

This is to test the internal strength of the hair (the cortex). Hair that has been damaged due to chemical services may have lost much of its natural strength. This type of hair may stretch over two-thirds of its original length and may even break off. It is important to carry out this test before perming. Hair that is in good condition will stretch and then return to its original length.

Take one strand of hair and hold each end firmly between the thumb and forefinger of each hand and gently pull. If the hair stretches more than half of its original length, then it is over-elastic and may snap or break during chemical processing.

Porosity test

This tests the condition of the outer layer of the hair shaft – the cuticle. If the cuticle is damaged, it becomes **porous**. Perming chemicals added to porous hair will be absorbed unevenly and may produce uneven curl results. This is why special perm lotions for tinted and highlighted hair are used. They are weaker in strength and are less likely to over-process the hair and give a poor result.

Take a strand of hair and hold it by the points (where the hair has been cut) between the thumb and forefinger of one hand. Run the forefinger and thumb of your other hand from the root (where the hair grows from) down to the point. If the hair feels rough and bumpy, the cuticle scales are raised and open and this is an indication of porous hair. If the hair feels smooth, the cuticle is flat and closed and the hair's cuticle region is in good condition.

Incompatibility test

Some products do not work well together (they are **incompatible**) and may have a bad reaction if one is used over the top of another. Some colours, for example, contain metallic salts, which are incompatible with other chemicals. You should carry out an incompatibility test before perming if you are unsure of the colouring products already on the hair or if the hair has a doubtful history.

- Mix together (preferably in a glass bowl) 40 ml of 20 volume hydrogen peroxide and 2 ml of alkaline perm lotion.
- Place a small cutting of hair in the solution and wait. If heat is given off, the lotion fizzes and the hair breaks, dissolves or changes colour, then this is a positive reaction and the hair should NOT be permed or coloured with a product containing hydrogen peroxide. The hair contains metallic salts.

Pre-perm test curl

When handling fragile, porous hair or hair with a doubtful history, it is advisable to wind, process and neutralise one or more small sections of hair. The results will be a guide to the best rod size, processing time and lotion strength to use. This test will also give a good indication of the condition after the perming process and will determine whether the hair is suitable for this service.

Porous

Able to absorb substances. The condition of the cuticle determines how porous the hair is. If the cuticle scales are closed or lie flat, the hair will have good porosity; if they are tightly closed, penetration of products will be more difficult. If the scales are damaged and open, raised or missing, the hair will be over-porous and absorb chemicals too easily and quickly.

Incompatible product

A product that does not work well with other products. It may cause a reaction that could damage the hair and skin.

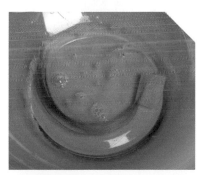

The incompatibility test

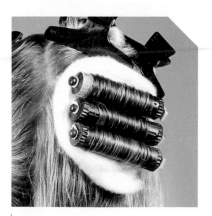

A pre-perm test curl on the head

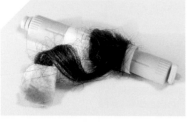

A pre-perm test curl tested separately

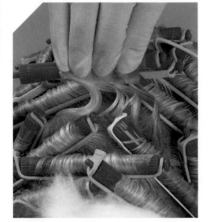

A development test curl

It is not always suitable or possible to carry out a test curl on the head, so a cutting of hair may be taken and tested separately, but remember there will be no scalp heat to help the processing.

- Wind two or three rods of your chosen size in the hair.
- Apply perm lotion suitable for the hair condition and leave to process for the manufacturer's specified time.
- Carry out a development test curl to see whether processing is sufficient (see below). If so, rinse, neutralise for the time specified by the manufacturer, remove rods and evaluate curl result.

Development test curl

This test is carried out during the processing of the perm to check whether the desired development has been reached. Always wear gloves to carry out this test.

- Hold the perm rod and undo the rubber fastener.
- Unwind the perm rod one and a half turns or until you see the start of the perm paper, holding firmly.
- Push the hair up and then in towards the scalp, allowing it to relax into an 'S' shape movement. Be careful not to pull the hair as it is in a very fragile state.
- When the size of the 'S' shape corresponds to the size of the perm rod, the processing is complete and the hair should be rinsed with warm water to avoid over-processing and neutralised following the manufacturer's instructions.

Always take test curls on different areas of the head as one area may be ready before another and this would cause an uneven curl result. The temperature of the salon will make a difference; perms will process more quickly on warm days than on cold days.

Skin test for perming

This test is carried out to check for allergic reactions or skin sensitivity to perm lotions and neutralisers.

Clean an area behind the ear and apply a small amount of the intended perm lotion and neutraliser to the skin using a cotton bud. The test should be left on the skin for 24–48 hours before the perm is carried out. If the skin becomes red or sore then the perm should not be carried out. Record the date and the result of the test on the client's record.

Once you have carried out the necessary tests and you are satisfied with the results, continue with the service.

When not to perm

- When the scalp is damaged or the skin is broken/damaged.
- When the hair is in poor condition.
- When the overall porosity of the hair is too high (over-bleached).
- If hair has evidence of metallic salts from previous colours.
- When the hair has poor elasticity.

Fact or fiction?

Is this statement fact or fiction?

It is important to ask your client questions during the consultation before perming and to record the client's responses to these questions.

To check your answer see page 500.

Top tips

Always test the hair to check that it is safe to carry out perming.

Task 5

Write down the six tests you have learned about in this perming unit and describe how to carry them out and why they are necessary.

A worksheet for this task is provided on the website for you to complete and add to your portfolio.

Perm and neutralise hair

Seeking assistance about contraindications and test results

We have discussed contraindications and the hair tests that may be necessary before a perm is carried out if you are doubtful about the hair or skin for any reason. Once you have identified a contraindication or have a problem test result, you need to know who you can ask for assistance in your salon. It is important that this person knows how to assess both contraindications and hair test results, and will normally be a more senior member of your salon team. If you are unsure what to do when you have one of the problems listed on page 350, you can ask this colleague to help you decide what action to take with your client.

Perming and neutralising products

Acid perm lotion

Acid perm lotion has been developed as a kinder alternative to the original alkaline perm lotion. Fewer bonds are broken in the cortex of the hair by acid perms and they are gentler to use on damaged hair or hair that processes very quickly (for example, porous hair).

Acid perms have activators that are added to them immediately before use. They rely on heat to open up the cuticle scales so that they can penetrate the cortex region. They generally have an acid pH of 6–7 and are made of a chemical called glycerol monothioglycollate.

Once an acid perm is mixed with its activator it only has a short life span and, consequently, any remaining lotion should be discarded. This makes pre-perm testing with acid perm lotions difficult, as you would not want to mix up a whole bottle of perm lotion to test one small piece of hair – this would not be cost-effective for the salon.

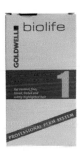

Acid perm lotion

Alkaline perm lotion

Alkaline perm lotion is generally stronger than acid perm lotion and comes in different strengths for different hair types. It has a pH of 7.1–9.5, which opens up the cuticle scales and allows the perm lotion to enter the cortex region of the hair. The higher the pH of the perm lotion, the more damaging it is to the hair (see Facts about hair and skin, page 13). This is why alkaline perms have conditioning agents added to them and acid perms are becoming increasingly popular. The chemical ingredient in alkaline perm lotion is ammonium thioglycollate.

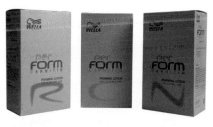

Alkaline perm lotions

Exothermic perms

Exothermic perms have the benefit of producing their own heat. Once the activator has been mixed with the perm lotion, you will be able to feel the lotion getting warm as you hold the bottle. Because they are self-heating, no added heat is necessary to open the cuticle or help the perm during processing.

Exothermic perms are generally made for use on all types of hair; however, you may need to leave them for less time on porous hair – always check the manufacturer's instructions. They can be a mixture of acid and alkaline or acid/alkaline depending on the manufacturer. The only way to check is to look at the chemical ingredients on the packaging and compare them with the acid or alkaline perm chemical ingredients.

Top tips

You should always recommend that your client has a perm before a colouring service, as the neutraliser is likely to fade or lighten the colour.

Suitability of perm lotions for different hair types

Neutralisers

Neutralisers come in many different forms: some are ready to use out of the bottle; some need to be mixed with warm water; some need to be foamed up in a bowl and applied with a sponge; some neutralisers are instant. The chemical ingredient in neutralisers may be either hydrogen peroxide or sodium bromate, both of which can lighten or fade hair colour.

Task 6

What are the active ingredients used in alkaline perm lotions? Write down this information and keep it in your portfolio for evidence.

Perm lotion	Hair type
Normal	Virgin hair that has not been treated with chemicals.
Resistant	White or greying hair, or very tight and compact cuticle scales.
Tinted	Hair that has been treated with permanent colours.
Bleached	Bleached or high-lift tinted hair including highlights (perm with great care if at all).
Porous	Dry, porous hair that has a poor cuticle area (perm with great care if at all).

Task 7

Find out about the perming products available in your salon. This will give you confidence when having to choose a perm lotion for your client's particular hair type.

Preparing and protecting your clients

It is vital to the well-being of your clients that you follow your salon's rules for preparing and protecting them during the perming and neutralising processes. You must always consider the effects of the chemicals you are using and their potential for harming your clients. This will help you evaluate any risks and prevent accidents happening.

Preparing the hair for perming

Begin by correctly gowning your client. Next, prepare the hair for perming by shampooing, using a soapless base shampoo with no additives, to ensure no residue is left on the hair as a barrier between the perm lotion and the hair.

When shampooing before a perm, use only cool/tepid water and do not massage vigorously to avoid over-stimulation of the scalp, as this can lead to sensitivity during the chemical process.

Barrier cream

This is a thick protective cream that should be applied all the way around the client's hairline before applying perm lotion (including the nape area) to avoid irritation of the skin. Care must be taken to avoid putting the cream onto the hair as this will cause a barrier between the perm lotion and the hair and will result in straight areas. Clients with sensitive skin will be more likely to have a skin reaction from the perm lotion so always take the utmost care to prevent this happening.

Top tips

Some clients use a lot of styling products that can leave white deposits on the hair even after shampooing. This build-up could cause a barrier between the perm lotion and the hair and should be removed with a clarifying shampoo. A second shampoo using a soapless base shampoo should then be carried out.

Applying pre-perm service

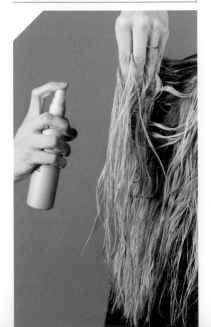

Pre-perm treatments

Pre-perm treatments are applied to the hair after shampooing and before the perm rods are used. They are used to:

- even out the porosity along the hair shaft to help the perm lotion penetrate at an even rate, which results in an even curl along the hair
- form a protective barrier along the cuticle region and close any cuticle scales that are raised
- make the hair more pliable when winding the perm rods into the hair.

Pre-perms come in either individual bottles or sprays and are applied to shampooed, towel-dried hair. Some companies make in-perm additives that are mixed with the perm lotion immediately before application to the hair. These types of products contain ingredients which lubricate and strengthen the hair prior to perming.

Post-perm conditioners

Special anti-oxidant surface conditioners are produced for use after perming. They have special properties.

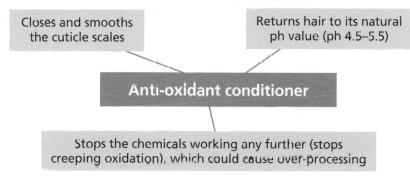

Closes and smooths the cuticle scales

Returns hair to its natural ph value (ph 4.5–5.5)

Anti-oxidant conditioner

Stops the chemicals working any further (stops creeping oxidation), which could cause over-processing

How to perm and neutralise hair

Perming can be one of the most rewarding hairdressing services, as you can achieve dramatically different results on a client's hair. For example, by perming you can add large, subtle curls to give root lift and support to styles, or you can turn long, straight hair into tumbling, curled tresses. You can also completely change the shape of a hairstyle by adding curls. Perming aids the appearance of the texture and movement of the hair by slightly swelling the hair shaft.

When you first begin perming it can seem like a very daunting and challenging practical skill to learn. It takes a huge amount of practice to learn the art of perm winding and the only way to master the techniques is to practise as much as possible (remember the old saying 'practice makes perfect').

Perming is one of the technical units of the Level 2 qualification, which requires you to practise in order to improve your winding technique, learn the correct placing of perm rods and improve your timing. Once you have practised and developed these areas, you will be ready to perm a client's hair, while remembering and putting into practice all that you have learned so far in this unit.

Question your client about any contraindications to perming and neutralising and record the responses

Carry out any hair tests you feel are necessary from your consultation

Choose your perm lotion and neutraliser from the results of your consultation

Ensure all products and equipment are close to hand and hygienic

Prepare your client thoroughly and make sure you prepare the hair ready for perming by using the correct shampoo. Towel-dry the hair to remove excess water

Apply a pre-perm treatment if necessary from the results of your consultation

Apply barrier cream around the hairline before applying perm lotion and neutraliser to stop hairline irritation

Apply an anti-oxidant conditioner after neutralising to stop the chemicals working any further (always read the manufacturer's instructions to check if this is recommended)

Preparing for perming and neutralising

Once you have mastered perm winding you need to improve how quickly you can wind a whole head of perm rods. This is because you need to be deemed 'commercially competent' at perming, which means you have 45 minutes to wind a whole head! Try timing yourself each time you practise perming as this will help you evaluate your progress.

In this section you will be learning how to carry out a perm from the beginning right through to the end, curled result.

Preparing the hair for perming

Begin by correctly gowning your client (see page 344). Next, prepare the hair for perming by shampooing, using a soapless base shampoo, to ensure no residue is left on the hair, which could act as a barrier between the perm lotion and the hair.

Factors influencing the service

These are sometimes known as critical influencing factors and are anything that could affect the perming process, for example hair condition. They must be taken into account for each individual client during the initial consultation before the perm is attempted.

You have already learned what needs to be assessed during a consultation for perming, but how can you be sure that you understand the curl size the client requires? Only by taking the time to discuss thoroughly the required results of the perm can you be certain you have gathered all the necessary information. Often a client will come in with a style book or picture of permed hair asking for the same result. You should explain that you can do something similar, but the model in the picture may have more or thicker hair, so the results will look slightly different.

Other factors that influence perming, which you need to take into account are:

- temperature of the salon
- hair condition
- hair texture
- hair length
- direction and size of the curl required
- previous chemical services
- haircut
- hair density.

Once you have considered all of the above, you will have the necessary information to choose the correct strength perm lotion, correct size perm rods, correct winding technique, application of perm lotion technique, and whether it is necessary to use added heat to aid processing.

The perming procedure

Sectioning and perm-winding techniques

There are three basic sectioning and perm-winding techniques that you need to master. They are:

- *Brick winding* – this is done to avoid any partings resulting from the perm and is ideal for fine hair.
- *Directional winding* – this is carried out when the hair needs perming in a specific direction and is ideal for clients requiring a parting within the hairstyle.
- *Nine-section winding* – this is the most commonly used perm wind when training as it is easier to learn how to fit all the rods onto the head shape using this technique. It is suitable for any hairstyle.

Step-by-step brick winding

1 Start at the front hairline taking a section of hair as wide as the perm rod but not longer than the rod (this will prevent 'baggy' ends) and wind to the scalp.

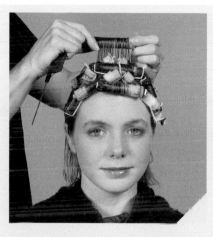

2 Now start the brick effect by sectioning underneath the perm rod, in the centre, to stop a channel line appearing. Wind another perm rod the other side and the brick wall effect will start to appear.

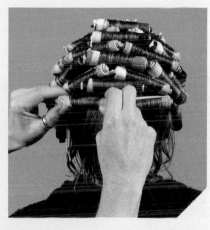

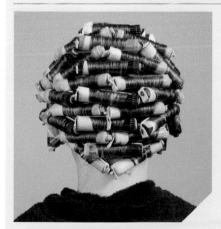

3 Try to slightly angle the section of the hair to be wound, as this will help the straight rods fit into the rounded shape of the head. Once all the hair is wound, check the rods are comfortable for your client.

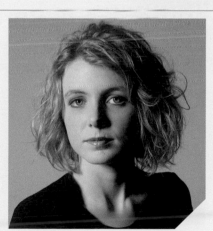

4 The finished result.

Top tips

When perm winding, you are trying to place straight perm rods onto a round head shape. This is not easy and takes practice – sectioning the hair first will help.

355

Unit

GH14

Perm and neutralise hair

Step-by-step directional perm winding

1 Firstly, section the hair where you wish the parting to appear. Wind from the top of the section away from the parting, finishing at the ear section. Repeat on the other side.

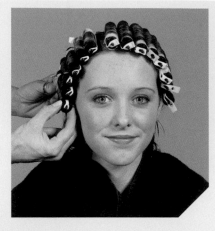

2 Wind the crown section in a directional movement to complement the finished hair style.

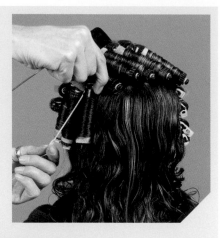

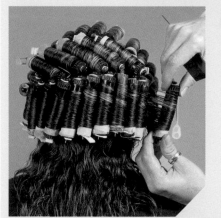

3 Keep good tension throughout winding and ensure there are no gaps by winding each rod as close as possible to previous rods.

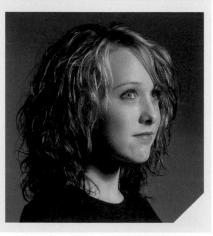

4 Once you have completed a section, evaluate the amount of hair left to ensure the intended winding plan for that section will work.

5 Once the wind is completed, apply barrier cream and cotton wool before applying perm lotion. Process the perm (following the manufacturer's instructions) then rinse and neutralise.

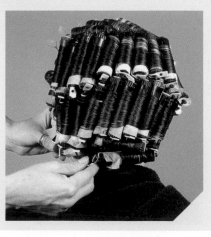

6 Dry the hair using the parting area as a focal point for the finished result.

Nine-section perm winding

This involves dividing the hair into nine neat sections (see overleaf) in readiness for perm winding. You should copy this technique on a head of hair using a perm rod to measure each section and check that a perm rod will fit in each section across the whole head. Once this is complete, you can start to wind each section. When training, it is easier to start winding the perm rods from the nape area, beginning in the central section and then winding left and right nape sections.

When sectioning, you need to follow the same principle as for roller setting by taking the same size section as the length and width of the perm rod. The section of hair should then be held at a 90-degree angle (straight out) from the head, the end paper placed on the hair and, keeping good, even tension on the hair, both hands used to wind the perm rod towards the scalp. Secure the perm rod close to the scalp by placing the perm rubber securely over the end of the rod.

Top tips

Try having perm rods wound into your hair so you can feel what your client is experiencing during a perm.

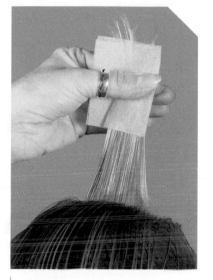

End papers are specially designed absorbent papers which make winding easier and help to prevent fish hooks or buckled ends

357

Unit

GH14

Perm and neutralise hair

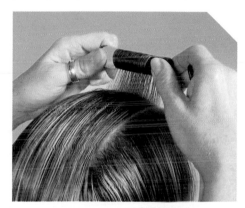

How to position perm rods correctly

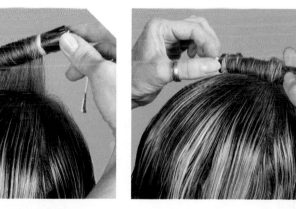

Incorrect positioning of perm rods

Task 8

Write down the three different perm winding techniques you have learned about and state why you would use each of them.

A worksheet for this task is provided on the website for you to complete and add to your portfolio.

Step-by-step nine-section perm winding

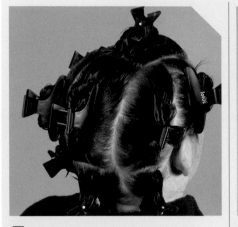

1 Divide the hair into nine sections, starting centrally in the front hairline. Use a perm rod to measure the width of each section as you work. Secure each section neatly.

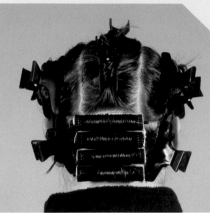

2 Wind the chosen perm rods into the hair starting at the top of the nape section. Then wind both sides of the nape sections. Move up the head, winding the central section first and then both of the middle sections. Lastly wind the very top section and then both side sections. This winding pattern is useful to help you learn how the rods need to be angled so they fit the head correctly — remember you are trying to fit straight perm rods onto a round head shape.

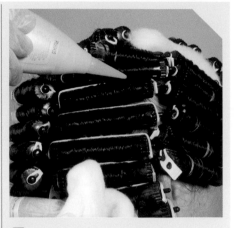

3 When you have wound all the perm rods correctly you need to get your wind checked by your assessor. Protect your client by applying barrier cream and cotton wool around the hairline to stop any perm lotion entering the face or eyes. Apply to the top and bottom of each rod until all the hair has been covered sufficiently. Process the perm by following the manufacturer's instructions, ensuring great client care throughout. Regularly check on your client's well-being throughout the perming process.

Top tips

After applying barrier cream and before applying perm lotion, always remember to place a strip of cotton wool securely around the client's hairline. The cotton wool will stick to the barrier cream and will fully protect the client from perm lotion entering the eyes or running into the ears or down the face.

Application of perm lotion

Protecting technique

This involves either applying pre-perm lotion to the hair to protect any porous areas from over-processing or applying barrier cream to protect the scalp and hairline from any possible chemical burns from the perm lotion.

Post-damping technique

This is where you apply perm lotion to hair that has been sectioned and wound around perm rods. When you are training and taking more than half an hour to wind a whole head of perm rods, this is the safest way of applying your perm lotion and will ensure that all areas of the head process evenly.

Pre-damping technique

The pre-damping technique involves applying perm lotion to hair that is resistant before sectioning or winding the perm rods. This technique is often used in salons where the stylist or perming technician is highly competent and able to wind a whole head of perm rods in a very short space of time. It is not recommended that you carry out a whole head of pre-damping technique while you are learning to perm hair, as you will find it takes longer to wind the whole head than it does for the perm to be processed. This would result in an over-processed head of frizzy hair. Protective gloves should always be worn when pre-damping.

When applying the perm lotion to the hair, always have a piece of cotton wool in your other (gloved) hand to remove any splashes. Keep the bottle close to the hair and always apply to the top and bottom of each wound rod. Start your application at the most resistant area and continue in a methodical manner until all the rods are covered. Be careful not to overload the hair so that the perm lotion soaks your client. Once the application is complete, remove the soiled cotton wool and replace with fresh cotton wool to avoid hairline irritation and burning. Read the manufacturer's instructions to see whether you need to cover the rods with a plastic cap while the perm is processing.

Monitoring curl development during processing

Heat speeds the development of the perming process and should only be used if advised in the manufacturer's instructions.

There are two types of heat:

- *body heat* – this is trapped by a plastic cap which will retain heat lost from the head
- *hairdryers and climazones/accelerators* – these can be used to speed up the processing time (usually by halving the time; check the manufacturer's instructions). Because these use dry heat, you may need to use a plastic cap as this will prevent the perm lotion from drying out and subsequently not processing (check manufacturer's instructions).

The processing time is very important and can be monitored accurately by using a timer. You must refer to the manufacturer's instructions to work out the length of processing time needed. This will also be dependent on the client's hair type, texture and condition. When it is necessary to check the development of the perm, carefully unwind a couple of perm rods from different areas over the head. Be careful not to disturb the curl too much as the hair is in a very fragile state. When the perm has processed sufficiently, it will look 'S'-shaped and resemble the size of the rod being used when gently pushed towards the scalp (see page 350 for the development test).

The neutralising procedure

Neutralising is a permanent process that re-joins the sulphur bonds into their new curled position. If neutralising is not carried out correctly, the perm will be unsuccessful and the client will be disappointed.

Preparing for neutralising

Always read the manufacturer's instructions before beginning to neutralise hair. You must comply with the Personal Protective Equipment at Work Regulations by wearing an apron and gloves.

It is advisable to check the client's gown and towels before beginning to neutralise in case they need replacing.

Water temperature and flow

You must wear gloves when rinsing the perm lotion from the hair, so it is important that you keep checking with the client that the water temperature is comfortable. It is easier to rinse the hair free of perm lotion if the water flow is not too strong, as too great a flow will soak both you and the client. Always rinse with warm water, as the scalp may be tender and the hair delicate. The hotter the water the tighter the curl will become; the cooler the water, the looser the curl will become.

Top tips

- For your own protection, you must always wear gloves to apply perm lotion to avoid the risk of dermatitis.
- A perm will process more quickly in a warm salon (summer) than in a cold salon (winter).

359

Unit

GH14

Perm and neutralise hair

Top tips

Some neutralisers need mixing with water before use. Always read the manufacturer's instructions. Apply the neutraliser to each perm rod so that you are confident all the rods have been covered. If even one rod is missed, it will result in a straight section of hair, which will look very obvious.

Perm and neutralise hair

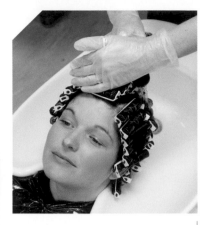

Rinse the perm for at least five minutes

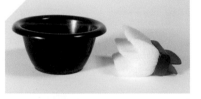

A neutralising sponge and bowl

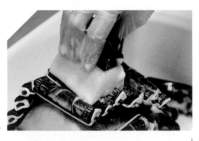

Applying neutraliser

Top tips

Never treat the hair vigorously at this stage of the process – this could weaken the curl result as the bonds have only just re-formed into their new shape.

Once all the rods have been removed, apply a second application of neutraliser

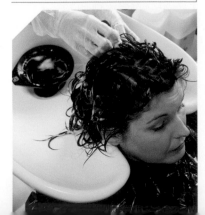

Why rinse thoroughly?

It is vital to the success of the perm that you rinse all the perm lotion from the hair. If any lotion is left in the hair, it will stop the sulphur bonds from re-forming fully and will result in a looser curl than expected that could even drop to completely straight.

After rinsing for about five minutes, check for any residue of perm lotion. When you have rinsed sufficiently to remove all traces of perm lotion, blot the hair gently with a towel. This will allow you to sit the client up at the basin and apply a fresh strip of cotton wool around the hairline for protection. Use a pad of cotton wool to further blot any excess moisture from the hair, which could dilute the strength of the neutraliser. You are now ready to apply the neutraliser.

Applying neutraliser

After reading the manufacturer's instructions, you will know whether to apply the neutraliser straight from the bottle (the same technique as applying perm lotion) or if it is necessary to tip the neutraliser into a bowl, foam up and apply to the hair using a neutralising sponge.

Eye care when neutralising

If neutraliser sponges are too soaked, the product may drip down the client's face and go into her eyes. If this happens, you should rinse the eyes carefully with cold water and seek the help of a first aider. If there are further problems, advise the client to see her GP. You will need to fill in an accident report sheet. You will also need to notify your salon manager and make a note on the client's record.

The importance of accurate timing

Once the first application of neutraliser is complete, you should start accurately timing the development. This timing will be dependent upon the manufacturer's instructions but is usually about five minutes. Since this is when the chemicals in the neutraliser (either hydrogen peroxide or sodium bromate) are re-joining the sulphur bonds to their new partners, it is important the chemicals are given sufficient time to function. If you rush the neutraliser, not all the bonds will re-join and the hair may be left weak and straight-looking. If the neutraliser is left on too long, this could result in over-processing the hair into a straight frizz.

Removing perm rods correctly

The removal of the perm rods is the next step once the time for the first application of neutraliser has elapsed. You should then gently unwind each perm rod, removing the end paper as you work. When all the rods have been removed, apply a second application of neutraliser to the hair, paying particular attention to the ends of the hair, which may not have been fully covered while wound around the rod. This is a more common problem when neutralising long hair. Once again, timing is important and you must be guided by the manufacturer's instructions.

Task 9

What are the three functions of anti-oxidant conditioners? (If you need a reminder, look back at page 353.)

Removing all neutraliser

When the time for the second application of neutraliser has elapsed, rinse the neutraliser thoroughly from the hair. Again, it is important to make sure all traces of the neutraliser are removed as the chemical ingredients may carry on working if left in the hair. This is called **creeping oxidation** and can affect the success of the perm. To prevent this happening, a surface conditioner containing anti-oxidant properties is commonly applied, gently massaged into the hair and then removed by rinsing.

> **Creeping oxidation**
>
> This occurs when residues of chemicals are left in the hair (not rinsed correctly) and the chemical reactions they produce carry on working. This can cause damage to the hair.

Coping with perming and neutralising problems

Perming problems and how to deal with them

Problem	Reason	Action
Perm slow to take	Cold salon temperature; wrong selection of perm lotion; lotion evaporated; insufficient lotion applied.	Use added heat – dryer/climazone; re-damp with stronger lotion; re-damp with same lotion.
Perm processing too quickly	Hair too porous, allowing lotion to enter hair shaft too quickly; hair too dry when lotion applied; very hot salon.	Remove any extra heat; remove cap if used; rinse hair.
Hair breakage	Too much tension; lotion too strong for hair type; over-processing.	Use restructurant or deep penetrating conditioner.
Rubber banding marks	Wound too tight.	Use restructurant
Hairline and scalp irritation	Cuts, abrasions on scalp; cap and wool left around hairline; too much lotion applied.	Rinse immediately using cool water.
Fish hooks	Hair ends buckled or bent during winding.	Remove by cutting.
Frizziness	Over-processing; lotion too strong; rods too small.	Cut if possible; use restructurant or deep penetrating conditioner.
Uneven curl formation	Lotion applied unevenly; rod tension uneven	Re-perm if hair is in good condition.
Too-tight curl	Over-processed; rod size too small.	Deep condition; assess hair condition for relaxing.

Neutralising problems and how to deal with them

Problem	Reason	Action
Frizziness	Over-processing.	Cut if possible.
Uneven curl formation	Neutraliser applied unevenly.	Use restructurant or deep penetrating conditioner; re-perm if hair in good condition.

Task 10

Write down the 11 problems you have learned can happen during perming and neutralising. Write down the reasons the problems happen and the action necessary to rectify the problems.

A worksheet for this task is provided on the website for you to complete and add to your portfolio.

361

Unit

GH14

Perm and neutralise hair

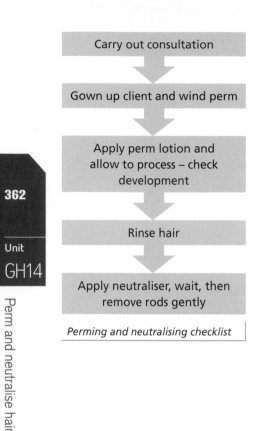

Carry out consultation

Gown up client and wind perm

Apply perm lotion and allow to process – check development

Rinse hair

Apply neutraliser, wait, then remove rods gently

Perming and neutralising checklist

How to provide aftercare advice

It is important to give your client good aftercare advice by recommending the most suitable products to use at home in order to maintain the life of the perm. It is also important to recommend your client does not shampoo her hair too soon after the perm as this may loosen the curl slightly. Do not assume your client has as much information on caring for her hair as you do. Offer as much advice as you can on the correct use of styling products, styling tools and heated styling equipment.

The client's lifestyle is important to consider and you should give advice on the time needed to maintain the perm and lifestyle factors such as swimming and how they can affect perms. You should also offer advice on the correct time intervals between other hairdressing services, as permed hair needs regular cutting, and the fact that the hair is permed will need to be taken into consideration before colouring services.

Advice	Reason
Do not shampoo hair for 24–48 hours after the perm	The curl may loosen or drop if hair is shampooed too soon after the perm.
Use styling products for permed/chemically treated hair	These will put moisture back into the hair which the perm may have removed and help maintain the curl.
Use professional styling tools	Use tools suited to maintaining the curl and maintaining the condition of the cuticle.
Take care when using heated styling equipment	Do not over-use heated styling equipment as this will damage the hair. Always use a heat protector before using heated styling equipment.
Have regular haircuts in between perms	Regular cuts will keep the hair healthy by removing dry ends from the previous perm.
Do not swim in chlorinated water straight after having a perm	Chlorinated water may affect any residue of perming/ neutralising chemicals left on the hair shaft. Wait until after hair has been shampooed before swimming.
It is important to maintain the perm	Perms are not a magic answer to all hair types and need maintaining with specialist shampoos and conditioners in order to keep the curl at its best.
Take care when colouring permed hair	Permed hair may become dry and lack moisture so it is important that this is taken into account before colouring, otherwise the end result could be damaged and unmanageable hair.

Your questions answered

Question	Answer
How long do I have to complete my perm on assessment?	You have 45 minutes to complete the winding only.
Will I be asked questions on what the chemicals do to the hair when I'm perming?	Yes, you need to fully understand what the perm lotion and neutraliser do to the hair when you are perming to be competent in this perming unit.
Will perm winding get easier?	Yes, like any new skill, it gets easier with a lot of hard practice. Remember, practice makes perfect!
How many perms do I have to do on assessment?	You have to successfully complete three perm assessments and at least two must be carried out on a full head.

Salon life

To perm or not to perm – that is the question!

Shelley's story

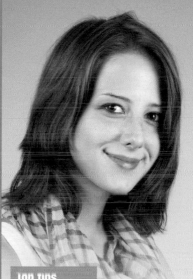

I once did the most disastrous perm and gave my poor client a head full of cotton-wool-like hair! This was due to my inexperience with consultations. Although I realised the client had coloured hair, because I could clearly see artificial colour, I did not bother to do any elasticity, porosity or pre-perm test curls. If I had, I would not have ended up with such a devastated client. The reason the perm turned out so badly was because the client had a full head of bleached hair but had recently put a darker colour on top. I chose a perm for coloured hair which was too strong for the bleached hair and it over-processed really quickly. When I was removing the perm rods after neutralising, I knew the hair was damaged and my heart sank. The client cried when I tried to blow-dry her head full of fuzz! I cut as much as I could off and gave her complimentary conditioning but nothing could repair such bad damage. If only I had asked more in-depth questions during the consultation and carried out the hair tests, I could have avoided such an awful situation.

Top tips

- Always read the manufacturer's instructions as not all perm and neutralising instructions are the same for each product.
- Always carry out a thorough consultation and repeat back to the client so you are both clear about the required results of the perm.
- Always give clear and accurate aftercare advice to enable your client to care for their freshly permed hair at home. This will help prolong and maintain the life of the curl.

Ask the expert

Q *How will I know if the client has bleach under coloured hair?*

A Your consultation is vital to finding out as much as possible about the client's hair's chemical history. If you are still not sure, you can carry out an elasticity test to check the internal strength of the cortex or a pre-perm test curl to see the condition of the hair once it has been permed. Remember: do not carry out the perm if you think the hair is not strong enough, as this could cause considerable damage to your client's hair. Never compromise your professionalism – you will regret it!

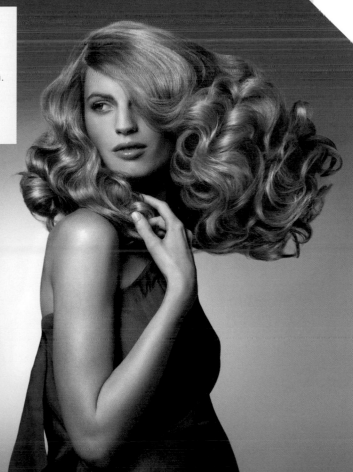

Check your knowledge

The following questions will help you to check your understanding of this unit.
The answers can be found on pages 500–1.

1 What personal protective equipment should you wear during the perming and neutralising processes?

_____

2 What perming information should be recorded on your client's record?

_____

3 Why is it important to keep your work area tidy during the perming and neutralising processes?
   a) To impress your client
   b) To impress your boss and your client
   c) For health and safety reasons and to avoid accidents

4 Why is it important to minimise wastage of perming and neutralising products?
   a) To be cost-effective and keep salon profits up
   b) So you can save the leftover perm lotion for the next client
   c) So you can prove you only ever need to use half a bottle of perm and neutraliser

5 Name two perming tests that should be carried out before perming.
   a) Pre-perm test curl and development test curl
   b) Pre-perm test curl and elasticity test
   c) Development test curl and elasticity test

6 Name a perming test carried out during the perming process.

_____

7 State five factors that influence perming.

_____

_____

8 State three different types of perm lotion.

_____

9 What two things are used to protect the client's hairline during perming?

_____

10 Which three perm winds do you need to perfect for this qualification?

_____

11 Why should you always check water temperature and flow during rinsing of perm lotion and neutraliser?

_____

_____

12 What types of heat can be used to help the perm process?

_____

13 Why is it important to use personal protective equipment?

_____

14 Why is accurate timing important during the perming and neutralising procedures?

_____

15 How do you know how long the perm lotion should be processed for?

_____

16 Why is it important to section accurately when winding a perm?

_____

_____

17 What result could perm rod rubbers positioned too tightly have?

_____

_____

18 How could you resolve the problem of a frizzy perm result?

_____

_____

19 Name the three stages of the perming process and explain what happens at each stage.

_____

_____

_____

20 How long are you allowed for winding a perm on assessment to be commercially competent?

_____

Getting ready for assessment

You will be assessed using a combination of assessment methods, as described below. Remember that within each of the services you carry out with a client, you will cover different units. For example, when perming and neutralising hair (GH14), you will also have to be aware of health and safety (G20) and advise and consult with clients (G7). If you are not sure what you have covered in your service, always ask your assessor or supervisor for advice.

	NVQ	VRQ
Credit value	8	7
Guided Learning Hours	70	60

	NVQ	VRQ
Practical demonstrations, to be observed by assessor	For this unit you will be observed practically carrying out at least three perms, of which two have to be full head perms. You must not have any help winding the perm or any advice or guidance from anyone in order to be classed as competent. You will need to prove that you have given good aftercare advice to your client to help her maintain the perm.	Your assessor will observe these aspects of your performance on at least three occasions. These observations must cover: • two observed perms, which must be on a full head VTCT – At least 75 per cent of observation outcomes must be on real clients. C&G – Simulation is not allowed for any performance evidence. From the range, you must show that you have: • used all products • questioned clients on all the areas of contraindication • carried out all tests in the range • taken into account all the factors • carried out all the types of sectioning techniques • given all the advice.
Service timings	All perm wind techniques – 45 minutes (winding only)	All perm wind techniques – 45 minutes (winding only)
Additional evidence	The evidence of the observed assessment will be recorded in your assessment book and you will need to provide other evidence to authenticate the work carried out by either written evidence (for example an analysis sheet signed by your assessor and your client), client record details or photographic evidence. You will need to prove you have the knowledge necessary for this unit by answering oral questions and completing a written assessment paper.	It is likely most evidence of your performance will be gathered from the observations made by your assessor but you may be required to produce other evidence to support your performance if your assessor has not been present. There is an external paper requirement for this unit.

Task mapping

When you have completed the tasks in this unit, check the table below to see which Performance Criteria (purple), Range (red), Knowledge (green) and Key Skills (blue) you have covered within GH14 to use as additional evidence within your portfolio. Information about which Functional Skills you have covered is available on the website.

Task and page reference	Mapping to Performance Criteria, Range, Knowledge and Key Skills
1 (page 344)	Performance Criteria: Practising 2f, 2g Range: Practising 1c, 1d, VRQ R1d, 2b Knowledge: 39, 40, 41, 47, VRQ 1i, 2i, 2l Key Skills: C1.2, C1.3, C2.3, N1.1, N1.2, N1.3, N2.1, N2.2, N2.3
2 (page 345)	Performance Criteria: Practising 1b, 1g, VRQ 1a, 2g Range: N/A Knowledge: 8, 10, 12, 13, 16, 18, VRQ 1a, 1h, 2q Key Skills: C1.2, C1.3, C2.3
3 (page 346)	Performance Criteria: Practising 1g, 1h, 2e, VRQ 2b, 2g Range: 2a–e, VRQ Rf–j Knowledge: 6, 18, 22, 37, VRQ 1d, 1f, 2q Key Skills: C1.2, C1.3
4 (page 346)	Performance Criteria: Practising 1g, VRQ 2e Range: Practising 1a–e Knowledge: 43, VRQ 1h Key Skills: C1.2, C1.3, C2.3
5 (page 350)	Performance Criteria: Practising 2c, 3h, VRQ 1b, 2b, 2q Range: 3a–d, VRQ Rk_o Knowledge: 25, 26, 27, 28, 46, VRQ 1g Key Skills: C1.2, C1.3, C2.3
6 (page 352)	Performance Criteria: Practising 2g, 3a, VRQ Practising 2b Range: 1c, VRQ Rc, d Knowledge: 41, VRQ 1i Key Skills: C1.2, C1.3
7 (page 352)	Performance Criteria: Practising 2g, 3a, VRQ Practising 2b Range: 1c, VRQ R c, d Knowledge: 41, VRQ 1i Key Skills: C1.2, C1.3
8 (page 357)	Performance Criteria: Practising 3b, VRQ Practising 2c, 2d Range: 5a–c, VRQ Rv, w, x Knowledge: 44, VRQ 2n Key Skills: C1.2, C1.3, C2.3
9 (page 360)	Performance Criteria: Practising 3g, VRQ Practising 2e Range: 1e, VRQ Re Knowledge: 34, 42, VRQ 2l Key Skills: C1.2, C1.3, C2.3
10 (page 361)	Performance Criteria: Practising 3n, 3o Range: N/A Knowledge: 48, 49, VRQ 2p Key Skills: C1.2, C1.3, C2.3

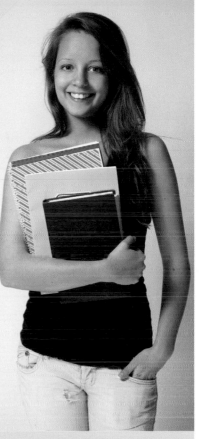

367

Unit

GH14

Perm and neutralise hair

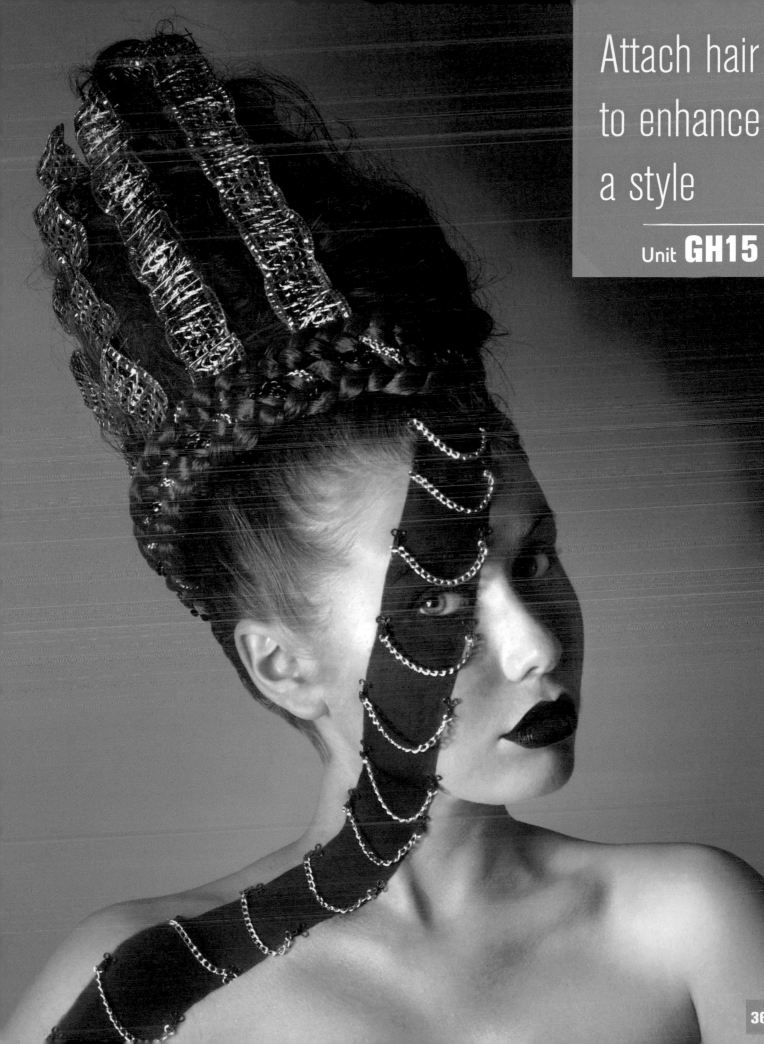

Attach hair
to enhance
a style

Unit **GH15**

369

What you will learn:

- **How to maintain effective and safe working methods when attaching hair**
- **How to plan and prepare to attach hair**
- **How to attach and blend pieces of hair**
- **How to remove pieces of hair**
- **How to provide aftercare advice**

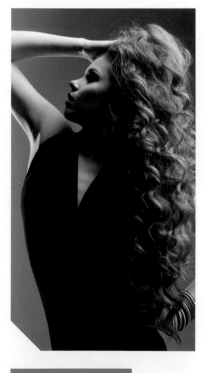

Pre-consultation

A discussion between a client and the stylist to determine the service. This is carried out before the actual service so that cost, tests, length of service and colour matching of added hair can be confirmed.

Introduction

Added hair has been used over many centuries, to be decorative, to hide baldness and to follow fashion. You can achieve instant length, volume and even add a splash of colour that can be taken out the very next day. In this unit you will learn how to carry out a **pre-consultation** and consultation taking into account all factors; complete the appropriate tests; take into account all health and safety requirements; prepare the product, tools and equipment for the service; attach and remove hair extensions; and offer a full aftercare package.

How to maintain effective and safe working methods

It is important to work in a safe manner and ensure your working environment is free from any risks or hazards. In this unit (and with reference to others) you will learn how to work in a safe manner to address all the health and safety requirements for this unit.

Preparing for the service

Gowning and personal protective equipment (PPE)

Protective equipment is important for all hairdressing services. By using the correct PPE you will ensure the safety and comfort of yourself and the client. Your client should be wearing a gown and towel secured at the neck. The stylist should be wearing gloves and an apron.

Health and safety

A risk assessment should be carried out for this service. COSHH regulations must be followed for storage, handling and disposal of all products, tools and equipment used for the extension process.

All electrical equipment must be tested by a qualified electrician every six months. A record should be kept of the inspection date and any work carried out on the equipment. (Refer to G20 for information on COSHH, risk assessment and the Electricity at Work Regulations.)

Task 1

Carry out a risk assessment in your salon or training establishment, taking into account all factors involved in attaching additional hair. Refer to G20, page 47, for information on completing a risk assessment.

A worksheet for this task is provided on the website for you to complete and add to your portfolio.

Positioning

The correct positioning when applying extensions will produce a better end result. It is important to have your shoulders and elbows down, keeping your arms relaxed. By maintaining this posture you will ensure even tension and the correct angle and positioning of the extensions. This in turn will prevent fatigue, strained muscles and backache. You need to make sure you position your tools and equipment on your workstation for ease of use, so that you do not overstretch.

Your client needs to be sitting squarely in front of your mirror with the base of her back to the back of the chair and both feet flat on the floor. This will ensure that you are able to attach the extensions so they are level and balanced in the hair.

Keeping your work area clean and tidy

In order to work quickly, hygienically and effectively, you need to make sure you prepare your work area before you receive your client and tidy away at the end of every service. Any hair fall from a previous service needs to be swept up from the floor to prevent it from becoming a hazard.

Brushes and combs need to be cleaned and sterilised using the most appropriate method (refer to G20, page 63, for sterilising methods).

Sequencing your work

Working in a methodical manner will allow you to work quickly and efficiently around the head, making best use of your working time. To begin:

- brush the client's hair to remove any loose hair and tangles
- section the hair at the back, just below the occipital bone (see page 7), and secure the top section of hair so that it does not get in the way of the application process
- measure the **weft** across the head and cut to size
- attach the hair by securing the middle clip first. Check for any lumps or gaps – if positioned incorrectly, open the clip and reapply in the correct position.

Minimising the risk of damage to tools and equipment

All tools and equipment should be stored in a safe place when not in use. Any unused hair should be kept with the clips holding the hair in place to prevent tangling and kept in a bag to keep the hair fresh.

Minimising waste

At the pre-consultation you should have determined with the client how many extensions are required and ordered the correct amount of hair to carry out the service. By spending time planning the service you will minimise the possibility of wastage. You should also ensure you have enough added hair to be able to complete the service.

Minimise the risk of cross-infection

Every hairdressing service begins with a face-to-face consultation. This is the time that you check for any diseases or disorders that would prevent you from carrying out the service. If a client has had an infestation of head lice, you must ensure that these have been cleared from the head completely before the service can be carried out. (For more information on diseases and disorders refer to G7, pages 144–48.)

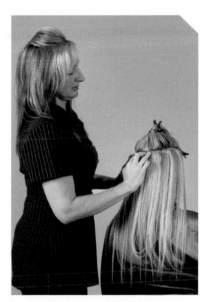

Correct posture for both the stylist and the client

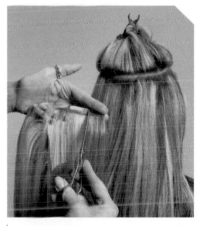

Cutting weft to size

371

Unit
GH15

Attach hair to enhance a style

Top tips

When cutting weft to size, use a pair of normal household scissors as the weft is thick and may damage your hairdressing scissors.

Weft

Sections of added hair, either real or synthetic, that can be attached using a variety of attachment systems.

Unit
GH15

Attach hair to enhance a style

Fact or fiction?

Is this statement fact or fiction?

You are required by law to take a non-refundable deposit from the client for a hair extension service.

To check your answer see page 501.

Top tips

If you as a stylist have very long hair, it is advisable to tie it back to ensure it does not become tangled or stuck to any of the adhesives you may be using.

Traction alopecia

Hair thinning or loss due to excessive tension on the hair follicle.

Traction alopecia

All tools and equipment must be cleaned after every client, using the most appropriate sterilisation method. (See G20, page 63.)

Effective use of working time

You will need to carry out a pre-consultation prior to the actual appointment. This will allow you to complete a preliminary check of the hair to make sure it is suitable to have the hair extension service. You can conduct the necessary tests (see page 374), make a plan of the amount of hair to be attached, decide where it is going to be positioned and match up the texture and colour of the hair to be ordered for the service.

By being prepared to receive your client you will be able to work more efficiently. All products, tools and equipment should be prepared before the client arrives. Equipment should have been cleaned and sterilised after your last client, in readiness to begin the service.

You should have discussed at the initial consultation any pre-cutting that might need to be carried out before the extensions are applied to ensure even blending. You will also have discussed where you are going to be placing the extensions, and should have established a plan that you and your client have already agreed to work to.

Personal hygiene

To portray a professional image, good personal hygiene is essential. You need to make sure that your uniform is washed and ironed, long hair is tied back and minimal jewellery is worn. Use a good deodorant, and breath fresheners if you have had very spicy food the night before. (Refer to G20, page 73, for more information on personal hygiene.)

Minimise the risk of harm or injury

To prevent the risk of harm or injury to the client, you must make sure that all of the relevant tests are carried out before beginning the service, to make sure the client is not allergic to any of the adhesives or removal solutions that are used. You also need to carry out pull and elasticity tests to see if the hair can withstand the process. If these tests are not carried out you will run the risk of **traction alopecia** (see also page 374).

A thorough consultation is important to make sure the client does not have a previous history of any medical conditions that could cause further problems during the service. For example, the adhesives that are used could aggravate skin allergies or breathing problems such as asthma. (See also page 373 on client consultation.)

All of these tests should be carried out during the initial consultation.

Keeping accurate and up-to-date client records

During your consultation you will gather a lot of information that can be used to create notes for your client record card. You will then have a written record of all of the medical history required, and can add information on how successful the service was, any changes you would make in the future, and what aftercare advice you have given the client. This will safeguard you in the future if a client has not maintained her extensions; you will be able to look back and confirm what was discussed.

ELEMENTS ❋ HAIRDRESSING

Date	Stylist name
Client name	Address/telephone number

TESTS	**COMMENTS**
Elasticity	
Porosity	
Pull	
Skin	

INFLUENCING FACTORS	
Direction and fall of added hair	
Porosity	
Length of hair	
Hairstyle	
Head and face shape	
Hair texture	
Hair density	
Hair damage	
Lifestyle	

CONTRAINDICATIONS	
Skin sensitivities	
Previous allergic reactions	
Hair or scalp disorders	
Previous medical history	

APPLICATION	
Amount of added hair	
Attachment method	
Colour analysis	
Target colour	
Aftercare advice	
Products	
Hair care	

Client signature

Task 2

Using the information above, produce a mind map or spider diagram listing in order of importance the initial steps you need to take to prepare for an extension/attachment process. Compare your notes with your colleagues to see if you agree with one another.

How to plan and prepare to attach hair

Client consultation

A thorough consultation forms part of every hairdressing service. When completing a hair extension service the consultation will be slightly longer than for most other hairdressing services. This is because all of the tests need to be carried out to make sure the service can proceed, and because the hair colour and texture need to be matched up so that the hair can be ordered in advance of the service.

When the consultation has been carried out, a deposit is taken and the hair is ordered. The hair ordered is specific to that client and it is extremely unlikely that you would be able to use it on another client, so it is important that you discuss in detail all of the client's requirements.

Fact or fiction?

Is this statement fact or fiction?

The client is required to pay for the full service at the initial consultation.

To check your answer, see page 501.

Tests prior to the service

The table below lists the three tests you will need to perform before attaching hair.

Test	When and why?	Method
Pull test	This test is carried out before the service to check that the hair will be able to withstand the extension attachment process.	A few strands of the hair are selected and gently pulled at the root. If the hair can be pulled out easily, extensions would not be suitable because the extra stress that the weight of the added hair would put on the natural hair could result in large amounts of hair loss.
Skin test	This test is carried out prior to the service (usually completed at the first pre-consultation). It tests whether the client is allergic to any of the adhesives or removal solutions used in the service.	Clean an area behind the ear using a cotton wool bud (or something similar). Place a small amount of the adhesive or removal solution on the cleansed area. This needs to be carried out 24–48 hours before the service. A positive reaction may produce reddening of the skin, a rash or general sensitivity. If any of these reactions occur, you cannot go ahead with the service.
Elasticity test	This test is carried out at the initial consultation to check the inner strength of the hair.	Select a few strands of hair and hold them between the thumb and forefinger. Gently pull the hair to see if it will stretch up to a third of its length and return to its natural state. If the hair breaks, the internal bonds may be weak and further discussion needs to take place with your client to ascertain whether an extension service is suitable.

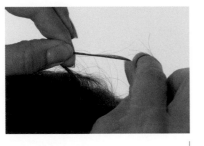

The elasticity test

Task 3

In pairs, carry out a pull test, skin test and elasticity test and record your findings. Would your partner be able to have an extension service carried out on their hair? If not, what would you recommend as an alternative?

A worksheet for this task is provided on the website for you to complete and add to your portfolio.

Hair type and condition

As well as carrying out the necessary tests on the hair, you will also be making a visual analysis of the hair to determine the general condition. You will need to decide if the hair is normal, dry/damaged or oily, as this will affect the result and lasting ability of the hair extensions. If the hair is excessively oily you will need to use a clarifying shampoo to remove the oil and sebum from the hair (refer to GH8 for more on shampooing and conditioning hair).

You will also need to decide whether the hair is brittle, normal or if there is obvious breakage. If you find you are ticking the box for brittle hair, you may suggest that the client has a course of specialised treatments leading up to the extension service. If you are ticking the 'breakage' box, you need to discuss this further with your client as it may mean that the service cannot be carried out.

Hair type	Shampoo type	Specialised treatments	Is the service advisable?	Further recommendations
Normal	Soapless shampoo that will not deposit any oils onto the hair	Not required	Yes	None
Oily	Clarifying shampoo	Not required	Yes, provided the hair is not so oily that it would cause the extensions to 'slip' from the hair	24-hour extensions as the hair can be shampooed on a more regular basis and the extension reapplied
Brittle	A shampoo to replace lost moisture	A course of penetrating, moisturising treatments to replace lost moisture	If there is an improvement in the hair's condition after the treatments	Advise the client to continue with the treatment until the hair reaches the stage where the service can be carried out
Breakage	A shampoo to replace lost moisture	A course of penetrating, moisturising treatments	No	Until the hair's condition improves, the service should not be carried out

Consequences of not carrying out tests

By law you are required to carry out all tests as specified by the manufacturers. Failure to do so may result in legal action being taken against you by the client. You may cause severe damage to the client's hair and scalp, and in addition the salon may receive a bad reputation which in turn will affect business and profits.

Contraindications to the service

- *Hair and scalp disorders* – for example, hair loss (alopecia), excessive thinning, eczema, psoriasis If the client displays any of these conditions, you cannot carry out an extension service as the extensions will put extra stress on the root area and will speed up any hair loss that the client is experiencing.
- *Previous allergic reactions* – because of the fumes released from the adhesives and solvents used in extensions, the risk is that an allergy could trigger breathing problems. An alternative to using glue or adhesive attachment processes would be to offer clip-in extensions.
- *Pregnancy and breastfeeding* – if a client has recently given birth, hair loss can occur until the pregnancy hormones have settled down or when the client is no longer breastfeeding. The client may think that the increase in hair loss is due to the extensions and not the pregnancy hormones. You should therefore advise a client to wait until up to eight months after having the baby before they consider an extension service.
- *Cancer treatment* – if a client is receiving treatment for cancer, this can cause complete hair loss. Because extensions are applied to the root area, they put added tension on the hair and could cause the hair to fall out more quickly. When the treatment is complete and the hair has begun to grow again, if all of the relevant tests are carried out and the hair is strong enough, extensions can be applied.
- *Breakage at the root area* – this is where the extensions are applied (fixed), so any extra strain on already weak, fragile hair could result in further hair loss.
- *Asthma or other breathing difficulties* – because of the products used and the fumes given off, all work should be carried out in a well-ventilated area.

Considering the hair type and condition prior to the service

375

Unit

GH15

Attach hair to enhance a style

Unit
GH15

Attach hair to enhance a style

Top tips

Give your client all of the facts, the good as well as the bad. They will appreciate your honesty – after all, you are the expert!

Managing client expectations

It is important that both you and your client agree what is expected from the service you are going to carry out. If a client is going from short to long hair in one process, this will impact on the day-to-day maintenance of her hair.

You must be clear about your client's expectations – why does she want extensions? Is it to:

- add more volume
- add more length
- change the style completely
- add colour to the hair?

You need to listen carefully to the client's requirements and give the best possible advice. You must decide if hair extensions are suitable for your client. Diagrams can be used to show where the extensions are going to be placed in order to flatter the client's head and face shape.

Points to discuss with the client

- The extensions may feel heavy in the hair at first and a little uncomfortable.
- The amount of hair that the client has added will increase the time spent on shampooing and blow-drying the hair.
- The client may have to have her hair cut before the service to remove solid, blunt lines.
- Lifestyle – if the client attends the gym regularly and likes to use the swimming pool, then extensions should not be advised as chlorine will leave the extensions looking dry and dull and will cause them to become tangled. If the client does horse riding, the safety helmet may weaken and pull the extensions away from the hair.

Referring problems to the relevant person

If you have carried out a thorough consultation and given the client adequate aftercare and maintenance advice, hopefully there won't be any problems to refer. In the event that problems do occur, you need to be aware who you should go to for help to report a general problem or concern. Most salons have a chain of command; you need to check with your senior stylist, manager or training provider who you should report to in case of an emergency.

Selecting added hair

Suitable texture

You need to assess the client's natural hair and decide if you think the hair texture falls into one of three categories: fine, medium or thick. You can do this by selecting a few strands of the hair and laying them across the palm of your hand. (If the hair is very light and difficult to see, you may prefer to use a piece of dark coloured paper so the hair contrasts and can be seen well.) When you have decided on the thickness of one individual hair, you then order the extension hair in the same texture. You will also need to use wavy extension hair to match naturally wavy hair and straight with straight. It isn't possible to create a curly hairstyle with extension hair if a client has straight hair.

Suitable colour

You need to colour-match extension hair to natural hair. You will need to use a shade chart/colour swatches provided by the manufacturer. Place the natural hair against the colour swatch. By selecting two or more extension colours and alternating them (usually one lighter and one darker), you can achieve a more natural colour match.

Suitable length

Generally the length of hair applied as extension hair is double the length of the natural hair. The natural hair needs to be shoulder length or just above. (The hair needs to be long enough to hide bonds and attachments that hold the extensions in place.)

Suitable width

Many of the weft extensions come in a strip. Clients' heads are all shapes and sizes. You may have to cut the weft to fit the width of the client's head.

Task 4

Working in pairs, use a shade chart/swatch and match your partner's hair to the chart to determine the most suitable colour match for them. Record your findings and make additional notes on the texture of their hair, and the amount of curl, wave or straightness present.

A worksheet for this task is provided on the website for you to complete and add to your portfolio.

Preparing the client

- If your client is having any chemical processes, ensure these are carried out before the extension service.
- Check that you are happy with the hair you ordered for the client.
- To be able to begin an extension service, you need to make sure the client's hair is shampooed using a clarifying shampoo and is free of any products. Most adhesives will only stick to the hair if it is free from oil, grease and dirt. (Make sure you don't apply any conditioners before an extension service, as these will put a barrier on the hair.)
- Do you need to carry out any pre-cutting to the hair to remove solid, blunt or straight lines? By completing the cut before the extensions are applied you will not be putting any extra tension on the hair immediately after the service.
- To remove bulk from the hair you should be using texturising techniques (point, castle, chipping; see GH12, pages 300–1 and 310–11, for cutting tools, methods and techniques). By using these techniques you will be removing bulk from the hair but not the overall length.

You should now be ready to section the hair to apply the extensions.

Top tips

Extensions cannot be applied within 2 cm of a client's natural hairline, parting, crown or occipital bone. If extensions are applied to these areas the bonds will be visible.

Task 5

In groups, compile your own checklist of questions that you would ask a client before carrying out an extension service, then a separate checklist of factors you would be looking at to ensure it was safe to carry out the service.

A worksheet for this task is provided on the website for you to complete and add to your portfolio.

How to attach and blend pieces of hair

Consultation for temporary extensions

If a client wants to add colour, volume or length to specific areas, you may only need to carry out partial extensions, i.e. attaching hair only to areas of the head where the client may be thinning or just wants additional length. Temporary bonding systems are adhesive strips that 'stick' to the hair or scalp or use added hair (wefts of hair or ponytails that are clipped into the hair and removed before sleeping). All of these can either be natural or synthetic hair (false hair).

These techniques are used when a client wants to change her style or enhance the shape of her own haircut for a short period of time, for example for a special occasion such as a wedding or prom. If the client is looking for a more permanent service you would choose bonded hair extensions that are attached to the hair with an adhesive and will last up to three months if the correct aftercare is used.

Ponytails

To create instant length, a ponytail which clips into the hair can be used. First, secure the natural hair into a ponytail or bun. The added hair is then attached by clipping or wrapping a bendable wire around the natural hair.

Wefts

Wefts come in lengths that can be cut to fit the width of the client's head and are secured with clips that are already attached to the weft. They can also be sewn into a braid (cornrow) already placed in the client's hair. If wefts are clipped into the hair, they can be removed at the end of an evening or important function.

Self-adhesive wefts

There are several attachment systems available to secure wefts to the hair and scalp. The weft may have a liner tape that is attached to the root of the hair and will last up to six weeks. Self-adhesive weft is also available with two thin adhesive strips; the hair is sectioned and effectively sandwiched between the two strips.

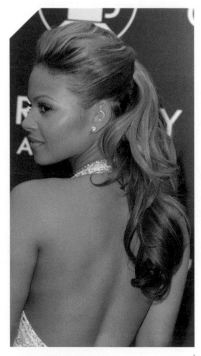

An added ponytail

Sectioning and tension for temporary extensions

Clean and even sectioning is the key to working in a neat, methodical and efficient manner. Time spent on correct sectioning allows you to make the best use of your working time.

Sectioning for a ponytail extension

When you are sectioning the hair to apply hair extensions, you first need to decide on their placement. A ponytail can be fixed to the crown area, low in the nape or slightly off centre, to the side of the head. The sections need to be taken accordingly. They need to be neat, making sure that stray hair is not caught up where the ponytail is to be attached. If this happens it will pull on the client's hair, causing discomfort.

Sectioning for weft

The sectioning should follow the natural contour of the head, from side to side, creating a U-shaped parting. The look you want to achieve will determine how close the next section is taken to the previous one. If a thicker look is required, you will take the sections much closer to the weft.

Tension

It is important to have the correct posture when carrying out an extension service. You need to be relaxed so that shoulders and arms are dropped, otherwise you will put tension on the hair, causing root lift. If the extension does not lay flat and shows signs of root lift, it will have to be removed and replaced.

Braided wefts (cornrows)

The correct amount of tension needs to be used for the plait. Don't braid wefts too tightly as this can cause headaches, itching, pulling and discomfort.

Securing added hair

Attachment systems designed to last from 24 hours to 3 months

There is a wide variety of hair attachment systems that enable the stylist to create individual looks to suit all occasions and budgets. You need to follow manufacturers' instructions on attachment techniques. Many of the attachment methods can be reused. It is therefore important to ensure that you provide your client with the correct information about looking after her extension hair and have chosen the correct system to suit the client.

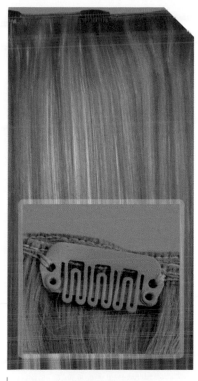

A weft

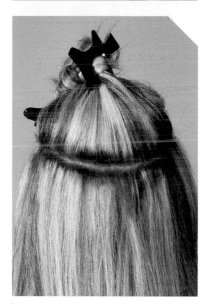

Sectioning for weft creates a U-shape

379

Unit
GH15

Attach hair to enhance a style

Attach hair to enhance a style

Step-by-step securing a ponytail

1 Brush all of the hair, ensuring there are no knots or tangles, and section the hair into two parts (back and front). Secure the hair in a ponytail with a covered band. The ponytail can be secured onto the hair using the clip provided.

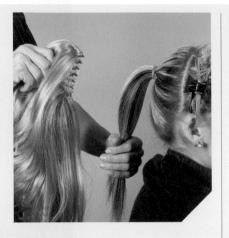

2 An alternative method would involve placing grips around the base of the ponytail in a criss cross formation to stop them from slipping.

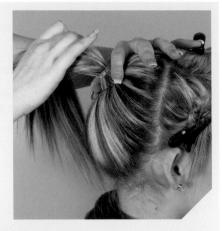

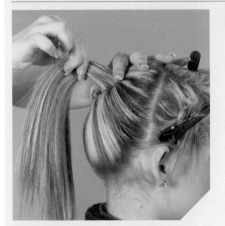

3 The band can be removed from the hair once you are happy that the grips will hold the hair in place.

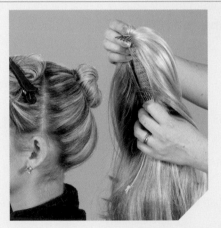

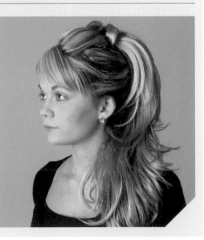

4 The ponytail is fixed into a bun position. The added hair is removed from the clip, placed over the bun and secured into place. The front section of hair is released and used to blend the added hair.

5 The hair is styled and dressed to suit the client's requirements, and the appropriate aftercare advice is given.

Step-by-step clip-in weft to last 24 hours

1 The hair is divided into workable sections – backcombing is used at the root area to give a secure base to attach the weft to.

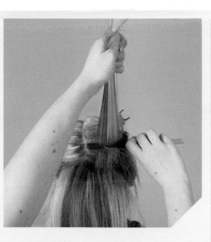

2 The weft is measured across the head and cut to size.

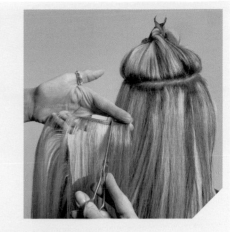

Attach hair to enhance & style

3 The weft is held in place and secured with the middle clip followed by the two side clips.

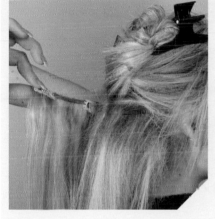

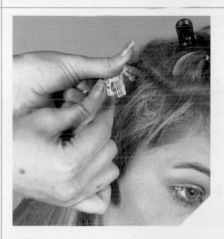

4 You can ask the client to tilt her head to help with the application.

5 The finished result.

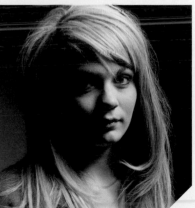

Step-by-step braided weft to last 1–3 months

1 Carry out an in-depth consultation to determine the length and amount of added hair to be used.

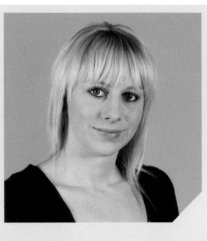

2 Brush through the hair to remove tangles and section the hair in a horseshoe section just below the occipital bone.

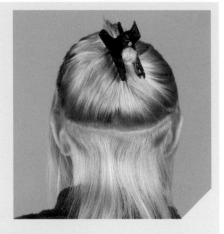

3 Taking a small section of hair, begin to plait the hair into the middle of the head working in from either side. Add extension hair into these plaits to give them strength.

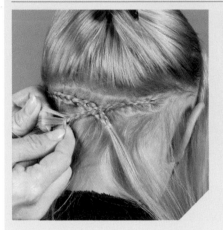

4 Measure and cut the extension to the correct length and stitch onto the plait using a blanket stitch. Use a curved needle for ease.

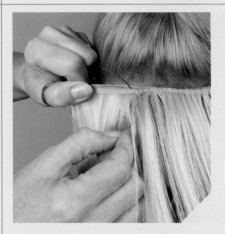

5 Use this method to work up the head and join the sides in. Make sure you do not add directly onto the hairline. Do not put extensions on the occipital bone as it will look lumpy.

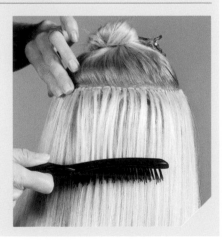

Step-by-step adhesive wefts

1 Section the hair where the wefts are going to be attached. Measure and cut the weft to size.

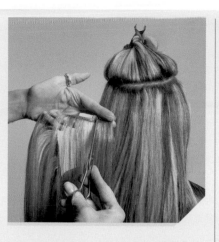

2 Place the hair on a secure workstation and apply a small, even amount of adhesive along the length of the weft.

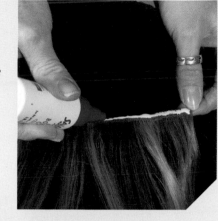

Attach hair to enhance a style

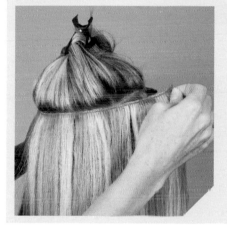

3 Secure the weft to the root area, ensuring the hair above is not caught in this section as this will cause discomfort to the client.

4 Style the hair to suit the client's requirements and provide the appropriate aftercare advice.

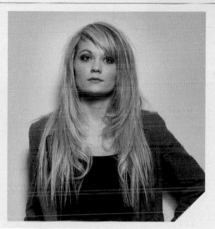

Advantages and disadvantages of different hair extension systems

24-hour extensions (e.g. ponytail and clip-in weft)		4-week extensions (e.g. adhesive or cornrow extensions)	
Advantages	**Disadvantages**	**Advantages**	**Disadvantages**
• They are quick and easy to apply. • A skin test is not necessary. • Minimal upkeep is required. • The client can learn to attach them herself.	• If not attached correctly they could come away from the hair. • The client may find the extra weight uncomfortable. • They are only for a one-off event.	• Once applied the client has a new look for up to 4 weeks. • An instant transformation occurs that is more permanent than 24-hour extensions. • Can be used to hide thinning or add volume, length or colour on a more permanent basis.	• A full head service can take up to 4 hours. • Not suitable for swimmers or horse riders. • Difficult to wear hair up without the extension showing.

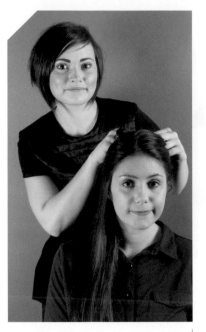

Assessing where the hair naturally falls

Influencing factors – attachment method

Direction and fall of the added hair

It is important that you work with the hair's growth patterns and natural fall. You need to look at how the client wears her hair and where natural partings sit. Extensions cannot go against natural hair fall because the cuticles sit the same way and the hair would become matted.

The quantity of added hair

If you have a client who has very dense hair, you can sew two wefts together to create the correct amount of thickness for the hair type. If attaching a ponytail you need to take into consideration the texture and density of the existing hair. If a client has very fine hair and not a lot of it, a ponytail thick in texture and density would not blend very well.

The need to blend the client's hair with added hair

With any added hair you will need to make sure that you have colour-matched the hair to the natural colour by using a shade chart/swatch provided by the manufacturer. Two or more colours can be combined to produce a more natural look. You also need to make sure that the hair is the correct texture and holds the same degree of curl or straightness as the natural hair. You can pre-cut the hair using texturising techniques to remove any straight, blunt lines around the perimeter of the hair; this will enable the added hair to blend more effectively.

Head and face shape

In all hairdressing services the head and face shape has to be taken into consideration when choosing the most appropriate style for a client. The length, volume, colour and balance need to complement the client's features. At the consultation you need to decide what shape face the client has and the most suitable style to enhance her features (refer back to page 140 for details of head and face shapes). Added hair can be used to enhance or disguise any features that a client may not be happy with. For example, if the client's head is flat at the back (occipital bone), added hair can be used to bulk out this area and give volume.

Hair texture

By determining the hair's texture, you will be able to judge how much added hair to use. (See also page 376.)

To determine the degree of curl or straightness of the hair, it is best to shampoo it first. A client may straighten their hair, so waves or curls may not be obvious.

Hair density

This refers to the amount of hair the client has per square inch on the head. If a client has experienced hair loss through medication or illness, you need to take this into consideration when deciding on the type of added hair you are going to use.

- If the hair is sparse you may choose to braid the hair and apply wefts to build up the density.

- If the hair is very sparse, extensions may not be suitable as they will show and look unsightly. A full wig is also an option that can be considered.

Elasticity

The hair needs to have good elasticity for any added hair attachment as the weight of the added hair will put strain on the natural hair. If the elasticity is poor, added hair could lead to breakage and a very unhappy client!

Hair damage

Extensions are applied to the root area. If there is any evident damage you should not apply them as this will cause further damage and may result in the client losing hair.

Traction alopecia

Traction alopecia is hair loss resulting from such excessive pulling that the hair follicles are unable to produce new hairs to replace the old ones. If traction alopecia is evident, you cannot apply bonded hair extensions and careful consideration must be given to whether any other form of hair attachment is suitable and will not cause the problem to worsen.

Lifestyle

Chlorine and salt water can cause matting of the hair. If your client swims on a regular basis, the extensions should be worn in a high bun on the top of her head, tied back or plaited. It is advisable to secure the hair with a soft covered band, as uncovered bands will tangle in the hair. If your client rides a horse or wears protective headgear on a regular basis, some of the extension bonds may soften and be flattened by the constant pressure of the headgear.

Hairstyle

If the hair is too short the extensions may not be able to be attached. The style needs to be suitable for the added hair to enhance. If the client has a very blunt look, the hair may not blend easily and will need to be texturised so the extensions blend with the natural hair.

Client comfort

Depending on the extension service being carried out, you may need to give your client a rest. A full extension service can take up to 4 hours, and neither you nor the client can be expected to sit/stand for that length of time without having regular breaks.

If you are using weft or clip-on added hair, you need to make sure that any clips or grips are not causing the client any discomfort.

Adapting cutting techniques

Straight or blunt cuts will make hair extensions look false. It is important to blend the hair extensions with the natural hair to achieve a seamless join. Freehand cutting techniques and razoring techniques will remove bulk and harsh, blunt lines from the hair without putting extra tension on the added hair. You need to constantly cross-check the haircut for balance, fall and movement to ensure the hair integrates (fits in) with the extensions.

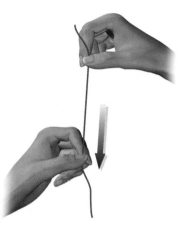

The elasticity test

385

Unit
GH15

Attach hair to enhance a style

Coping with problems

Tangles

If a client has a problem with matting or tangles, you need to check that the correct aftercare advice has been given. The client will need to separate the added hair from her natural hair and any loose hair that has escaped from the extensions needs to be replaced back into the weft.

Incorrect application

If you have incorrectly placed an extension (with root lift, lumps or gaps), you will need to remove the extension, cleanse the hair to remove all traces of adhesive and replace with a new extension.

Confirming the end result

During, and at the end of, the service, you need to affirm that the client is happy with the end result. You need to show the client her hair from all angles using a back mirror.

How to remove pieces of hair

Using the correct products, tools and equipment

Following manufacturers' instructions

The removal solution is highly flammable so should be used in a well-ventilated area. Do not allow anyone to smoke when the solvent is being used and always use the correct PPE for yourself and your client.

Removing pieces of hair to minimise damage to the hair

The way in which the extension is removed will depend upon the type of extension. All removal techniques must be followed using the manufacturer's instructions. Each extension company may use different techniques, tools, equipment or products to remove extensions, so to prevent any problems occurring read the manufacturer's instructions carefully.

Some salons will factor the removal expense into the cost of the complete service. This is done because many clients may consider removing the extensions themselves, which can lead to damage and breakage to the hair.

Leaving your client's hair prepared for the next service

You need to ensure that any glue or adhesive is completely removed from the hair as further damage can be caused if this is 'picked off' the hair. You should recommend that your client uses a good conditioner to help restore the hair's condition, especially at the root area as this would have been avoided when the extensions were present.

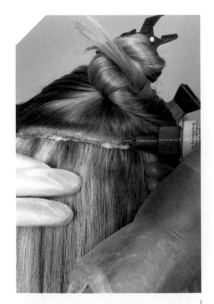

Removal solution for glued in weft

How to provide aftercare advice

When a client agrees to having an extension service, she is taking on a big commitment. It is important from the outset that you inform the client of the advantages and disadvantages of having and maintaining hair extensions.

Homecare products

Each manufacturer will recommend that you use their aftercare products. Many manufacturers will have specialised products to complement their attachment system. You need to ensure you recommend the correct aftercare products to maintain the added hair. The client should have a large-toothed comb to detangle the hair and a soft bristle brush for day-to-day brushing. Heavy conditioning treatments or conditioning masks should be avoided as these will weaken the adhesive and may cause the extension to slip in the hair.

Hair care

Once the client is armed with the correct range of aftercare products, you will need to give advice on styling. Care must be taken not to be too vigorous when drying the hair. Electric tongs and straighteners can be used on real added hair – you should advise your client to use a heat protector spray and avoid using the heat on too high a setting. If the hair is synthetic, heated electrical equipment cannot be used as it will melt the hair.

How to maintain the style

The hair should be brushed every day and detangled from point to root. Advise the client when working close to the roots/wefts to put her hand on them to prevent pulling, and to brush carefully.

You should advise clients to tie their hair up before sleep, either with a soft covered band or the hair can be plaited. A silk or satin pillow case is recommended so the hair slides around rather than rubbing, which can cause matting.

How lifestyle affects clients' choice of style (active sports, career requirements)

If clients have active lifestyles, they may not be able to spend the time required on the upkeep of the extensions. You therefore need to question your clients carefully during the consultation to see how the extensions will fit in with their lifestyle. For example, if a client does a lot of swimming then clip-in extensions would be a better option than sewn-in extensions.

Salon life

Hair delight or hair disaster?

Sammie's story

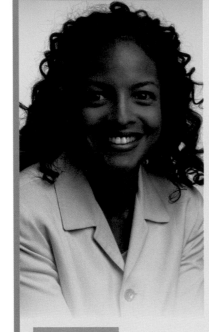

I'd wanted extensions for ages so as soon as I'd saved up the money I found a relatively cheap salon and booked an appointment for permanent extensions. I had a 5-minute consultation, during which they colour-matched my hair, and I paid half of the money upfront as a deposit.

When the big day arrived I was so excited! It took ages to put the extensions in. At one point I had three people working on my head. When they finally finished and I looked in the mirror I didn't recognise myself! I wasn't sure if I liked them – it felt like there was a carpet of hair on my head. I decided to give myself time to get used to them.

A week later, I hated them! They gave me headaches because they were so tight to the scalp, they itched and I still looked like I had a carpet of hair – they had no shape. When I phoned the salon they said they would have to charge me to have them removed. They weren't concerned at all that I was unhappy with the service. So I went to a different salon. They told me that the extensions had been put in incorrectly. Because three different people had applied them, the tension across my head was inconsistent. Also, the extensions should have been pre-cut to complement my hairstyle, and I should have had at least a half-hour consultation before the service to decide on the amount of hair to be added and the density. When the application was completed, I should have been given clear aftercare advice.

I learned a lesson the hard way. I was trying to save money but it ended up costing me more and I didn't get the result I wanted. I will always carry out a full consultation with my clients and explain the boths the pros and cons of any service, so they know what they are getting themselves into!

Top tips

Time spent on a thorough consultation at the beginning of a service will ensure both you and the client know what to expect before, during and after the service. This will save valuable time and money by ensuring that none of your clients are disappointed.

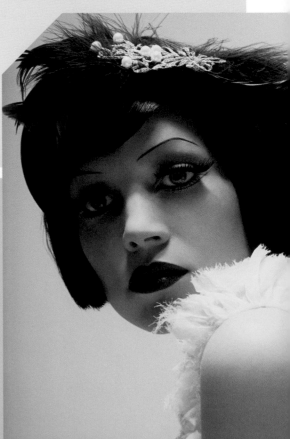

Ask the expert

Q   *If a client is determined to have more permanent extensions and I don't think it is right for her, what should I do?*

A   You need to make sure that you give the correct advice. If you have advised a client to have clip-in extensions as an alternative but the client still wants to go ahead with a longer-lasting service, then you need to record the conversation and the advice that you have given to your client. Ask the client to sign this record and then you will be able to refer to it if the client is subsequently unhappy with the service.

Check your knowledge

The following questions will help you to check your understanding of this unit. The answers can be found on page 501.

1 By maintaining the correct posture when applying extensions, you:
   a) can apply the extensions quicker
   b) prevent backache and incorrect positioning of the extensions
   c) use less extension hair
   d) can avoid asking your client to move her head.

2 To prevent the hair from becoming tangled, you must brush or comb the hair from:
   a) the mid-lengths first
   b) root to point
   c) point to root
   d) it doesn't matter as long as the hair is brushed.

3 The hair is sometimes pre-cut before added hair is applied:
   a) to save time at the end of the service
   b) because you can't cut the hair once added hair is in place
   c) to create a definite style that added hair can be applied to
   d) to remove any hard, blunt lines from the hair.

4 To avoid incorrect application of added hair:
   a) ensure the correct positioning and tension when applying the added hair
   b) try not to let your client talk during the process so she doesn't move her head
   c) don't talk to your client so you can concentrate
   d) make sure you are being assisted by a junior.

5 A contraindication to a service for applying added hair would be:
   a) if the client has had her hair coloured
   b) breakage at the root area
   c) if the client's hair was a thick density
   d) if the client only wanted the added hair to last one evening.

6 What does the term 'pre-consultation' mean?

_____

_____

_____

7 How should your client be positioned for the service?

_____

_____

_____

389

Unit

GH15

Attach hair to enhance a style

8 What impact would regular swimming have on hair extensions?

_____

_____

_____

9 What is traction alopecia?

_____

_____

_____

10 How is a pull test carried out?

_____

_____

_____

Attach hair to enhance a style

Getting ready for assessment

You will be assessed using a combination of assessment methods, as described below. Remember that within each of the services you carry out with a client, you will cover different units. For example, when attaching hair to enhance a style (GH15), you will also have to be aware of health and safety (G20) and advise and consult with clients (G7). You may also shampoo and condition hair (GH8) and cut hair (GH12). If you are not sure what you have covered in your service, always ask your assessor or supervisor for advice.

	NVQ	VRQ
Credit value	3	N/A
Guided Learning Hours	22	N/A

	NVQ
Practical demonstrations, to be observed by assessor	At least two. You must cover all of the points listed in the range for this unit. You must demonstrate both of the attachment systems, and one of your performances must include the removal of extensions. Simulation is not allowed for this unit.
Service timings	• Attachment of hair designed to last up to 24 hours (clip-in weft) – 30 minutes • Attachment of hair designed to last from 24 hours to 4 weeks – up to 120 minutes
Additional evidence	You will be required to complete an independent written paper to support the underpinning knowledge required for this unit.

Task mapping

When you have completed the tasks in this unit, check the table below to see which Performance Criteria (purple), Range (red), Knowledge (green) and Key Skills (blue) you have covered within GH15 to use as additional evidence within your portfolio. Information about which Functional Skills you have covered is available on the website.

Task and page reference	Mapping to Performance Criteria, Range, Knowledge and Key Skills
1 (page 370)	Performance Criteria: 1a, 1b, 1c, 1d, 1e, 1g, 1h, 1i, 2d Range: N/A Knowledge: 3, 4, 6, 7, 8, 9, 13, 14, 16 Key Skills: C1.2, C1.3, C2.3
2 (page 373)	Performance Criteria: 1f, 1j Range: N/A Knowledge: 34, 35, 36, 37 Key Skills: N1.1, N2.1, C1.2
3 (page 374)	Performance Criteria: 2a–e Range: 4a–c Knowledge: 21–28 Key Skills: C1.2, C1.3, C2.3
4 (page 377)	Performance Criteria: 2a, 2b, 2c, 3f, 3j Range: 2a–m Knowledge: 29 Key Skills: C1.2, C1.3, C2.3
5 (page 377)	Performance Criteria: 2f Range: 2g, 2h Knowledge: N/A Key Skills: C1.1, C2.1A

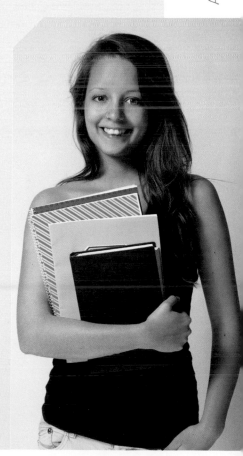

Create an image based on a theme within the hair and beauty sector

What you will learn:

- **How to plan an image**
- **How to create an image**

Introduction

Within the hairdressing industry there are many opportunities for stylists to express themselves through their work. With this unit you will be able to build on the skills you have already learned and explore other technical skills in order to complete a 'total' look. This will incorporate hair, make-up and nail art.

You will be required to complete a mood board that documents your ideas and tells the story of your journey from the start through to completion.

You will showcase your work in the form of a presentation to a target audience and communicate effectively to outline the purpose of your mood board and present your 'total look'.

Finally, it is important that you can work both as part of a team and as an individual following all salon and health and safety requirements.

How to plan an image

How to identify media images to create a theme

In our everyday lives we are constantly exposed to, and influenced by, media images. These may be on the TV and the internet, or in books, magazines, newspapers, films and photographs.

You need to explore these avenues so that you have a wide and varied range of material to work with. Don't forget to document the sources you have used to gather information so that you can compile your **bibliography**.

Your theme

You may begin with an idea for one theme, and then as you investigate other forms of media images, decide on another or even combine several types of images to produce a fantasy theme. Your only limit is your imagination!

Bibliography

A list of the sources that you have used when researching a topic.

Top tips

You may have a very clear idea of the type of image you wish to create but as you progress with the idea you might find you cannot express your creativity as much as you would like. Be prepared to change track!

Task 1

Research some images to show several different themes. To get you started you may like to use a mind map like the one opposite to explore different ideas at the first stage.

The easiest way to begin is to think of something that you enjoy. It could be a particular pop artist, a classic or current film, or even a book. You might choose to base your theme on a wedding or a prom or even a catwalk event.

Whatever you choose, put this in the middle of your mind map and have branches coming off ready to brainstorm other ideas that spring to mind when you look at your heading. You may find that talking your idea through with family, friends and colleagues will give you a different slant on your original idea.

When you are planning your image it is also important to know the assessment criteria that you are working towards in order to gain your assessment.

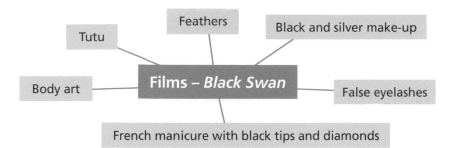

The purpose of a mood board

A **mood board** is a tool used by many different professions. Interior designers will gather swatches of material, paint samples, images and drawings when they are thinking of ideas for how to dress a room.

Hairdressing manufacturers will go out into town and city centres to see the current trends and influences 'on the street'. The inspiration they gather helps them to put together mood boards so they can bring out new colour ranges or design a collection of new-season looks.

The mood board should tell a story, from your initial idea to how you developed it, and what you plan your end result to be. It needs to be bright, colourful, eye-catching and original.

> **Mood board**
>
> A mood board can include images, text, objects and textiles. It is a tool to express and display your ideas and feelings and the thought processes behind them.

Image of a mood board that represents hair, make-up and nail art = total look!

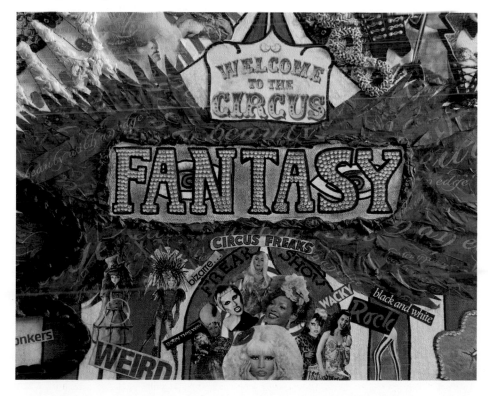

Create an image based on a theme within the hair and beauty sector

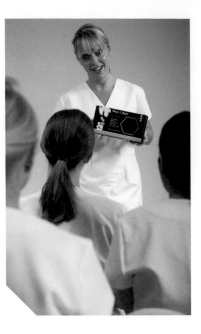

How to present a mood board to others

When compiling, making or building your mood board, think about how you are going to present it to others.

You may like to compile a checklist by thinking of the things you would like to see on a mood board if it was presented to you.

- Does it have a beginning (initial design), middle (how you have developed the idea) and end (is there a definite end result to your story)?
- Is there text to support your images – do you need text or do the images give enough information on their own?
- Is it clear – or is it a jumbled mess? It is fine to have one or more mood boards. The original one that you start with could include so much information that it looks confusing. However, once you have a firmer idea of your theme, you may dismiss much of the information, so a second mood board still containing your original ideas may be more suited to a presentation.
- How well have you used colour? A mood board needs to be eye-catching and hold the imagination of the people looking at it.
- Have other types of resources been used or is it all magazine cuttings? You could practise some nail art on false nails and attach those to your mood board.
- Is it realistic and achievable – can you recreate the 'look'?

You must also be aware of who you will be presenting to. Different age groups will have different expectations: a young audience will be interested in films or magazines, whereas a more mature age group may find the media of newspapers and documentaries more appealing.

When carrying out your presentation, plan how and where you will be to get your information across to your target audience. Make a checklist that you can refer to as your safety blanket. This will be particularly helpful on the day of your presentation when you are sure to be feeling nervous.

A suggested checklist would include:

- *Mood board* – don't forget it!
- *Prompt cards* – these can just be headings which you can check to make sure you have given all the information you planned to.
- *Resources/props* – you may have costumes/clothing, jewellery and accessories that you would like to show your audience.
- *Handouts* – some students like to keep a diary of events to record their progression. These need to be interesting and to the point for your audience.
- Where will you be giving your presentation? It's a good idea to view the room before the presentation to familiarise yourself with the surroundings.
- What will you need to take with you or arrange to be there? If you want to use a PowerPoint™ presentation, make sure the appropriate equipment can be set up in the room.
- Invite your audience to ask questions; it allows you to expand on information.

Personal learning and thinking skills –

Reflect upon the ways that you manage yourself and your time within your working day. Make a list of any areas that could be improved upon. Is your self management effective?

Making the presentation

When faced with giving a presentation, most people feel nervous or apprehensive. However, if you have prepared adequately by practising at home, and have a good knowledge and understanding of your topic, your confidence will grow and your presentation will go smoothly.

Points to consider include:

- Speak clearly and check that you are talking loudly enough to be heard at the back of the room. Close any windows if there is a lot of noise outside as this can be a distraction to both you and your audience.
- Think about your body language – try not to fidget! It can be very distracting to watch someone if they are constantly playing with their hair.
- Make your presentation standing up. It projects your voice and enables you to move around to address different members of your audience.
- Don't allow your presentation to go on for too long or make it so short that the audience don't have time to digest your information. Ten minutes is a good length of time to present your theme. This then allows time for questions and answers at the end.
- Be ready to answer questions at the end. Think about what inspired your theme, the journey you have travelled to reach your end result and the factors that influenced your decisions along the way.
- Enjoy yourself! If the audience can see you have passion and knowledge and have enjoyed the experience they will react more positively towards you.

Task 2

In small groups discuss presentations that you have seen, looking at the good and bad points that you may have noticed.

Using the task sheet provided on the website, list the positives and possible negatives of a presentation. This may highlight areas that you need to avoid or other areas that you need to focus on.

The concept of advertising to a target audience

Your initial idea for the theme of your image is your '**concept**' idea. As well as planning the concept of your mood board, you need to plan its delivery.

Advertising is used in all aspects of our everyday lives. We are not even aware of some of it. Your mood board is what you will be advertising; this is your marketing tool. If you think about what attracts you to making a purchase, or what makes you have a general interest in something, you will probably find that there is a common theme that appeals to you.

Concept

Your first idea, used as a starting point to base your presentation/ theme on.

Create an image based on a theme within the hair and beauty sector

It is important to target the right audience with your promotion. This can be an invited audience of local dignitaries, teachers, lecturers, your peers, colleagues and prospective employers. The type of people in your audience will influence your choice of marketing tools. If you are looking to reach a young market you may use YouTube or Facebook and your product needs to have credibility and be marketed using appropriate images and tone. A more mature market is more likely to read local newspapers or flyers that come through the door, or listen to local radio.

Task 3

In groups, think of the many different ways in which you can advertise. Put these into a mind map. Decide what methods of advertising are suitable for the following age groups:

- 13 to 19 – teen marketing
- 18 to 23 – college marketing
- 22 and above – young adult marketing
- 50 and above – older adult marketing.

Your advertising methods need to have a positive outcome. If they are not effective you will be wasting money which could have a detrimental effect on the business or product you are promoting.

The salon's requirements for preparing the client, yourself and the work area

Before you get down to the business of creating your 'total look', don't overlook these essential preparation guidelines.

Prepare yourself

Most colleges and training establishments require you to wear a uniform. Try to have everything organised the night before.

- Your uniform needs to be clean and ironed and your footwear should be appropriate (closed-in and low-heeled shoes).
- Shower or bathe before your assessment, make sure your teeth and nails are clean and clip your nails if they are too long. Don't wear overpowering perfume – a discreetly perfumed deodorant is enough.
- If it is a requirement to have your hair tied back for an assessment, ensure you either do this in the morning or have something with you to tie up your hair when you are about to begin. Make sure your hair is clean.
- Don't wear lots of jewellery.
- Apply suitable make-up.
- Bring the correct PPE (for example, gloves and an apron – refer to G20, page 55). You can fail an assessment under health and safety if you don't follow the correct procedures.
- Are you required to display your mood board? If so, is it to hand and positioned safely?
- Switch off your mobile phone! You will be concentrating, so this is easy to forget.

Top tips

How many students are there in your class? If every one of them received either a message or phone call during a lesson or assessment, think how irritating this would be for the lecturer, other students or clients! Turn off your phone.

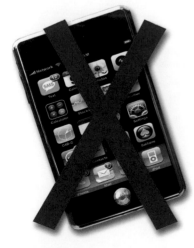

Client preparation

In all hairdressing services, the client is gowned and additional PPE is used to protect the client and her clothing for the duration of the service.

When you are creating your image you might use coloured hairsprays. If these stain the hair they will also stain the client's clothing and skin! Make sure your client is correctly gowned and protected throughout the service.

If you are shampooing your client you will need to use:

- a gown
- a plastic disposable cape
- a towel secured with a clip.

The cape can be removed after shampooing for client comfort and the towel replaced with a dry one if it has got wet during the shampooing service.

If you are using temporary or coloured sprays you will need to use a chemical gown if one is available, with a towel. If your training establishment provides face shields, use one to protect the client from the spray. You must also make sure you use sprays in a well-ventilated room. Refer to G20 and the COSHH regulations on pages 56–57.

Finally, to increase your client's comfort, make sure she is in a relaxed and comfortable position and has removed any excessive jewellery before you begin your services.

Preparing your work area

Your work area must be clean and tidy to receive your client/model. All equipment should be clean and sterile (refer to G20), page 63, for the best methods of sterilisation). This will prevent the risk of cross infection/infestation and portray a professional appearance.

Make a checklist of all the equipment you will need so that you are ready to begin working immediately. When you are being assessed it is important to be prepared and look professional while following all health and safety rules and regulations.

As you will be covering three technical services (hair, make-up and nails) you will be surprised at the amount of equipment you will need. You need to think about what you will be using and when it will be required as it won't be practical to have all of your equipment out at the same time. It is important that you don't create any hazards by having your work area 'littered' with lots of clutter.

Salon requirements for preparation – follow safe and hygienic working practices

For any hairdressing service you must follow all health and safety legislation to ensure the well-being of yourself, your clients and others. Your salon/training establishment will also have its own workplace polices that all staff must follow. This not only ensures the smooth running of the salon and increases the profitability of the business, it also promotes professionalism amongst staff and reduces the possibility of accidents occurring.

399

Top tips

Make a list of all the tools and equipment that you will need in order to complete your total look.

Create an image based on a theme within the hair and beauty sector

Create an image based on a theme within the hair and beauty sector

Refer to G20 for full details of health and safety practices in the salon and relevant legislation that must be followed. Some essential things to bear in mind are outlined below.

Electricity at Work Regulations 1989

If you are using electrical equipment you are required by law to make safety checks. You need to check that plugs and wires are safe and that all electrical equipment has had a current PAT (portable appliance test) test. (Refer to page 57 of G20 for more details of the Electricity at Work Act.)

Methods of sterilisation

To prevent the risk of cross-infection/infestation you should sterilise all tools and equipment after each client. There are various methods of sterilisation and some are more effective than others.

Refer to the chart on page 63 of G20 for the best methods of sterilising tools.

Disposal of waste

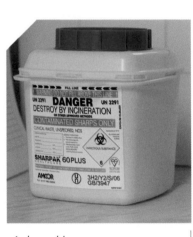

A sharps bin

To keep your work area clean and tidy and avoid the risk of cross-contamination you should dispose of waste products as you work. Any chemical products used will need to be disposed of following the manufacturer's instructions. (Refer to pages 56–57 of G20 and the COSHH regulations.) All other waste products can be disposed of in a waste bin, which should be emptied when it is full.

Remember to place any used sharps in the yellow sharps bin (see page 65 of G20).

COSHH

Under COSHH regulations you must make sure you know where the manufacturers' data sheets and COSHH assessment sheets are kept. This is especially important if you are using products that you are not familiar with. These will give information on the correct way to handle, use, store and dispose of any products.

You also need to make sure you are working in a well-ventilated area if you use substances that give off strong fumes or could create breathing difficulties. (Refer to page 56 of G20.)

Personal Protective Equipment (PPE)

You are required to use and wear PPE for both yourself and your client. Think about the service you will be carrying out and make sure both you and the client are adequately protected.

Task 4

In pairs, think of all the services that are involved in creating your theme and decide on the type of PPE that will be required. Compare your findings and discuss their importance. What could happen if the correct PPE wasn't used?

A task sheet has been provided on the website for your answers.

How to create an image

Now that you have completed the research and planning of your image, the fun starts – you can begin to create it.

Communicate and behave in a professional manner

Throughout each of the services that make up your image, you will need to communicate clearly and effectively – this includes both verbal and non-verbal communication. Communication is part of our everyday lives and sometimes it is easy to fall into bad habits.

Remember not to shout across the room or 'butt' into a conversation. It may be that you only need a quick 'yes' or 'no' so you can carry on with what you're doing but if everyone did this it would soon be very disruptive to the whole group and unhelpful to your trainer.

You also need to be able to communicate effectively to achieve your assessment. If you have someone assisting you, you will need to give clear instructions. You also need to be able to follow instructions. You need to check your client/model is comfortable and happy throughout the assessment. Be professional and make sure your body language is positive.

Task 5

Think of all the different types of ways in which you will communicate in a salon and when and why you will use them. Use the task sheet provided on the website to record your findings.

An example would be verbal communication used during the consultation with the client to gather information or explain a service to the client.

Top tips

Research the different types of nail art products that are available.

Technical skills required for creating a theme-based image

When you have decided on the image that you want to recreate you need to look at the technical challenges that lie ahead of you.

You will be using all of the hairdressing skills that you have learned and experimenting with new ones. Because this unit requires a total look you will also be completing make-up, nail art and dressing your model for a complete finished look.

Nail art

The qualification that you are undertaking will determine whether you are already working with nails. Most hairdressers have some experience in this field – either from doing their own nails or practising on family and friends.

You must do your research. There are a lot of products available on the market that you could use. You can use false nails and design your own nail art by using self-adhesive gems, jewels, crystals and 3D nail art. It is important to know your strengths and weaknesses so that you don't put yourself under any unnecessary stress on the day. If you work within your own abilities, you will be confident and comfortable with the work you are carrying out.

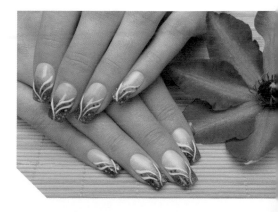

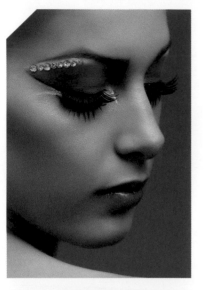

402

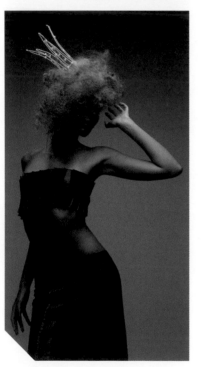

Make-up

Most of us use make-up every day so we already have a basic knowledge of application and technique. However, it is vital that you research and practise your techniques before you complete your final look.

If you have images, either from magazines or photos you have taken of one of your practice runs, you will have a good reference to help you recreate the look.

Make-up can make a bold statement and with the added use of false eyelashes or face gemstones you can turn an ordinary look into an edgy or avant-garde image. It is important to patch test your client if you are introducing new products and complete a thorough consultation to check the client doesn't have any allergies.

Fashion

The way in which you 'dress' your model can bring a total look together. This doesn't have to be expensive and by asking your model, family and friends, as well as raiding your own wardrobe, you should be able to find most things that you need.

Take into account how you will dress your model when you begin your initial research. If you choose something that requires a very specific look, for example a peacock theme, you may find that the resources are difficult to get hold of or could be too expensive. Great effects can be achieved with the use of fabrics being draped or tied and the use of added accessories can help you to achieve your desired outcome.

Hair

This is your opportunity to use all the hairdressing skills you have learned to date. You may be covering many different technical areas and have the chance to showcase your work. There is the opportunity to cluster some units. If you have decided to cut and colour the hair you may be able to achieve this on assessment. You may be incorporating plaiting techniques or setting the hair before styling. Speak to your lecturer and ask what can be used for assessment.

If the hair is the main focus for your final look, make sure you have set yourself a realistic goal and practised beforehand. Recap on backcombing and backbrushing techniques and make sure you have enough styling and finishing products. The hair, make-up, nail art and dress should all work together to produce something that is eye-catching and reflects your skills and personality.

Salon life

My journey

Abi's story

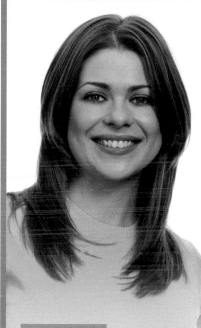

I have just completed my first year as a Hair and Beauty student and taken part in our end-of-year competition. We were given a choice of themes and as I had a keen interest in art I decided to enter the 'fantasy' category where I could really put all of my skills to the test. I chose my theme based on a film I had recently watched called *Black Swan*. I was inspired by the film but discovered that this was a popular choice so I changed direction slightly and looked at *Swan Lake*. I also have a cousin who dances for the Royal Ballet School so was hoping for some help in the costume department.

I prepared my model on the day, having been put through from the heats. I used a corset and tutu, and bought several feather boas which I took apart and then spent hours sticking on hundreds of feathers. For the hair I used a multitude of barrel curls with the sides of the hair slicked back close to the head. This was to keep to the theme of a traditional ballet dancer but incorporating a swan-like theme within the hair design. I sprayed her face and body white and used silver self-adhesive gems on her lips with a heavy body glitter on her cheeks. It was all about the sparkle! I used the whitener from a French manicure set on the whole nail bed and used a clear glitter nail varnish over the top and gemstones for more sparkle.

The day approached quickly and although I was slightly nervous I was also excited. I had planned and prepared for so many months leading up to the competition that I felt ready to showcase my work to an audience of over 400 people.

I was in shock when my name was called for first prize. I was stunned and amazed. My family went mad! I gained so much confidence from the competition and felt this unit helped me to prepare for such a big event.

Top tips

Planning and preparation are essential in the lead up to any event where you are showcasing your skills.

Ask the expert

Q *I would like to use a mask for my theme. Will this mean I won't achieve my assessment?*

A I would suggest that you used a hand-held mask if it is important as part of your theme. Your assessor can then still see the make-up underneath the mask and you will achieve both your assessment and the total look.

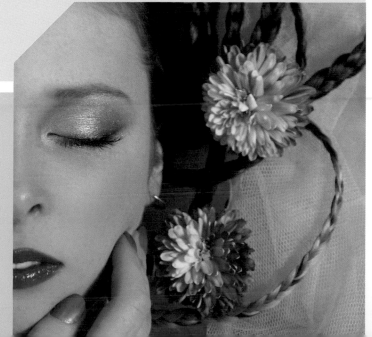

Create an image based on a theme within the hair and beauty sector

Methods of evaluating the effectiveness of your theme-based image

In our day-to-day lives we are constantly evaluating but don't always realise we are doing so. You may buy a new mascara and when you use it you will have an opinion on its effectiveness. Does it make your lashes thicker and fuller? Is it the right colour? You are evaluating it. It is important that you do this with your work and take on board the evaluation of other people too.

Verbal feedback

You will receive feedback from a wide range of people during your journey to creating your final image. Your family and friends may offer advice on your initial idea. Your model will give you feedback as you are working on her and on how the final result looks. Your peers will give you their opinions as you are practising your look. Your target audience will comment on your presentation of your mood board. Your assessor will give you your final verbal feedback on your assessment, highlighting the positives and giving encouragement on any weaker areas that need to be built on.

It is important to take all of this feedback on board as you may use it to make 'tweaks' as well as gaining personal development.

Written feedback

This feedback is usually recorded on an analysis/consultation sheet by your assessor, which is supported by the verbal feedback. This forms part of the evidence required for your portfolio.

You may have used questionnaires to gain relevant information from your presentation. It is important to evaluate the answers to see if there is a common theme. It could all be very positive feedback or it may give you ideas on how you can develop your image. All feedback is valuable and important so make sure you take the time to read it!

Positive and negative feedback

Both are equally important. Without negative feedback you will not be able to identify weaker areas and build on your skills. Most people want to improve and be the best they can be. Taking on board negative feedback will allow you to focus on specific areas. This has a very positive effect. If you have had difficulty with a particular technique, you may find there is only one area of negative feedback; once you have improved it, it means you can achieve your end result.

Positive feedback makes it all worthwhile. It will make you feel proud of your work and give you confidence to tackle new challenges as well as highlighting your strengths.

Photographic evidence

Photographic evidence is an excellent tool for recording your journey. You can keep it, not only for assessment purposes, but as something to look back on to see your progression.

You may choose to take photographs ranging from your first concept to the final image and have a diary of your work. This can also be used to show prospective employers together with a portfolio of all your hairdressing work.

Top tips

When you produce a questionnaire it is a good idea to use both open questions that require a written response and closed questions that only require a 'yes' or 'no'.

Examples of suitable questions include:

- What was the most eye-catching part of the theme? (This requires a longer written response.)
- Was the presentation clear with relevant information? (Yes/no?)

Self-evaluation

This is an important process to go through. At the end of every hairdressing service you will be evaluating your work. This needs to be an in-depth and critical evaluation. The purpose of the evaluation is to assess:

- Were you happy with the end result?
- What were your strengths or weaknesses?
- Did you achieve what you set out to?
- What was your favourite part of the process?
- What new methods and/or techniques did you learn as a result of the process?
- Is there anything you would do differently next time?

Choose one positive outcome to take forward as a result of the process.

This is not an exhaustive list and you may like to make up your own evaluation form.

Why evaluation is important

Evaluation is important because it allows you to build on existing skills and identify any gaps in your knowledge or skillset area. It shows that you care about the work you are carrying out and are not afraid to be self-critical.

Aftercare advice

With every hairdressing service it is important to provide the client with aftercare advice. This is an assessment and professional requirement.

Methods of removal

The type of advice that you need to give to a client will depend on the look that you have created. If you have carried out a 'hair-up' look with the use of backcombing/backbrushing, hair grips and hairsprays or gels, it is important that you advise your client on the best way to take her hair down.

The table below gives some recommendations for methods of removal.

Technique used	Method of removal
Hair up	Remove hairpins/hairgrips gently without tearing the hair. Brush the hair through from points to roots.
Backcombing/backbrushing	Use a soft bristle brush. Beginning at the nape area, brush the hair from points to roots to gently remove the back brushing/combing.
Crimping	Section the hair and begin in the nape area. Use a soft bristle brush and brush from points to roots.
Plaiting/twisting/braiding	Remove the covered band used to secure the hair. Unwind the hair beginning at the ends and working up towards the root area.
Application of products	All products used will be water-soluble. They need to be brushed out first and then shampooed for complete removal.

Top tips

- In pairs, think of all the looks that are created and the advice you would give to a client for removal. Add this to the table provided so you can refer to it.
- If you have used false nails you also need to provide your client with the correct information for removal. You don't want the client to 'pull' the nails off as this will damage the nail bed. Always refer to the manufacturer's instructions for the correct removal techniques.

Create an image based on a theme within the hair and beauty sector

Product recommendations

What if your client wants to recreate the look at home? It is important that you give her information about the products you have used. You need to understand the different effects the products achieve. It is important to keep up to date on what your salon stocks and know the benefits of each product.

You should only make a recommendation about a product if you know it will be suitable to achieve the desired outcome.

Refer to page 246 of GH10.

Further treatment needs/maintenance

If you have used colour to enhance your client's hair, you will need to advise her about the timescale between services. You may also have identified that your client requires further treatments as a result of several practice sessions, to return the hair back to its natural state. Offer deep conditioning treatments if appropriate.

Maintenance advice

For all hairdressing services you will be giving your client maintenance advice.

As you are covering three different disciplines, you need to make sure you provide aftercare advice across all three areas. If you have created a hair-up look you may want to provide grips for the client to take home and show her the correct way to use them if required. You can advise on the use of shine spray and hairspray to help maintain the look. With nails and make-up you can encourage the client to purchase the lipstick or nail varnish so she can repair chipped nails and maintain her lip colour.

Task 6

In pairs or groups think of all the services you may cover to complete this unit and discuss the maintenance required.

Check your knowledge

The following questions will help you to check your understanding of this unit.
The answers can be found on pages 501–2.

1 What is the purpose of a mood board?
  a) To record the development of your initial idea through to your final concept
  b) To stop you from feeling angry
  c) To provide evidence for assessment
  d) To gauge the mood of your client

2 What is meant by the term 'media images'?
  a) Images from the internet, books, cinema, magazines, etc.
  b) The photographic evidence that you have taken
  c) A written description of the image used for your total look
  d) Pictures of televisions

3 What is the recommended length of time for your presentation?
  a) Two minutes
  b) Ten minutes
  c) Half an hour
  d) One hour

4 What should you use to protect your client from coloured hairsprays?
  a) A chemical gown, a towel and a face shield
  b) Sunglasses and an outdoor coat
  c) Plastic goggles, a gown and a towel
  d) Use your hand to screen the client's face from the spray

5 Why is feedback important?
  a) To prevent hunger pains
  b) To identify strengths and weaknesses
  c) To allow your client the opportunity to chat
  d) So that everyone in the salon knows how good you are at your job

Create an image based on a theme within the hair and beauty sector

Getting ready for assessment

You will be assessed using a combination of assessment methods, as described below. Remember that within each of the services you carry out with a client, you will cover different units. For example, when creating an image based on a theme, you may also shampoo and condition hair (GH8) and set or dress hair (GH11). If you are not sure what you have covered in your service, always ask your assessor or supervisor for advice.

	NVQ	VRQ
Credit value	N/A	7
Guided Learning Hours	N/A	60

	VRQ
Practical demonstrations, to be observed by assessor	In this unit you must demonstrate competent performance of all practical criteria on at least three occasions. Simulation should be avoided where possible and evidence gathered in a realistic working environment. All outcomes, assessment criteria and range statements must be achieved.
Service timings	There are no maximum service timings for this unit.
Additional evidence	Where possible your assessor will assess knowledge and understanding criteria alongside practical criteria through oral questioning. There is no written independent paper for this unit.

Task mapping

When you have completed the tasks in this unit, check the table below to see which Performance Criteria (purple), Range (red), Knowledge (green) and Key Skills (blue) you have covered within this unit to use as additional evidence within your portfolio. Information about which Functional Skills you have covered is available on the website.

Task and page reference	Mapping to Performance Criteria, Range, Knowledge and Key Skills
1 (page 394)	Performance Criteria: 1a Range: R1a, R1b Knowledge: N/A Key Skills: N/A
2 (page 397)	Performance Criteria: 2a, 2b Range: R1a–c, R3a Knowledge: 1d Key Skills: N/A
3 (page 398)	Performance Criteria: — Range: R1c, R3a Knowledge: 1e Key Skills: N/A
4 (page 400)	Performance Criteria: 2c Range: R3b Knowledge: 2g Key Skills: N/A
5 (page 401)	Performance Criteria: 2a Range: R3a, R3b Knowledge: 2h Key Skills: N/A
6 (page 406)	Performance Criteria: N/A Range: R3b, R4d Knowledge: 1f, 2g Key Skills: N/A

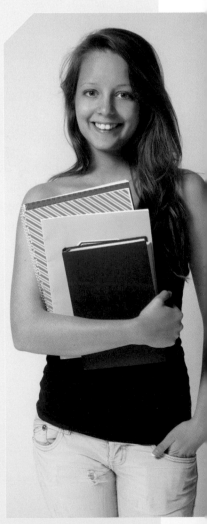

Create an image based on a theme within the hair and beauty sector

Section

3

Practical skills –

barbering

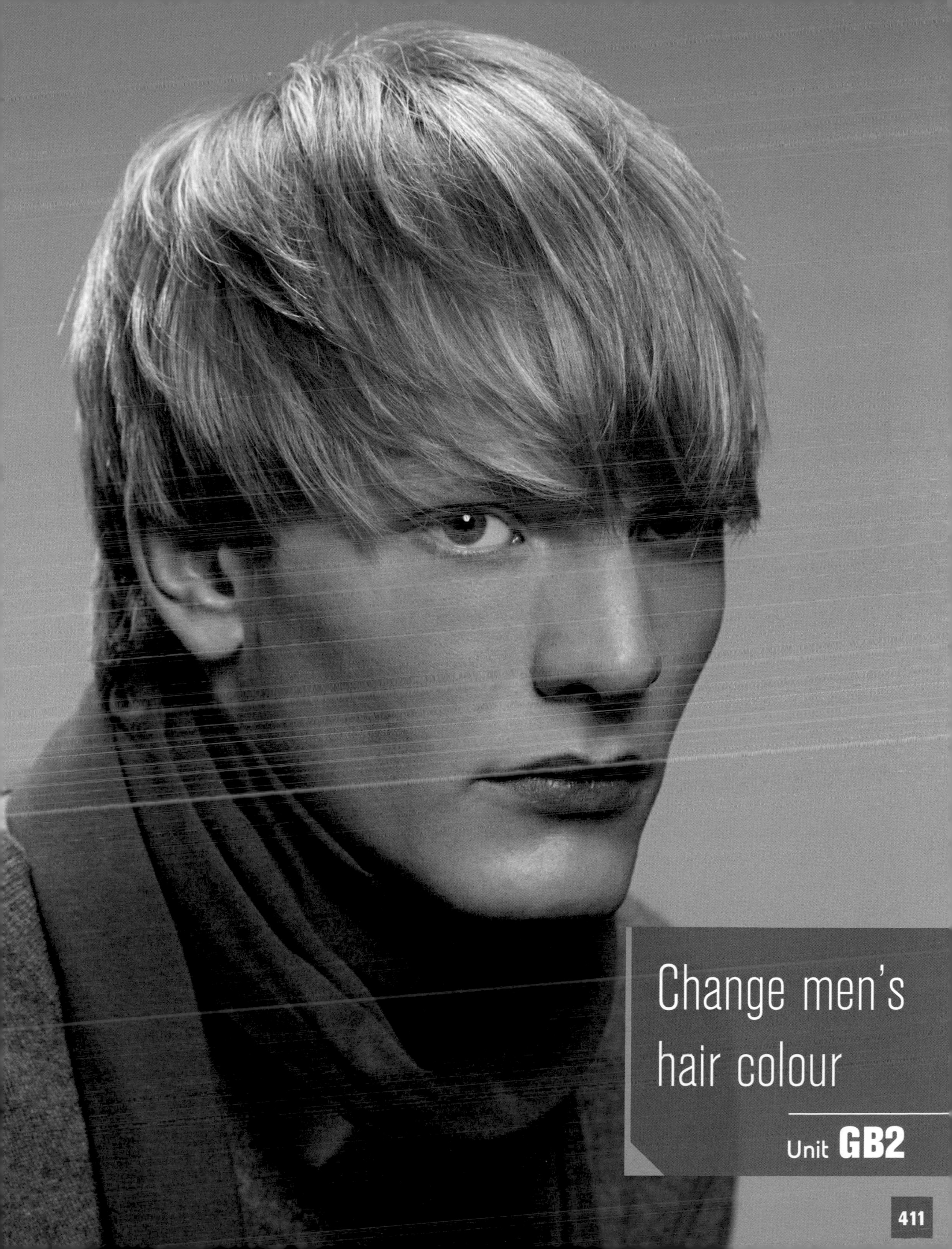

Change men's hair colour

Unit **GB2**

What you will learn:

- **How to maintain effective and safe methods of working when colouring and lightening hair**
- **How to prepare for colouring and lightening hair**
- **How to colour and lighten hair**
- **How to provide aftercare advice**

Introduction

Colouring forms part of a service that men have now come to expect within the salon. Colour aids the appearance of texture, depth and movement of the hair. There are many different techniques involved in colouring; this unit will cover semi-permanent, quasi-permanent, permanent and lightening effects, working on a full and partial head, regrowth areas and using highlighting and lowlighting effects.

Because you are working with chemicals you need to work in a safe manner, following manufacturers' instructions and using the correct personal protective equipment (PPE) for both yourself and your client. You need to ensure safe working practices and adhere to health and safety regulations.

How to maintain effective and safe methods of working

Health and safety considerations

Gowning

It is important to ensure the correct gowning for a colouring service so that product does not come into contact with the client's clothing. This is the correct gowning procedure:

- Use a chemical gown (if one is available; if not use an ordinary cutting gown).
- Place a plastic disposable cape around the client.
- Place a colouring towel over the top of the cape and secure.

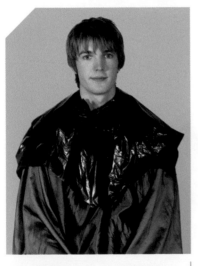

It is important to ensure the correct gowning for a colouring service

Task 1

You have a duty to protect yourself when carrying out a colouring service. Refer back to GH9, pages 200–1, and make a list of the protective equipment that should be used during a colouring service. Write a brief statement on the importance of each.

A worksheet for this task is provided on the website for you to complete and add to your portfolio.

Using barrier cream

Barrier cream is used to prevent any tint sitting on the client's face – dark tints will stain the skin. Some clients have very sensitive skin, which can become inflamed if a barrier cream is not used.

Apply the barrier cream, either with your finger or using a cotton wool bud. Make sure that the cream is evenly and thickly applied as close to the hairline as you can get without depositing any on the hair itself, as this will act as a barrier to the colour.

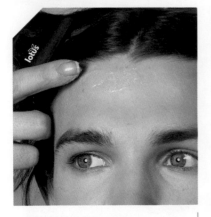

Applying barrier cream

It is recommended that you remove the barrier cream before you remove the colour. It is a good idea to do this before you shampoo so you do not spread the barrier cream onto the hair; if this happens it will make the hair oily in appearance and will need to be removed using neat shampoo on the hair to break down the oil/waxes contained within the barrier cream.

Task 2

Your client has arrived for a root retouch permanent colour. The last time he had a colour he had a reaction to the barrier cream which made the skin around his hairline very red and sore. The colour he has is a very dark base so will stain the skin without any barrier cream. What alternative can you use as a barrier cream? (You may like to refer to GH9.)

Positioning

Why is the position of your client important when colouring hair?

Good client position will enable you to work freely and effectively around your client.

Will you have to adjust your client's position during the colouring process?

Yes, in order to reach more difficult areas of the head when working. Do not be afraid to ask your client to tilt his head backwards or forwards so that you can apply the colour easily, and remember to place your tools and equipment within easy reach.

You also need to consider your own posture and position. Read back through page 73 to remind yourself of this.

Keeping your work area clean and tidy

Clients expect to see a professional environment where all tools and equipment are maintained to a high standard. They don't want to be sitting amid chaos; this will make them feel that the finished result of their hair service will also look chaotic!

To prepare your work area to receive your client, you need to:

- wipe over the work surface to remove dust and hair cuttings
- make sure that all hair cuttings from previous clients that have fallen onto the floor are swept away
- check that all equipment not required for your next client is put away
- have your client's record card to hand along with all the protective equipment and colouring equipment that you will need for the service
- make sure all hair is removed from brushes and combs and that equipment is sterilised after every client.

Minimising the wastage of products

- Never mix colours before you have carried out a consultation. Even if you're sure your client will have the same as last time, there is always the chance that he may change his mind!
- Only mix small amounts – you can always mix up more as required.
- Always use a measuring device to mix your colours to ensure the correct measurements and end result.

Fact or fiction?

Is this statement fact or fiction?

A skin test should be carried out before every colouring service.

To check your answer see page 502.

413

Unit
GB2

Change men's hair colour

Top tips

To ensure the health and safety of yourself, your client and your colleagues:

- always read the manufacturer's instructions
- always follow the COSHH Regulations 2003 for storage, mixing and disposal of colouring products
- always clean up after yourself
- always report hazards to the relevant person
- check that your equipment is in good working order and the portable appliance test (PAT) sticker is current.

Minimise the risk of cross-infection

- You need to carry out a thorough consultation to prevent any infestation or infection being passed from one client to another.
- **Cross-infection** can occur through towels, gowns, cutting collars, brushes and combs, so never reuse these without sterilising first. (Refer to G20, pages 63–64, and G7, page 144, for the best methods of sterilisation for your various tools and equipment.)

Minimising harm or injury to yourself or others

When carrying out a colouring process, you may need to use extra equipment; it is your responsibility to make sure that the equipment is in good working order.

> ### Task 3
>
> What safety considerations do you need to consider for equipment that will be used during a colouring service? Discuss in groups and record your findings.

Safe use of products

The golden rule when working with any product is to read the manufacturer's instructions. This is especially important with colouring, as each manufacturer's products may be different. You must follow all of the health and safety guidelines set down by the manufacturers and your salon or training institution. Here are some guidelines:

- Complete a skin test on the client before carrying out any colouring process (with the exception of a temporary colour).
- Mix only the amount of product that you think you are going to need – mixing too much is wasteful and uneconomic.
- Mix the product immediately before use – tint starts to oxidise (develop) as soon as it makes contact with the air.
- Place lids back on products as soon as you have measured out the amount that you require.
- Use the correct PPE.
- Store chemicals correctly when they are not being used – refer to manufacturers' COSHH sheets for information on handling, storage and disposal of products, the harm they could cause and how to treat in case of an accident.
- Always mix in a well-ventilated room, especially when using powder lighteners as these can be ingested and cause breathing difficulties.

Personal hygiene

Good personal hygiene will minimise the risk of cross-infection. It will also create a professional image and instil confidence in your client – no one wants a stylist with poor hygiene looking after them! (Refer to G17 for more on appearance and behaviour.)

Using your time effectively

Each salon allows a set amount of time for the different services that it offers. Time allocation allowed for colouring services differs, depending on the method of application and the products used. For example, applying a semi-permanent colour does not take as long as applying a full-head bleach.

It is important to be prepared to receive your client as this will cut down on time for the service overall.

Cross-infection

The transfer of infection from one person to another.

Top tips

You cannot carry out a colouring service if your client has not had a skin test 24–48 hours prior to the service being carried out. This is to ensure the health and safety of your client by checking that he doesn't have an allergic reaction to the colouring products that are going to be used.

Carrying out a consultation

By completing an in-depth consultation you should be able to determine what tools and equipment you will be using for the service, how you will be placing the colour and what colouring product you will be using.

Task 4

In pairs, choose a 'colour look' for men from a magazine and discuss the methods, techniques, tools and equipment used to achieve the look. Do you agree with each other or would you both tackle the job differently? Record your findings.

A colouring consultation sheet for this task is provided on the website for you to complete and add to your portfolio.

During the consultation you also need to take into consideration:

- critical influencing factors, e.g. any previous chemical services
- hair condition
- client requirements/lifestyle
- whether there is any white hair present.

415

Unit
GB2

Change men's hair colour

Shade chart for men's colouring service

Choosing suitable products and equipment

When you begin a colouring service you need to take into account the type of product you will be using, as this affects how you prepare the hair for the application of the colour.

Product type	Preparation required	Suitability
Semi-permanent	Usually applied to shampooed, towel-dried hair.	This product will not lighten the hair; it will only add depth and tone. Usually lasts 4–8 shampoos.
Quasi-permanent	Can be applied to either wet or dry hair. It is important to read individual manufacturers' instructions.	This product isn't supposed to lift the hair but prolonged use can produce a regrowth effect at the root area. Will add depth and tone and lasts for 8–12 shampoos.
Permanent	Applied to dry hair.	This product has the ability to lift and lighten the hair up to three levels and darken the hair as is suitable for the client's skin tone and requirements. This is a permanent product that has to grow out of the hair.
Lightening products	Applied to dry hair.	There is a range of lightening products to lighten the hair; they are permanent products that have to grow out.

Mixing and measuring

Some products don't require any mixing and can be used straight from their own packaging; other products are mixed either with developers or hydrogen peroxide.

When measuring out hydrogen peroxide and tint, make sure that you are accurate – do not guess. Read the amount in the measuring flask at eye level for accurate measurement. It is best to put the measuring flask on a flat surface, as holding it may result in an inaccurate measurement.

When mixing a quarter or half a tube of tint, note where the marks are on the side of the tube and only squeeze out the tint to these guidelines. Always squeeze the tube from the end (as you would with toothpaste at home).

If you are using more than one colour, first mix the two tints together in a bowl before adding the hydrogen peroxide. This will ensure thorough mixing of the tints.

Prepare the tint immediately before use. Do not allow the tint to stand for any length of time or it will lose its effectiveness.

Tools and equipment

The type of colouring effect that you want will determine the equipment that you use.

Task 5

Complete the missing information in the table below to identify the different types of tools and equipment available for colouring services. You may like to refer to GH9.

Tools/equipment	Suitability	Effects
Highlighting/ lowlighting cap		
	Ideal for all lengths of hair, apart from very short hair (less than 5 cm). Used when one or more colours are being applied.	
Block colouring		A solid block of colour(s) is applied to a section of the hair.
Wide-toothed comb	Ideal for short hair where other techniques cannot be used.	

A worksheet containing this chart can be found on the website for you to use to record your findings. This can then be used as additional portfolio evidence.

Task 6

There are many other techniques used when colouring men's hair. Discuss in your groups any other methods of application and techniques you have seen used in your training establishment. (Clue: shoe shining/frosting.)

Using equipment that is safe for the purpose

During the colouring process you may need to use other electrical equipment to aid the development of your colour. By using this equipment you will be adding heat to the hair. You will need to make safety checks on the equipment; refer to G20, page 57, for information on the Electricity at Work Regulations.

As well as making checks on your electrical equipment, you will need to make checks on all other tools. Check that combs do not have any broken teeth as this may tear the hair and cause discomfort to the client. After a certain amount of time your tinting brushes may lose their bristles and this will hinder the distribution of your tint and may affect the colour result.

Reporting low levels of stock

You may not be directly in charge of ordering stock, but you are part of a team of people who use the stock. You have a responsibility to report any low or missing stock items and to make sure you are prepared for the services you are giving.

In most salons and colleges/training institutions, you would report low stock levels to the person directly in charge of you. This could be your salon manager or tutor. If that person is not available, the best course of action is to leave a memo in whatever communication system you use. You would then have recorded that you identified that stock was low and notified the relevant person.

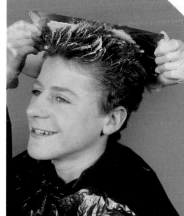

Shoe shining/frosting technique

417

Unit

GB2

Change men's hair colour

General allocation of time for colour application

As a trainee, the time allocations listed below are those you should be working towards and not what you are expected to achieve when you first begin.

Colouring service	Time allocation
Semi-permanent	30 minutes for consultation, preparation and application. Development time depends on the product you are using. Always read the manufacturer's instructions.
Quasi-permanent	30 minutes (as above).
Permanent regrowth	30 minutes for consultation, preparation and application.
Permanent full head (virgin hair)	45 minutes for the first application, then a further 20 minutes to complete the application.
Cap highlights/lowlights	30 minutes for consultation, pulling through the highlights and applying the product. Development time depends on the required end result and the product you are using.
Mesh/foil highlights or lowlights	Usually 45 minutes to a maximum of one hour (on hair below shoulder length). Fresh tint may have to be mixed halfway through as the product loses its strength after 30 minutes.
Frosting/shoe shining	18–20 minutes for mixing and application.

Keeping accurate and up-to-date client records

It is important to record all of the services that you carry out on a client for future reference.

This information will enable you to adjust the services, products or techniques used as required by the client, or maintain a colour if the client is happy with it.

Top tips

Remember that record cards come in many different formats. You may have access to a computerised record to log client information, or use handwritten record cards.

Task 7

Task 7

After any chemical hairdressing, you need to record what you did, the products you used, timings and the outcomes. There is other important information that needs to be included. Discuss in your groups the other information that you need to have on a client record card and record your findings.

How to prepare for colouring and lightening hair

In this section you will be looking at the hair and skin tests that you need to carry out before you begin the colouring and lightening process. You will also be looking at how critical influencing factors will have an effect on the colouring process and the correct preparation of your products.

Carrying out and recording all hair and skin tests

Before and during any colouring process, there are tests that need to be performed to make sure that you can carry out a colouring service. The test results may also influence your choice of products, tools and equipment. Below is a list of all the tests that need to be carried out. The information for each test can be found on pages 207–9.

- Skin test (also known as patch test and hypersensitivity test)
- Elasticity test
- Porosity test
- Incompatibility test
- Test cutting
- Strand test/colour test.

Recording the result

After every hair or skin test has been carried out, it is important that you complete the client's record card in full. Do not leave this until later – you could easily forget a piece of information that will be important for the client's next colouring service.

Identifying contraindications to a colouring/lightening service

Contraindication is a term that appears in all the practical hairdressing units. You need to be familiar with the term and what it means. If you fail to identify anything on the hair or scalp that will affect the hairdressing service, you may cause severe damage to the hair or scalp, or potentially pass on an infection or disease.

Fact or fiction?

Is this statement fact or fiction?

A porosity test is only carried out if the hair looks in bad condition.

To check your answer see page 502.

Contraindication

Anything present on the hair or scalp that will prevent you from carrying out a service.

Task 8

In pairs, list as many contraindications to a colouring service that you can think of. What advice would you give to the client on each of them and who would you refer to if it was a problem you couldn't deal with?

A worksheet for this task is provided on the website for you to complete and add to your portfolio.

Choosing products, application methods and equipment, taking into account critical influencing factors

Considering colour

When considering your choice of colour, you have to think about:

- the natural hair colour (the base colour)
- any colour that is already present on the hair
- the results of the hair and skin tests that you have performed
- the hair's condition.

You need to match up the client's existing hair colour to the shade chart to determine the client's base shade and to choose your target shade. Observe the following:

- the percentage (if any) of white hair your client has
- his skin tone (e.g. very pale, olive, flushed).

When you have established the 'base/depth' of your client's hair, you can then decide what products are suitable for the look that the client wants to achieve.

Choosing a method

Discuss and decide on the methods and techniques you are going to use and how the client will be able to maintain his colour. You also need to discuss the time duration between services and inform the client of the cost of the service.

The amount of white hair present will determine how much base colour is used, the percentage of hydrogen peroxide and where you begin the application. When adding colour to the hair (covering white hair), start at the most resistant area (where the white hair is most obvious). (Refer to page 210 for more information on white hair.)

Useful equipment

You can assist the development of the colour by adding heat. You can use:

- *a dry heat appliance (climazone)* – dry heat speeds up the development of permanent colours
- *a steamer* – moist heat is generally used for lightening products, for example bleaches.

Preparing the client and products prior to colouring

Checklist prior to colouring

- Check your record card for test results – what tests should have been carried out?
- Make sure you are organised to receive the client, with client record card, colour shade chart and colouring tools and equipment ready.
- Ensure the correct gowning procedure for your client to protect the client's clothing and the correct personal protective equipment (PPE) for yourself.
- Apply barrier cream to the client's skin.

Top tips

If the client already has colour on his hair and wants to lift the colour, you need to be aware that permanent colour (tint) cannot lift another permanent colour (tint).

Fact or fiction?

Is this statement fact or fiction?

A client may have 'hot' and 'cold' spots on his head that will affect the development of the colour.

To check your answer see page 502.

419

Unit

GB2

Change men's hair colour

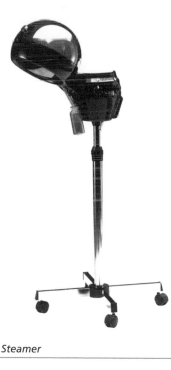

Steamer

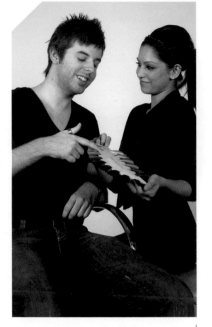

Consultation with a client

Checking manufacturers' instructions

Always read the manufacturer's instructions, as these will tell you whether you should apply the colour to wet or dry hair. They will also give you all the information that you require on how to mix your products and what peroxide strength to use, as well as any other relevant information. (Refer to pages 211–12 for the step-by-step preparation required to colour wet and dry hair.)

Consultation

It is a good idea to carry out the consultation before you gown the client, so that you can take into account his personality; for example, the way your client dresses is a good indication of the type of lifestyle he may lead.

You should also complete a full colouring consultation form and carry out porosity and elasticity tests during the consultation (see pages 207–9).

Refer to a colour shade chart (see page 217) to enable the client to see the colour choices available to him. It will also enable you to match up to the client's existing colour and choose one to enhance and complement his skin tone.

Principles of colouring

The principles of colouring are exactly the same for men's hair as for women's hair. Read the following sections in GH9:

- Principles of colouring; see pages 214–15
- Choosing the product and application; see pages 217–18
- Development and removal; see pages 220–21
- The finished result; see page 221

How to colour and lighten hair

When changing hair colour permanently, there is a wide variety of products and techniques that can be used – your imagination is your only limit!

Preparing the client for a permanent colouring service

The consultation

The consultation for a permanent colouring service should be slightly more in-depth because of the wider choice of products available and the effects you can achieve. For example, you can:

- lighten (permanently)
- darken (permanently)
- change tone (permanently).

First, you should check whether the client has an up-to-date skin test. This is to protect against any allergic reaction to the para dye that is contained in permanent colours. If the test is up to date (and there was no positive reaction), you are free to continue the consultation.

Top tips

Remember that you cannot lighten the hair when using semi- or quasi-permanent colours. You will be able to darken the hair or keep it on the same base and just change the tone.

Next, you should find out whether the client wants to:

- go lighter than his natural base colour
- go darker than his natural base colour
- stay at the same depth as his natural base colour but add a warm or cool tone.

The target colour to be achieved will determine the strength of hydrogen peroxide that you will use. During the consultation:

- use a colour shade chart
- match up the client's natural base shade to the shade chart
- decide whether you are lightening, darkening or adding tone
- decide on the technique that you will use
- agree with the client if it is a full head colour, partial or regrowth colour
- check whether the client wishes to have more than one colour in his hair
- find out if the client will be able to maintain the colour
- double-check with the client that you have chosen the right colour.

Permanent tint is permanent! If the client does not like the result, he will have to grow the colour out.

As well as the colour consultation, you will need to complete the standard client consultation form (refer to page 305).

Products, techniques, application and development

Semi-permanent, quasi-permanent, permanent and lighteners

All permanent colours are applied to dry hair. There are two main types:

- creams and gels – synthetic, organic
- metallic dyes – inorganic.

Synthetic dyes are known as para dyes. (For more information on para dyes, hydrogen peroxide, high lift tints and bleaches, and to find out where colour molecules sit on the hair shaft and their effects, refer to pages 214–23.)

Application of permanent tint or bleach to virgin hair

In order to get an even colour result, you need to take into account:

- the length of the hair
- the porosity of the hair
- body heat.

On hair that is over 2.5 cm long, the roots will develop more quickly than the ends of the hair. This is because heat that escapes from the scalp speeds up the development time. The hair that is furthest away from the scalp takes longer to develop because it does not have the benefit of body heat. Hair that is more porous will develop more quickly than hair that is in good condition.

On long hair, the ends (because the hair is older) will be more porous than the mid-lengths and will process more quickly.

Full head tint or bleach on virgin hair should be applied to the hair in the following order:

- mid-lengths
- ends
- roots.

When using lightening products, do not allow one application to overlap the other. This can cause breakage to the hair as you are effectively double-processing the hair.

Sectioning

In any hairdressing or barbering service it is important to section the hair evenly and cleanly. This allows you to work in a methodical method, securing any hair not required at the time out of the way. In colouring, using the correct sectioning will allow you to work close to the head and will ensure even coverage of colour.

Step-by-step application of a full head colour on virgin hair

1 Divide the hair into a hot cross bun (four sections) and apply the colour to the mid-lengths and ends first.

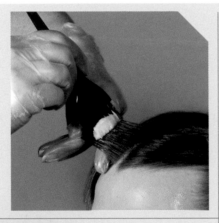

2 Avoid the root area as this will develop more quickly because of the body heat.

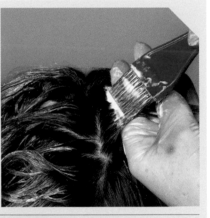

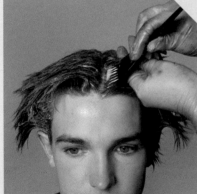

3 Once the colour has been applied to all sections of the mid-lengths and ends, go back to the area where the tint was first applied and begin your application at the root area.

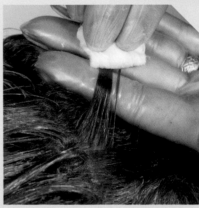

4 To check the development of your colour, use a piece of damp cotton wool and remove the excess tint.

5 Check that the ends and roots match to ensure an even colour result.

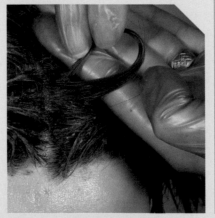

6 Apply shining products and style in the desired manner – give your client the appropriate aftercare advice.

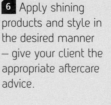

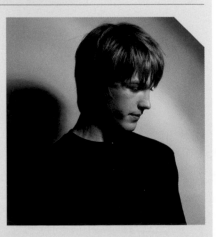

Salon life

Learning from others

Maria's story

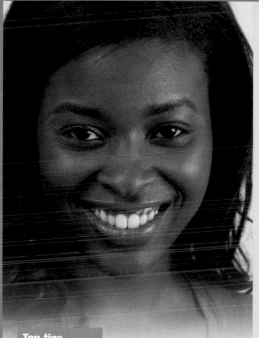

I have always had a great interest in colouring and have experimented a lot on myself and on any friends or family that I could get my hands on!

The first time I was supervised and instructed on how to apply foils to the hair, I was disappointed that I couldn't get mine to stay close enough to the roots. I have always picked most things up very easily, but holding the hair, the foil and the comb in my hand while applying the colour was getting the better of me. My tutor could see that I was frustrated, and suggested that I walk around the room and observe the techniques everyone else was using. I was amazed to see that even though we had all watched the same demonstration, we had all interpreted the method slightly differently. By watching what everyone else was doing, I could see exactly where I was having difficulties. I went back to my block (feeling much better for having had time out) and set to the task again. Success! I could do it! That lesson has always stayed with me and I now know the value of watching and learning from others. I can also complete a full head of foils in less than an hour!

Top tips

If you want to practise foils or mesh application at home, but you're not ready to use colour, mix up a small amount of flour and conditioner in a bowl. The consistency is thick enough to attach the foil to the hair, but can be removed easily by shampooing.

Ask the expert

Q I prefer to use mesh because the packets are self-adhesive. If I don't practise with foil as well, will this affect my chances of getting a job in a salon?

A This depends on the salon, but ideally you need to try to make yourself an 'all rounder' with both types of application. Using mesh all of the time can be quite costly, and foil may be needed for certain types of application. Ask your trainer to demonstrate the techniques again and, using the Top tip above, see if you can practise at home!

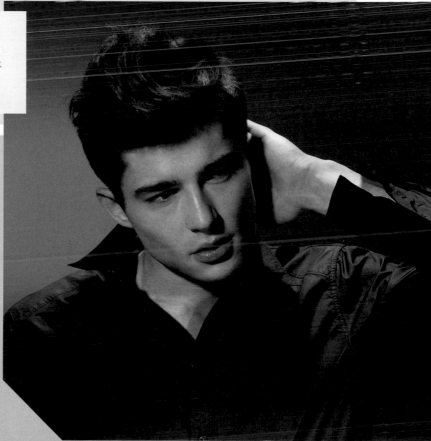

423

Unit

GB2

Change men's hair colour

Mesh and foils – partial head application

If you are adding one or more colours to the hair, you can choose to use foils or mesh. You will need to ask your client a number of questions to determine the amount of hair you are going to weave and apply colour to:

- Do you want to see more natural hair than coloured hair?
- Do you want to see equal amounts of natural hair to coloured hair?
- Would you like more coloured hair than natural hair?

By asking these questions you will be able to work out how much hair you will weave out of each section to colour. This is often referred to in percentages.

- If you are going to be carrying out a fine weave you will only be taking 25 per cent of the hair from the section.
- If you are going to split the hair so equal amounts are coloured and natural, you will be weaving 50 per cent of the mesh of hair.
- If you want more colour than natural hair, you will weave 75 per cent of the mesh of hair, leaving 25 per cent not coloured. This is only a rough guide as you may weave 20, 30 or 40 per cent, but it gives you a starting point to work from.

As with any colouring process, gown the client correctly then mix the colours required. Beginning at the nape area, drop a fine mesh of hair about 2 cm deep. Pick up this section of hair and, using the end of a pintail comb, select the strands you wish to apply colour to.

- If using two or more colours, you will need to alternate the colours as you apply them.
- If you require a lot of colour in the hair, you would weave every section.
- If the client did not want much colour in his hair, you would leave a section of hair in between each packet.

If you can place the packets in a brickwork pattern, this will avoid any channels or partings in the hair not being coloured (see page 281).

Step-by-step frosting/shoe shining

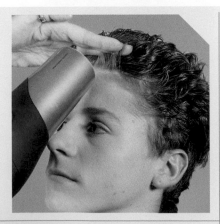
1 Blow-dry the hair into style.

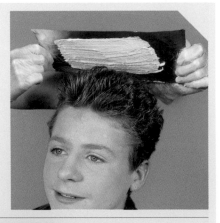
2 Apply your colouring product to a piece of foil.

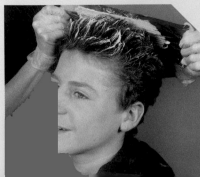
3 Using a side-to-side action across the top of the hair or area to be coloured, shoe shine the colour onto the hair.

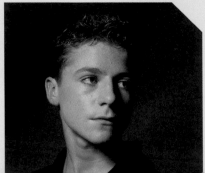
4 For subtle effects, reduce the processing time. This will create a very natural sunkissed look.

Critical influencing factors

When deciding on the product and technique to use, you will need to take into account the following critical influencing factors:

- temperature
- existing colour of hair
- percentage of white hair
- porosity
- length of hair
- test results.

Temperature

When colouring the hair, there are 'hot spots' in the nape area and the top of the head that you need to be aware of. In the case of a full head of foils, where you begin at the nape area, this hair will start to process as soon as you apply the product to the hair. By the time you reach the front of the head, the first section of hair may be near to the end of its development time. If this is the case, you need to apply the product quite quickly and you may need to think about using added heat on the last packets applied. You need to constantly check your packets as they are developing and use a water spray to remove any colour that has developed without disturbing the rest of the processing colour.

A heat appliance (see page 211) offers an excellent way of adding heat only where you require the heat to be directed. Because you turn off the arms that you do not require, you can process specific parts of the head, allowing the hair to process more evenly.

If using a product such as bleach, and the hair is not lifting as much as you would want, place the client under a steamer to help the bleach to develop. This form of heat will not dry your product out.

Existing colour of hair

When deciding on the target colour for the client, you should know the following:

- tint will not lift tint
- you can only achieve three shades of lift with a fashion colour
- high lift tint will give you 4–5 shades of lift if used on a base 6 or above
- if going darker than the base colour, it is only advisable to go three shades darker so that the colour will still suit the client's skin tone.

Percentage of white hair

The amount of white hair present will determine the strength of peroxide you use and whether a base colour needs to be added to the hair.

If the client wishes to go darker or stay at the same depth as his natural colour to cover white hair, you will be adding colour not lifting the hair. However, you will still need to use hydrogen peroxide to open the cuticle and allow the tint into the cortex.

Porosity

The porosity of the hair determines how well the colour takes. If hair is in good condition, the cuticle scales lie flat and the colour will coat the hair evenly, reflecting the light back to show healthy, shiny hair. If hair is in bad condition, the cuticle scales may be open, the colour will not take evenly and the light reflected back will bounce off in all directions, making the hair look flat and dull.

Length of hair

The length of hair plays an important part when deciding which technique and method of application to use. Also, the longer the hair is, the older it will be! The older the hair is, the more likely it is to be porous. This may not be from chemical services but day-to-day wear and tear.

Refer to pages 207–9 for information on how test results will affect application, colour choice, etc.

Application of products

Step-by-step regrowth application

1 Gown the client with the correct PPE, section the hair into four and apply barrier cream all around the hairline. Begin to apply the tint through the partings of the four sections, making sure that you do not put colour onto previously coloured hair.

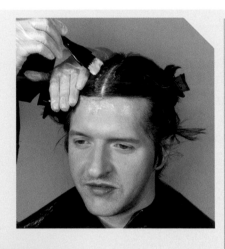

2 When all of the regrowth area has been covered, cross-check your application by going back through your sections in the opposite way to which you applied the tint to ensure complete coverage. Leave the product to develop according to the manufacturer's instructions. To ensure client comfort, offer him a magazine and a drink.

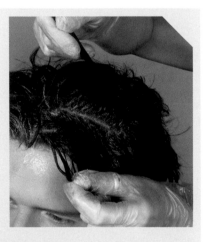

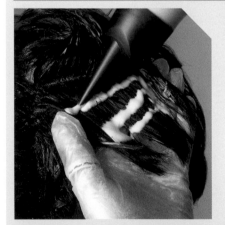

3 To refresh the colour on the ends that may have faded, a matching semi or quasi product can be applied to the mid-lengths and ends.

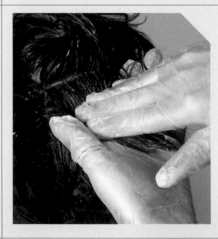

4 Work the product through with your fingers. If using an applicator flask ensure you are wearing the correct PPE.

5 When the colour has fully developed, take the client to the basin and emulsify the tint around the hairline and through the rest of the hair. Shampoo with TLS shampoo and condition with an anti-oxy conditioner (see page 186).

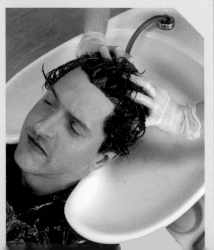

6 The finished result. Ensure all the product is removed and there is no tint on the skin, then style as desired.

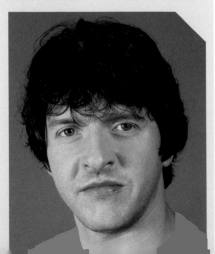

Changing tune

Some men do not want an obvious colour but want to blend in a few grey hairs. This is when you can consider using semi-permanent or quasi-permanent colours. They will add depth and can change the tone if desired.

Quasi-colours have a small amount of hydrogen peroxide in the developer. They allow the colour molecule to diffuse into the cortex and deposit the depth and tone.

Step-by-step changing tone using semi-permanent products

1 Consult with your client for the desired colour and use the colour swatches to hold against the skin for the colour choice. Gown yourself and the client. Section the hair into four and apply barrier cream to the hairline area.

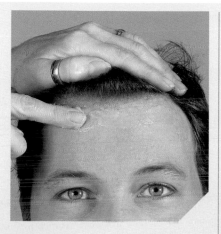

2 Apply the colour directly from the applicator flask to the hair, working from the roots straight through to the ends of the hair.

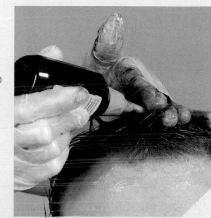

3 Check the development of the colour halfway through its development time by removing some of the product with damp cotton wool. Rinse the colour from the hair, checking the water temperature. Rinse until the water runs clear.

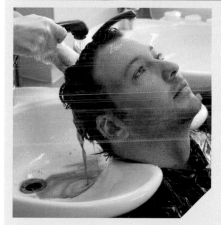

4 The finished result. Check the colour result with the client and style as desired.

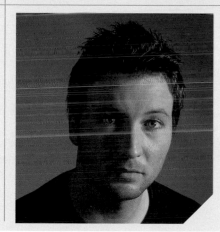

Developing the colour

When developing the colour, you should complete a strand test halfway through the development time. This will enable you to determine how well the colour is developing and whether added heat is required (see page 227).

When using added heat:

- check the temperature controls before you put the client under a heat source
- do not allow the product to dry out; this is especially important with bleaches and it is best to use a steamer for this reason
- use a timer
- monitor the development at regular intervals.

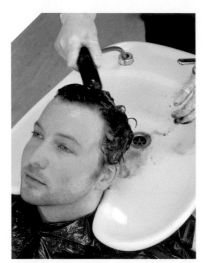

Colour removal

Product removal

When the colour is fully developed and you are happy with the result, remove the colour from the client's hair.

Step-by-step product removal

1   Take the client to the basin.
2   Remove any barrier cream
3   Moisten the tint with warm water and gently massage to loosen and emulsify the tint. Pay particular attention to the front hairline and nape area. Tint removes tint, so this is the best way of doing it.
4   Rinse the tint until the water runs clear.
5   Shampoo the hair twice using a soapless shampoo, again checking that you have removed all traces of tint from the nape area, behind the ears and the front hairline.
6   Condition with an anti-oxy conditioner to stop further oxidation and return the hair to its natural pH.

Development and removal for highlighting and lowlighting effects

Once you have finished applying the colour, check the following:

- Are the towel and cape protecting the client still in place and not covered in tint? If they are, change them.
- Is there any product spilt on the trolley you have been using? If so, clean it up.

If using foils or mesh, you should secure any that are around the client's face with a pin curl clip. Check the manufacturer's instructions for development times. You should monitor the development process all the way through. Take regular strand tests to check that the colour is developing evenly all over the head.

Step-by-step removal for highlighting/lowlighting effects

When the colour has processed, take the client to the basin. You should also remove any capes or towels that are no longer necessary to the client. You need to remove the packets in a methodical order so that the hair doesn't come into contact with remaining colour and so you don't end up with a tangled mess!

Begin by removing the packets from the nape area and working your way up. Try to remove dark colours before light colours; this will prevent any staining on the lighter coloured hair. Make sure you ask the client to close his eyes, or shield his face with your hand to protect it from splashes. Use a shampoo for coloured hair and apply an anti-oxy conditioner. Style the client's hair and confirm the look.

Rinsing full head or regrowth colour

Remove any unnecessary towels or capes. Remove any excess barrier cream. If you do not, you will leave a greasy residue around the hairline that could have an effect on the hair when you are blow-drying. You can remove any skin staining with a medi-wipe.

Coping with problems

If you identify a colouring problem but are unable to correct it, you should refer to the person in charge (either the salon manager or your tutor). Explain the problem and the course of action that you may have already taken. The manager/tutor will then be able to help you deal with the problem. If the problem is because of the client's hair and was unforeseen, you will need to make a note on the client's record card so that future stylists will be aware of potential problems. If the colouring problem was one caused by you, it will help you to see that all services must be followed in a logical order with great care and attention to detail, and it will be something that hopefully you will not repeat!

Coping with problems when highlighting/lowlighting

If some areas are processing more slowly than others, use added heat. When using foils or mesh, if you find that one part of the hair has processed more quickly than another, remove the product from the part that has developed while leaving the rest to continue developing. It is important that you remove the foils and colour from the hair without disturbing the rest of the colouring process. To do this, you will need:

- damp cotton wool/water spray – to remove the colour from the hair
- sectioning clips – to hold the packets out of the way as you work
- the correct personal protective equipment
- a bin close at hand – to dispose of cotton wool and used mesh/foils.

Removing product during treatment to avoid over-processing

- Section the hair away from where you will be working so that you can get to the packets that need to be removed.
- Open up the packets. Making sure you have a towel across your hand, spray the packets with a water spray and gently slide them out.
- Using damp cotton wool, wipe away the colour from the hair. Do not over-wet the hair as it will drip (think health and safety!).
- Continue in this way until you have removed all of the packets that have developed.
- Leave the rest of the hair to carry on processing, checking at regular intervals.

Confirming and recording the end result

You should be able to tell from your client's reaction whether or not he is pleased with the result, but you also need to ask such questions as:

- 'That's a really good result, what do you think?'
- 'Shall I book you in for a root regrowth colour in five weeks?'

As soon as possible, fill in the client's record card. For the service, you will need to make a note of the following:

- if bleach was used, how long the bleach took to develop fully
- the number of colours used and in what order for full-head foils
- any extra costs incurred for using more than one colour
- any problems encountered during the service.
- peroxide strength used
- developing times and sequence of application.

Unit

GB2

Change men's hair colour

How to provide aftercare advice

Every hairdressing and barbering service should include providing aftercare advice for your client on the maintenance and upkeep of the service you have carried out.

General recommendations

- Use a shampoo and conditioner for coloured hair – this will prolong the life of the colour.
- Protect the hair from direct sunlight as this will fade the colour.
- Inform your client how frequently he should return to the salon to have roots retouched or weaves redone.

Further advice

If your client has had his hair lightened (very light blonde), you will need to offer advice on the use of heated styling equipment. Overuse will not only affect the condition of the hair, which may be slightly dry if a strong lightening product has been used, but may also change the colour of the hair.

Personal, learning and thinking skills – Reflective learning

It is important to constantly evaluate your work. This needs to be critical and subjective. By using reflective learning you will be able to analyse your work, identify your strengths and build upon weaker areas. Look back at the assessments carried out for this unit and reflect on how they were carried out. What could be improved? What did you learn? Was there anything you would do differently next time?

Check your knowledge

The following questions will help you to check your understanding of this unit.
The answers can be found on page 502.

1 White hair is taken into account during a consultation because it affects:
   a) product choice and the application techniques used
   b) timings of the service
   c) whether added heat is used during the service
   d) the amount of product used.

2 When a tint is mixed up it will begin to:
   a) change colour
   b) neutralise
   c) pre-soften
   d) oxidise.

3 Block colouring is a technique where the hair is:
   a) coloured all over in a single solid block
   b) sectioned into two or more sections and coloured
   c) put into blocks of packets for colouring
   d) sectioned so the roots are block coloured at the beginning of the service.

4 The Electricity at Work Regulations are designed to ensure:
   a) the correct price is paid for electrical equipment
   b) that salons have the correct tools and equipment for the services they will be carrying out
   c) that equipment is fit and safe for use and all staff are trained in using it
   d) the correct storage and disposal of electrical equipment.

5 What is a 'hypersensitivity' test also known as?
   a) Elasticity test
   b) Porosity test
   c) Strand test
   d) Patch test

6 Why should powder lighteners be mixed in a well-ventilated room?
   a) So the smells can disperse quickly
   b) To prevent breathing problems
   c) You can see the mixture in a better light
   d) So powder particles can go out of the window

7 What tests are carried out before a colouring process?
   a) Porosity test, strand test, skin test
   b) Porosity test, test cutting, strand test
   c) Elasticity test, porosity test, skin test
   d) Skin test, development test, elasticity test

8 What are the natural colour pigments contained in the hair called?
- **a)** Melanie and melon
- **b)** Brown and black
- **c)** Eumelanin and pheomelanin
- **d)** Red and yellow

9 What part of the hair is affected by permanent colouring products?
- **a)** Cuticle
- **b)** Medulla
- **c)** Cortex
- **d)** All three of the above

10 How many levels of lift can be achieved when using 20 volume (6 per cent) peroxide?
- **a)** 0–1
- **b)** 2–3
- **c)** 1
- **d)** 3–4

If you would like to try additional questions about colouring hair, then have a go at the 'Check your knowledge' questions for GH9 (see pages 237–39).

Getting ready for assessment

You will be assessed using a combination of assessment methods, as described below. Remember that within each of the services you carry out with a client, you will cover different units. For example, when completing a colouring hair service (GB2), you may also shampoo hair (GH8). If you are not sure what you have covered in your service, always ask your assessor or supervisor for advice.

	NVQ	VRQ
Credit value	11	10
Guided Learning Hours	105	91

	NVQ	**VRQ**
Practical demonstrations, to be observed by assessor	Six performances, including: • one full-head application of quasi-permanent colour • one full-head virgin application of permanent colour or lightening product • one regrowth application of permanent colour or lightening product • four different techniques of partial head application of colour, one of which must use a lightening technique. Simulation is not allowed.	Seven performances, each on a different client, including: • one regrowth application of colour • one full head application of permanent colour • two applications of woven highlights/lowlights, one of which must be carried out on a full head. You need to use three of the four stated colouring products. You should cover all of the contraindications and carry out all hair tests. You should consider all factors and give appropriate aftercare advice.
Service timings	Mix and apply colour; full head, permanent colour or bleach – 45 minutes Mix and apply colour; regrowth, permanent colour or bleach – 25 minutes Pulled through highlights/lowlights (including preparation and application); full head – 35 minutes Woven highlights/lowlights (including preparation and application); full head 60 minutes	Regrowth application of permanent colour – 25 minutes Pulled through highlights/lowlights (full head) – 35 minutes Pulled through highlights/lowlights (minimum of 20 per cent of the head) – 15 minutes Woven highlights/lowlights (full head) – 75 minutes Woven highlights/lowlights (minimum of 20 per cent of the head) – 35 minutes
Additional evidence	You will be required to complete an independent written paper to support the underpinning knowledge required for this unit. The majority of evidence will be gathered from the observations carried out by your assessor.	Knowledge and understanding in this unit will be assessed by an external written paper.

433

Unit

GB2

Change men's hair colour

Task mapping

When you have completed the tasks in this unit, check the table below to see which Performance Criteria (purple), Range (red), Knowledge (green) and Key Skills (blue) you have covered within GB2 to use as additional evidence within your portfolio. Information about which Functional Skills you have covered is available on the website.

Task and page reference	Mapping to Performance Criteria, Range, Knowledge and Key Skills
1 (page 412)	Performance Criteria: 1a, 1b, 1e, VRQ 1a, 2j Range: N/A Knowledge: 1, 11, 12, 13, VRQ 1d, 1q Key Skills: C1.2, C1.3, C2.3
2 (page 413)	Performance Criteria: 1e, 1h Range: N/A Knowledge: 23, VRQ 1d, 2j Key Skills: C1.2, C1.3, C2.3
3 (page 414)	Performance Criteria: 1k, 2a–d, 2f–h, VRQ 2j Range: 1a–d, 2a–f, 3a–e, 4a–i Knowledge: 30, 31, VRQ 1d, 1o, 1q, 2k, 2o Key Skills: C1.1, C1.2, C1.3, C2.1A, C2.2B, C2.3
4 (page 415)	Performance Criteria: 1h, 3d, VRQ 1c, 2b, Range: VRQ R5a–e Knowledge: 37, 40, 48, 52, 57 Key Skills: C1.1, C1.2, C1.3, C2.3
5 (page 416)	Performance Criteria: VRQ 2b, 1n, 2b Range: N/A Knowledge: 3, 27, 34, VRQ 2k Key Skills: C1.2, C1.3, C2.3
6 (page 416)	Performance Criteria:1h, 2a, 2e, VRQ 2b Range: 2a–f Knowledge: 47 Key Skills: C1.1, C2.1A, C2.2B
7 (page 418)	Performance Criteria: 1n, 2b, 2d, 4a, 4b Range: 6a–c Knowledge: 3, 7, 27, 34 Key Skills: C1.1, C2.1A, C2.2B, N1.1, N1.2, N1.3, N2.1, N2.2, N2.3
8 (page 418)	Performance Criteria: 2e, 2h, 3c, 3i, 3m, VRQ 1c Range: 2a–f Knowledge: 5, 6, 47, VRQ 1g Key Skills: C1.1, C1.2, C1.3, C2.3

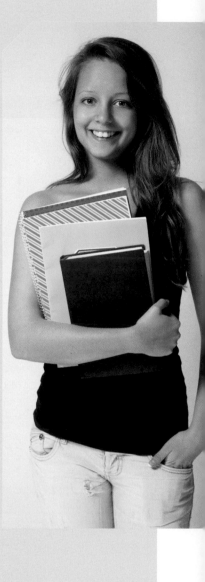

Cut hair using basic
barbering techniques

What you will learn:

- **How to maintain effective and safe methods of working when cutting**
- **How to cut hair to achieve a variety of looks**
- **How to provide aftercare advice**

Introduction

Many hairdressing salons are unisex and require stylists to have cutting skills in both ladies' and men's hairdressing. Many of the skills that you have can be adapted to suit both types of hairdressing.

This unit will help you to develop your cutting skills using clippers with attachments, clipper-over-comb and scissor-over-comb techniques, thinning and freehand techniques. It covers critical influencing factors, such as male pattern baldness, and considers the health and safety laws and regulations that you will need to follow when cutting men's hair.

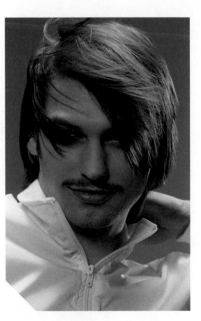

Sterilisation

The process of completely ridding material of live micro-organisms, leaving no forms of life.

Sharps

Sharp tools or instruments that must not be disposed of in a normal bin; correct disposal is in a yellow sharps container.

How to maintain effective and safe methods of working when cutting

It is essential to take health and safety into account when cutting men's hair. You should know which **sterilisation** methods to use to avoid cross-infection or infestation, and how to dispose of used **sharps** (blades). This section also looks at the tools and equipment suitable for men's barbering and how to maintain and care for your equipment.

Preparing the client for a cutting service

With any hairdressing service, you need to prepare the client for the service. Whether you are carrying out a haircut on dry or wet hair, you will need to protect the client and his clothing from hair cuttings.

For a dry cut:

- place a cutting gown around the client's neck — this is usually secured with a Velcro strip (make sure that all the client's clothing is covered)
- over the top of the cutting gown, place a cutting collar — this is to prevent hair cuttings falling down the client's neck.

For a wet cut:

- use a cutting gown, then place a towel over the top and secure with a clip
- after shampooing, towel-dry the client's hair and then remove the towel, replacing it with a cutting collar (see GH8 for shampooing procedure and product choice).

You also need to be aware of the hair cuttings that fall onto the client's face; these need to be removed throughout the service. You will require a neck brush so that you can gently brush away the loose hair cuttings as they fall. You should check that the gown is secure at all times, especially if you have moved the client from one seat to another. This, again, is to prevent any hair cuttings from falling down the client's back.

Positioning

The way in which your client is positioned in the chair is very important when carrying out a cutting service. You should make sure that he is:

- comfortable
- seated with the base of his back against the back of the chair
- seated with both feet flat on the ground or footrest.

By ensuring that your client is sitting correctly, you will be able to work comfortably for the duration of the haircut.

There are times when you will require the client to put his head forward or slightly to the side. You will need to ask him to do this and gently direct his head into the position you require. Never move or push his head forward without saying what you are doing.

You also need to consider your own posture and position when you are working at your unit. Some salons may have their workstations situated close together. You then have a trolley alongside you, which will take up space. If you work on a client without bending your knees, you may find that you will be bumping into your colleague and it will also put a strain on your back. This may result in back problems and fatigue.

Health and safety issues

As part of your professional image and in order to maintain a good service to your clients, you need to keep your work area clean and tidy at all times. First impressions count, so when you take your client to your workstation, he will want to see a clean and tidy working area. You will need to find the time between each client to tidy up your equipment, remove hair cuttings and generally present yourself in a professional manner.

It is important to remove hair cuttings from the floor as these pose a health and safety risk. If not removed, your client could slip, resulting in a nasty injury and a potential court case for the salon.

Potential hazards in the salon

- Hair cuttings not swept up from previous client.
- Trailing leads from electrical equipment.
- Client incorrectly gowned for a service.
- Rucksacks or coats left on the floor.
- Spillages from previous services, for example a water spray used during a cut might have left the floor wet.

Task 1

In groups, discuss if the hazards listed above are low, high or medium risk.

A worksheet for this task is provided on the website for you to complete and add to your portfolio.

Top tips

If hair cuttings are sticking to the client, a small amount of talc can be used to help you remove them. Dip your neck brush into the talc, making sure you do not overload the neck brush and engulf your client in talcum powder! The talc will absorb the moisture that is making the hair stick to the skin and will allow you to remove the hair cuttings.

437

Unit

GB3

Fact or fiction?

Is this statement fact or fiction?

Good posture is essential to portray a professional appearance and reduce the risk of injury or unnecessary fatigue.

To check your answer see page 502.

Cut hair using basic barbering techniques

Offset scissors

Standard scissors

Cut hair using basic barbering techniques

Thinning scissors

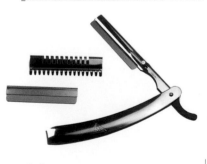

Safety razor

Graduation

Cutting hair at different lengths and blending them together.

Safe working methods

Tools and equipment

You will require a variety of tools and equipment to help you complete a haircut successfully. You need to understand their uses and how to care for your equipment, so that you will minimise the risk of damage to your tools, yourself or others.

Scissors

The most important piece of equipment for a hairdresser is scissors.

Scissors vary in design, size and price. The best way to find out if a pair of scissors suits you is to pick them up and see if they are comfortable to hold. Hands and fingers vary in size so holding them is the only way to tell if they suit you.

Thinning scissors

The purpose of thinning scissors is to remove bulk from the hair. There are two main types: those that have two notched (serrated) blades and those that have one ordinary blade and one notched blade. The spaces between the notches vary in size and determine the amount of hair that is removed.

Scissors with two notched blades will take off more hair than thinning scissors with one notched blade and one ordinary blade. Notched scissors with wide spaces between the notches will remove more hair than thinning scissors with smaller spaces between the notches.

Thinning scissors are also called:

- texturising scissors
- serrated scissors
- notched scissors.

Task 2

You have a new, junior member of staff beginning work at your salon. You have been asked to give him advice on the maintenance and safety aspects of caring and looking after scissors. What advice would you give him?

Razors

The most commonly used razors are open or cut-throat razors, shapers and safety razors. You should only use a razor on wet hair. The more modern razor has a disposable blade and a guard over it so only a small amount of the hair is cut. This also gives added protection and prevents cuts.

The disposable razor is easy to use. Once the blade becomes blunt it can be replaced quickly and easily, ensuring you do not tear the client's hair.

Electric and rechargeable clippers

Clippers are generally used for short, **graduated** styles and for removing unwanted hair in the neck area. They are used on dry hair only. For graduated looks they can give the effect of a scissor-over-comb cut and are used in both men's and ladies' hairdressing.

Clippers work by the bottom blade remaining fixed while the top blade moves at a very high speed. You can add clipper attachments to vary/alter the length of the cut, depending on the size of the grade that you attach – the higher the number is on the grade, the longer the hair will be left; the lower the number on the grade, the shorter the hair will be cut.

Rechargeable clippers are generally smaller than electric clippers and give a closer haircut. They can be used to trim behind the backs of the ears and other hard-to-reach areas. Different heads are available for these clippers for use in hair sculpting. After use they should be cleaned and replaced on their stand for recharging.

You should oil both types of clippers after every use to maintain them and to make sure that they run smoothly. This will help to prolong their life.

Clipper attachments

Clipper attachments, also known as grades, are added to your clippers to allow you to cut the hair at different lengths. They are available in different sizes ranging from a grade 1 (the smallest) up to a grade 8 (the largest). They are available in black or colour-coded.

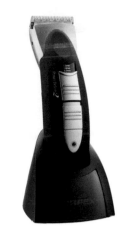

Rechargeable clippers

Cut hair using basic barbering techniques

Grade size	Length that the hair is cut to
One	3 mm
Two	6 mm
Three	10 mm
Four	13 mm
Five	16 mm
Six	19 mm
Seven	22 mm
Eight	25 mm

Clipper attachments are attached to the clipper head, making sure that they are sitting firmly and correctly on the clippers. You are then ready to begin the haircut. Clipper attachments should not be used if they have missing or broken teeth as this will result in an uneven haircut.

You should confirm with the client the size of the clipper grade as you attach it to your clippers, to double-check that you heard correctly and are using the correct grade.

You can sterilise the clipper attachments by brushing off the hair cuttings then either using a sterilising spray or removing them from the clippers and immersing them in Barbicide® solution for the recommended time.

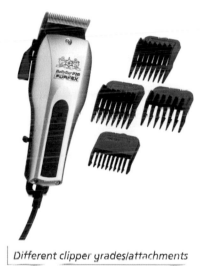

Different clipper grades/attachments

Tools – their uses and how to care for them

Tool	Uses	Care
Scissors	These are used for most cutting methods and techniques.	Wipe away hair cuttings, oil scissors frequently and sterilise using the most suitable method for your salon/training establishment. Store in a protective case.
Thinning scissors	These will remove bulk from the hair without removing length.	Wipe away hair cuttings. Oil scissors frequently and use the appropriate sterilising method. Store in protective case.
Razor	These are used mainly on wet hair to remove both length and bulk from the hair.	Remove hair cuttings and oil frequently. Sterilise using the most appropriate method for your salon. Store in protective case and out of the reach of small children.
Clippers	These are used for short graduated styles and to remove unwanted hair from outside the hairline.	Remove hair cuttings and oil after every use. Sterilise using sterilising wipes and sprays. Place protective cover across cutting edge when not in use.

Fact or fiction?

Is this statement fact or fiction?

A neck brush and water spray cannot be sterilised, only washed in warm soapy water.

To check your answer see page 502.

Tension

How firmly a mesh of hair is held when cutting. Tension should always be kept even, as uneven tension will produce an uneven cut.

Neck brush and water spray

A neck brush removes cuttings from the client and is necessary for the duration of the haircut.

Use a water spray to damp down hair that dries too quickly. If the hair is allowed to dry out halfway through, you will not achieve even **tension** throughout your cut.

Using equipment safely to minimise damage to tools

- Do not use electrical equipment with wet hands.
- Check plugs and wires are not loose or damaged before use.
- Use the correct piece of equipment for the job you want to do.
- Replace equipment carefully after use, ensuring it is clean and in good working order.
- Switch off electrical items when not in use and unplug to avoid trailing wires.
- When putting away electrical equipment, avoid folding flexes too tightly as this will cause them to short-circuit if they get damaged.

Task 3

Using the information on the Electricity at Work Regulations in G20, page 57, complete the gaps on the worksheet provided on the website. The worksheet can then be used as additional portfolio evidence.

Sterilisation and cleaning of tools and equipment

You need to be aware that tools must be sterilised to ensure that you minimise any risk of infection or infestation that can be passed on by your equipment. Refer back to G20, pages 63–64, for more details.

Task 4

For each of the tools and equipment listed below, identify the most suitable sterilising method. You may wish to refer back to G20, pages 63–64.

- Neck brush
- Water spray
- Sectioning clips
- Cutting comb
- Scissors/thinning scissors
- Razor
- Clipper and attachments (grades)

A worksheet for this task is provided on the website for you to complete and add to your portfolio.

Disposal of used sharps

'Sharps' is the term used in hairdressing to describe the blades used in safety razors. Salons should supply a yellow sharps bin for the disposal of blades. This is a hard plastic bin that cannot be pierced, which is collected by the local health authority and incinerated. If you put a disposable blade from your razor/hair shaper in an ordinary black bin liner, the person emptying the bin may be cut and put at risk of cross-infection.

Cut hair using basic barbering techniques

Task 5

Investigate the sharps bin in your training establishment.

- Where is it kept?
- How often is it collected?

Good organisation and time management

You need to be prepared for every client, which means you must have the right tools available to cover every aspect of the men's cutting services that your salon offers. Good organisation means:

- all equipment is clean and sterilised
- client records are at hand
- a tidy working area which is free of excess waste (cut hair) and has no slippery surfaces or potential hazards.

Using your time effectively

You should always be organised and ready for the client's arrival. Each salon has its own time allocation for services offered, for example most experienced stylists will allow only 20 minutes for a dry cut and a maximum of 40 minutes for a cut and blow-dry. As a trainee, you should be aware of the time it takes you to cut a client's hair. If you took two hours for a basic cut, your salon would soon be out of business!

However, it is expected that you will take longer than an experienced stylist for your first cuts. These are the usual timings allowed for the following services:

- wet cut = 20 minutes
- cut and blow-dry = 30 minutes
- dry trim = 20 minutes.

By breaking the service down into fragments, it should show you how much time you will have to spend on each stage and give you a timescale to work towards.

What you do not want to do is constantly watch the clock. This will not only get you flustered but will also make the client feel uncomfortable. All you need to do is be aware that you are on track and not running over on one part of the service, which will have a knock-on effect on the rest of the day's services.

Protecting yourself

For your own health and safety you need to be aware of potential hazards to yourself, for example the possibility of cross-infection from blood-borne diseases such as hepatitis and HIV.

Prevention is better than cure. You can have a vaccination for hepatitis A and B if you are in a high-risk group, of which hairdressing could be considered one. You are at risk because of the potential of cuts from scissors and sharps – this increases the risk of exposure to blood. If you have an open cut, make sure that it is covered with a dressing so that if you accidentally cut a client you will not be at risk from cross-infection of blood.

Cut hair using basic barbering techniques

Your personal health and hygiene needs to be of a high professional standard at all times. You need to make sure that all equipment that you use is clean and sterile for each client to minimise the risk of cross-infection or infestation between clients. You will need to make sure you have good personal hygiene standards; that is, the use of deodorants and breath fresheners, and ensure your appearance reflects your profession.

Identifying factors that may influence the service prior to cutting

When you carry out a consultation on your client, you need to be aware that there may be factors that may not let you carry out the service. You should be checking the hair and scalp for any infections or infestations and looking for any strong hair growth patterns or problem areas that could be classed as a critical influencing factor. (Refer to G7, pages 138–48.)

Influencing factors

An influencing factor is anything that you may have to take into account in order to get the end result that you hope to achieve. For example, if a client had extremely fine hair, you would not carry out thinning techniques on him. If the client had a crown that wanted to stand up on end, you would not want to cut the hair too short as it would make this feature worse.

These are all classed as critical influencing factors because they will have an influence on how you will carry out the service and what techniques and methods you will use.

Hair density

When you talk about the hair's **density**, you are referring to the amount of hair that an individual client has per square centimetre on his head. On some heads of hair you can see the scalp through the hair. This means that the client does not have very dense hair. On other heads there may be a lot of hair per square centimetre, meaning the client has very dense hair.

It is sometimes easy to get density and thickness of the hair confused. You will need to remember that density refers to the amount of hair on a head and **texture** refers to the thickness of an individual hair, not the amount of hair the client has.

Hair texture

You should examine the hair's texture very carefully during your consultation with the client because this may affect the cutting technique that you choose to use. If you decide on a particular cutting technique because of the hair's texture, you will have identified an 'influencing factor'. For example, if the client has very fine hair, you may choose the **club cutting** method to increase bulk in the hair. On the other hand, you would not want to increase bulk in thick hair, so you might choose a thinning technique for this hair texture.

You can determine the texture of the hair by separating a few strands of hair and placing them across the palm of your hand. The texture of the hair usually falls into one of three categories: fine, medium or thick. You will need to look at the hair closely and decide which one of these categories it falls into.

Hair density

The amount of hair a client has per square inch on his head.

Hair texture

The thickness of one individual strand of hair.

Club cutting

Cutting technique which leaves the ends of the hair blunt, removing length only.

Elasticity

You need to test the elasticity of the hair to see how good the internal strength of the hair is (remember, porosity testing determines the condition of the outside of the hair shaft). (Refer to G7, pages 141–44, for hair tests.) If the hair is in bad condition, you may choose not to use razoring techniques on it. This is because if the hair is very fragile it may not be able to withstand this method of cutting, which can put extra stress on the hair.

Head and face shapes

When consulting with the client before deciding on the length of the cut, you should take into consideration the client's head and face shape because these can become influencing factors in your choice of length for the cut. For example, if a client wanted a crew cut (very short), you would need to take into account the client's head shape – a bumpy head becomes more obvious with a crew cut.

The four most common face shapes are: square, round, oblong and oval. You will need to decide which face shape your client has to determine which style will best suit him. For example, to balance out a square face you will need to style the hair to make the 'squareness' of the face less obvious.

Task 6

Look at the four most common face shapes as represented by the celebrities below. Using the worksheet provided on the website, draw in the most suitable hairstyle that will disguise the areas that you would not want to draw attention to. Remember, you are aiming to make every face shape appear oval!

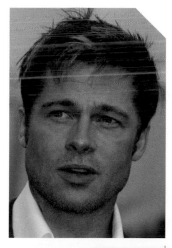

Brad Pitt has a square face shape

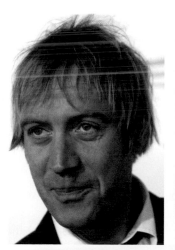

Rhys Ifans has an oblong face shape

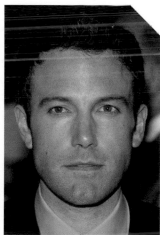

Ben Affleck has an oval face shape

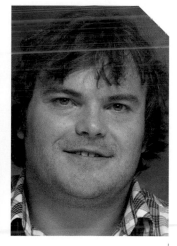

Jack Black has a round face shape

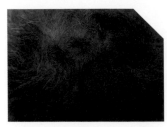

Double crown

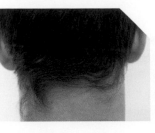

Nape whorl

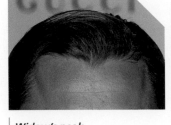

Widow's peak

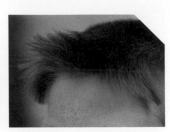

Cowlick

Cut hair using basic barbering techniques

Double crown

Two swirls of hair on the crown of the head, growing clockwise around each centre.

Nape whorl

A growth pattern at the nape of the neck where hair grows in circles or at angles rather than straight down or across. The hairline is uneven and care must be taken not to cut above it.

Widow's peak

A growth pattern where the hair at the front hairline grows downwards at the centre, forming a 'V' shape of hair and two half-circles of hair at either side.

Cowlick

A growth pattern where the hair grows strongly to one side of the forehead and may stick up.

Male pattern baldness

Hereditary condition where the hair recedes at the front hairline and thins at the crown. Eventually the whole hair may be lost, leaving short, downy hair.

Hair growth patterns

On some heads, the hair growth patterns are very obvious. For example, if the client has a **cowlick** in the middle of his fringe and the fringe has jumped or parted as a result, this will be obvious to you. The client may also have blow-dried his hair so well that he has disguised a **double crown** or strong hairline movement.

You need to look very closely at potential problem areas when the hair is dry and take a second look as a safeguard if you wet the hair. By deciding to leave length because of the client's hair growth patterns, you will be identifying an influencing factor.

Potential factors to consider when cutting hair with strong growth patterns are:

- the nape hairline may grow unevenly, meaning that the hair would need to be tapered into the neck
- there may be a cowlick in the fringe area so the fringe needs to be made heavier to help the hair stay down
- there may be a double crown, so the parting may have to be changed to distribute the hair more evenly either side of the head to disguise the double crown.

Where a client's hair recedes at the temples or may be slightly thinning at the crown area, you will need to take this into account as a critical influencing factor. The client may ask you to style his hair in such a way that you would be emphasising the **male pattern baldness.**

Male pattern baldness is the term used to describe a hereditary factor that can affect male clients at a very young age. Most men can look at their fathers or grandfathers to see how their hair will thin or recede (or not). Some clients may be sensitive to this so you should:

- be tactful
- suggest a variation on the style suggested by the client if you think his idea would emphasise the baldness
- leave the hair slightly longer to compensate for these areas.

Not every client who has male pattern baldness will be concerned about it and you may find that they wish to have a very short haircut, such as a crew cut.

A crew cut

Piercings

During your consultation you should also be checking to see if the client has any facial piercings. You can ask the client to remove any piercings if they are going to be difficult to work around. Alternatively, you can cover them with a plaster. It is important to consider all aspects of health and safety. If the piercing is caught with scissors or a comb, this could rip the piercing out or cause a great deal of discomfort to the client and lead to an infection.

In-growing hair

In-growing hair can be caused as a result of cutting the hair too close to the skin. This is a particularly common problem with dark skin and tightly curled hair.

Instead of the hair growing upward from the follicle, the hair bends back towards the skin surface, re-enters the skin and becomes trapped causing irritation, pain to the client and bumps on the skin. If left untreated it can cause infection and permanent scarring.

To treat the problem your client will need to allow the area of affected skin time to heal. He will then need to use gentle exfoliation to allow the hair to break free. This is not something that should be carried out by you, the stylist. If you think there may be cause for concern you should refer your client to his GP.

Salon life

Men are from Mars, women are from Venus

Sophie's story

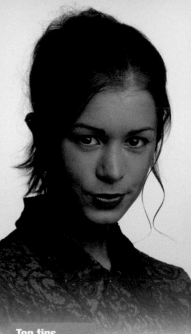

I love cutting hair but the thought of cutting men's hair and having to talk to them filled me with dread. I am fairly shy and usually more comfortable with women. I don't know a lot about football or other sports and thought I would be carrying out the whole haircut in complete silence!

It was such a relief when I completed my first gents' haircut – he was so nice! He reminded me a lot of my brother who is only one year older than me. We had loads to talk about – music and the local music festival that we'd both been to. The time flew, my confidence had grown heaps and I was soon looking forward to my next gents' haircut.

My advice to anyone who is worried is relax and enjoy, because there is always common ground. I have learned so much from all age groups and now really enjoy my barbering.

Top tips

- If you smile the client will smile back because smiling is contagious.
- Make sure you do a thorough consultation and repeat back to the client so you know exactly what you are doing. This will give both you and the client confidence.

Ask the expert

Q *What do you do if you have a client who doesn't want to talk to you no matter how hard you try?*

A Some clients use this time to relax and switch off, especially if they have a stressful job. Don't be alarmed! As long as you have established enough information during the consultation and give your client the appropriate aftercare advice, you have carried out a professional service. Just enjoy the opportunity to immerse yourself in your work and don't take the quietness of your client personally – he is enjoying the time to relax.

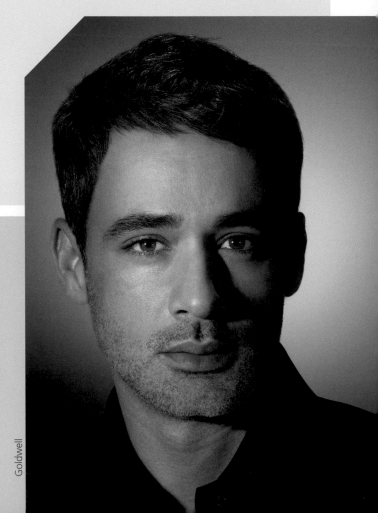

Goldwell

How to cut hair to achieve a variety of looks

This section covers the barbering techniques you will need to carry out to complete the unit. It looks at cutting techniques used specifically for men's barbering. You will need to take into account the presence of male pattern baldness and different hair growth patterns that will determine the neckline shape of the haircut. This section also looks at a wide range of cutting techniques and effects on different types of hair.

Preparing the client for a cutting service

Consultation

Before you can begin any service you need to complete a consultation with your client. This is to establish:

- the client's wishes
- the technique/method of cutting that you will be using
- the tools and equipment suitable for the job.

A suggested consultation checklist is given on page 305.

During the consultation, check for any infections or infestations that may prevent you from carrying out the service (see also G7, pages 144–48).

Hair preparation

You need to be aware of the advantages and disadvantages of both wet and dry methods of cutting – see the table below.

Advantages and disadvantages of cutting wet and dry hair

Wet hair		Dry hair	
Advantages	**Disadvantages**	**Advantages**	**Disadvantages**
- More precise lines can be achieved because tension is easier to maintain. - The hair is easier to comb, manage and control in its wet state. - The hair can be manipulated into style (pushed into place) during cutting to see if the desired result is being achieved.	- The client may be uncomfortable if the salon temperature is too cool. - You are not able to see weight/bulk lines in the hair, especially permed and naturally curly hair.	- Because the hair does not 'jump' up as it does when wet, the hair will be the same length when finished. - Dry, split ends are easier to see when the hair is dry.	- The hair can fly everywhere. - Because it is more difficult to keep even tension on dry hair (especially curly hair), the cut can be uneven. - The client may have greasy/dirty hair.

Accurately establishing and following cutting guidelines

When you are ready to begin your cut on the client, you need to make sure that you work in a methodical manner. You will need to section the hair so that you can see your guidelines clearly, making sure that they are neat and level. Hair that you are not working on will need to be secured out of the way. The sections (meshes) of hair you are working on need to be combed through so that even, clean tension is maintained throughout each section. The sections of hair should be no more than half an inch deep; this will help you use each section as a guideline for the next section of hair you are going to cut.

By following these guidelines, you will be able to work around the head, using your time to the maximum benefit and ensuring you achieve the required result.

> ### Task 7
>
> Research the answers to the following questions.
>
> - Why is club cutting a good technique to use on fine hair?
> - Can this technique be used on either wet or dry hair?
> - Does this method of cutting help to encourage curl into the hair?
> - What effect does this technique have on the ends of the hair?

Cutting techniques

Club or blunt cutting

This method leaves the ends of the hair blunt and level. It is sometimes called the blunt cut. The technique is most commonly used for removing length from the hair and is ideal for fine hair as it gives the appearance of increasing bulk. It can also help to reduce the tendency of the hair to curl.

Club cutting can be used on wet or dry hair. It is very suitable for curly hair because the sections are combed through and held with tension, ensuring that the ends of the hair are blunt and level. This technique can be used on any hairstyle that is cut with scissors.

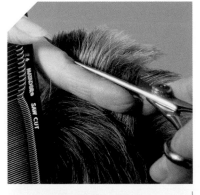

Club cutting

Freehand cutting

This technique is mainly used on straight hair. This is because curly hair will not sit in one place; the curl in the hair means it will lift and not remain in a way in which it can be cut **freehand**.

As the name of the technique suggests, you do not hold the hair with tension — the hair is combed into place and cut freehand. The freehand technique gives you a truer indication of where the hair will sit when dried, because you will not have used tension by pulling the hair down. This is an ideal method to use on fringes as they have a tendency to 'jump up' when dried and is also better suited to looks that are cut above the collar. Cutting hair above collar length requires a very blunt even line — by combing the hair down flat onto the neck and cutting freehand, you will be able to achieve this precise line. Freehand cutting can be used on wet or dry hair.

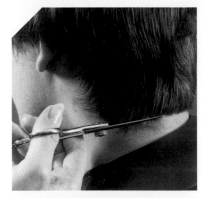

Freehand cutting

> **Freehand cutting**
>
> Cutting the hair without using any tension.

Scissor-over-comb

This technique is used to cut hair very short following the natural contours of the head. It is most frequently used in the nape area or around the ears and is often used in men's hairdressing to taper the hair into the hairline.

The technique can be used on wet or dry hair, although you will achieve a better result on dry hair as the cutting line is clearer.

Step-by-step scissor-over-comb technique

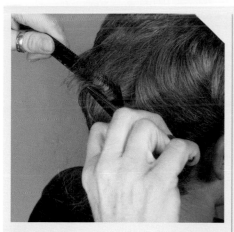

1 Comb all of the hair into style and place your scissors into the hair to pick up a mesh of hair for cutting.

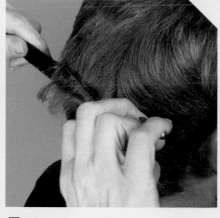

2 Replace the scissors with your comb to support the section of hair you are going to cut, holding the hair out at 90 degrees to the head.

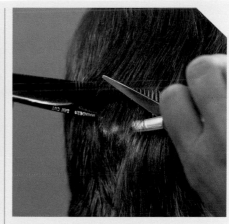

3 Remove the desired amount of hair, keeping your comb in position. Do not use your comb as a ruler to cut on – it is only there to lift the hair out from the head at a 90-degree angle to cut.

Clipper-over-comb

With the clipper-over-comb technique, clippers are used instead of scissors to give a similar effect to scissor-over-comb. Both techniques allow you to cut the hair shorter than if you were holding the hair between your fingers. It is important to note that clippers should only be used on dry hair.

Top tips

You should sterilise and oil your clippers after every client. Also make sure that you remove any remaining hair cuttings.

Thinning

There are various cutting techniques that can be used to thin the hair as well as using thinning scissors and razoring techniques (for information see page 438).

Some of the thinning techniques that you will be using are also referred to as texturising techniques. The thinning method of cutting removes bulk from the hair without removing the overall length. Thinning is normally carried out on dry hair because it is more obvious where the bulk/weight is in a haircut (the only exception is when using a razor).

Avoid using thinning techniques on front hairlines, natural partings or the crown area, as they will produce unwanted spiky effects.

Fading

This technique can be used when you want to fade the hair away to nothing. It is ideal for hairlines that grow in all directions, where you cannot always create a square or round neckline shape. You can achieve this look by using either scissor- or clipper-over-comb techniques.

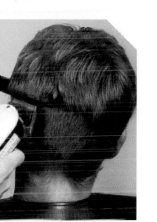

Clipper-over-comb technique. The comb is used to support the hair and then the clippers are used to remove the desired length of hair

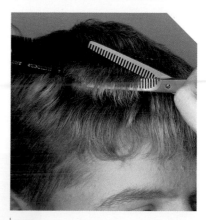

Thinning scissors remove bulk from the hair

Cut hair using basic barbering techniques

Technique	Suitability	Benefits
Weave cutting	Not suitable for the whole of the head. Good for flat areas requiring lift. Avoid natural partings, hairlines and crown areas. Can be used on any hair type.	The shorter pieces of hair will stand up, supporting the rest of the hair.
Pointing/chipping	Ideal for fine or straight hair, or hair that 'lines' easily.	Breaks up hard lines in the hair, removes weight and bulk without removing length, creating a soft edge.
Castle cutting	Can be used on all hair types.	Breaks up hard lines in the hair and removes weight from the ends. Creates a 'shattered' broken edge.
Razoring	Mainly used on wet hair. Not suitable for fine, coarse or dry hair.	This technique will encourage the ends of the hair to curl. Moves weight and length from the hair, leaving the ends soft and feathery.
Thinning scissors	Ideal for most hair types except very fine and very short hair (the shorter pieces may show and produce an unwanted effect).	Removes bulk without removing length. Overuse will result in the ends becoming wispy and the roots becoming bulky.
Club cutting	Ideal for fine- to medium-textured hair.	Will give fine hair the appearance of being thicker. Creates a blunt, even cutting edge.
Freehand cutting	Generally used on straight hair where a blunt even line is required.	Easy to use on difficult areas, around ears and necklines.
Scissor-over-comb	Used when the hair needs to be short and tapered and where the hair is too short to be picked up and cut.	Allows you to work closely into the natural contours of the head and create very short looks.
Clipper-over-comb	As scissor-over-comb, used where the hair needs to be short and tapered into the hairline.	Allows you to work quickly and close to the hairline.
Fading	Suitable for all hair types.	Suitable for a neckline that has nape whorls (hair growing in all directions) that needs to be blended away to nothing.

Thinning techniques

Tapering technique (slither cutting)

This method of cutting is a sliding movement that goes backwards and forwards along the hair. Hair is tapered by holding the section of hair in the crutch of the scissors (where the bottoms of the blades meet). Begin the sliding movement a third of the way down the length of the hair from the points, opening and closing the blades slightly as you slide the scissors.

Cutting effects

Uniform layer cut

This cut produces layers of hair the same length all over the head.

Step-by-step uniform layer cut

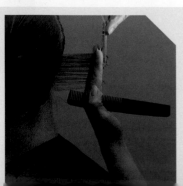

1 Begin by taking a section of hair at the middle of the nape area and hold out at 90 degrees to the head. Remove the required amount of hair by cutting above the fingers while keeping the hair at this angle. Work out to either side.

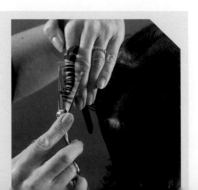

2 Using a piece of the hair from the first section as a guide, move up to the occipital area. Maintaining your 90-degree angle, work around the head in 'orange segments' before moving up the head towards the crown.

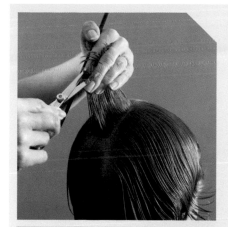 **3** Continue to work up towards the crown area, each time taking a piece of the already-cut section and using this as a guide to maintain your 90-degree angle.

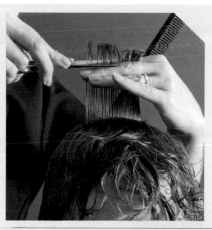 **4** At the top crown section, work across the head. Pull the hair up at a 90-degree angle, again using hair that was previously cut as your guideline.

5 Continue the section using your guide from the top crown area, working down towards the ear.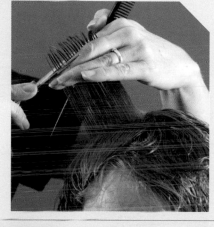

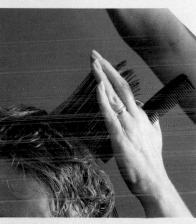 **6** Being careful not to lose your 90-degree angle, complete the same technique on both sides.

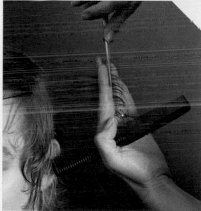 **7** As you work towards the ear, change your hand position so that the palm is facing up. Maintain your 90-degree angle.

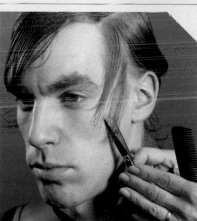 **8** Neaten your perimeter shape by combing the hair onto the face and cutting freehand. Follow through to the side and nape hase line.

9 Confirm the finished result with the client and provide the appropriate aftercare advice.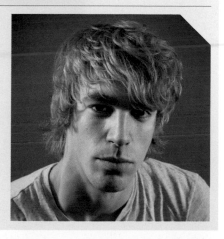

451

Unit

GB3

Cut hair using basic barbering techniques

Unit
GB3

Graduated layer cut

This cut produces a tapered look in the nape and at the sides, keeping more length and weight in the hair at the top of the head.

Step-by-step graduated layer cut on straight hair

1 Working from your baseline, take your first section at the centre back and elevate it out to a 45 degree angle. Remove the desired amount of length. Continue to do this section by section, working from the middle out towards the ear.

2 Working up towards the occipital bone, continue to use a 45-degree angle to connect each section to the previous section.

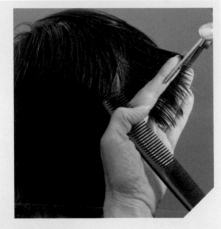

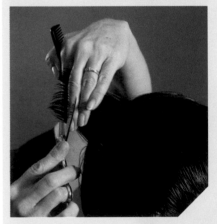

3 As you reach the crown area, change your hand position. Always begin in the centre, using hair from the previous section as a guide for continuing the 45-degree angle. Follow this out towards the ears, taking 'orange segments'.

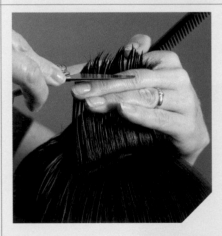

4 The top section is now completed by elevating the length straight up from the headshape. Proceed to cut all the way to the front, using the previous section as a guideline.

5 Connect the top to the perimeter fringe length using a 45-degree angle. The angle will help you to remove weight but maintain the length at the front fringe area.

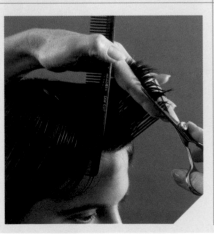

6 Check that the client is happy and that you have achieved a well-balanced result. Offer the appropriate aftercare advice.

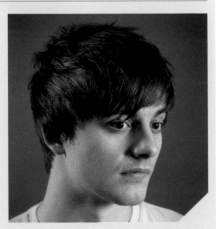

Adapting your cutting techniques to take into account influencing factors

You have looked at cutting methods/techniques and influencing factors – now you need to put the two together.

When you are going to carry out a haircutting service on a client, you need to establish during your consultation what critical influencing factors (if any) you have to consider. It is important to check through the client's hair before and after you shampoo the hair. This is because some influencing factors may be apparent only on wet hair and others only on dry hair. If a client has straightened his hair and you have carried out your consultation on straight hair, you may discover when you take him to the basin and wash his hair that he has a very strong natural wave which means you may need to use different cutting methods or techniques from the ones you had discussed.

Alternatively, if you do not carry out your consultation until the client's hair has been shampooed, you may not see potential problem areas that disappear when the hair is wet. It is important to carry out your consultation on dry hair and then re-check the hair when it is shampooed to make sure you have identified all the potential critical influencing factors.

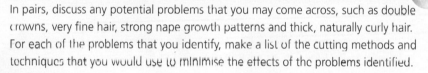

Task 8

In pairs, discuss any potential problems that you may come across, such as double crowns, very fine hair, strong nape growth patterns and thick, naturally curly hair. For each of the problems that you identify, make a list of the cutting methods and techniques that you would use to minimise the effects of the problems identified.

A worksheet for this task is provided on the website for you to complete and add to your portfolio.

Adjusting your position and cross-checking the cut

As you are progressing through the cut, you will need to adjust the position in which you are working in relation to the head. Although heads come in different shapes and sizes, they are all round. If you stand 'square' on to a head of hair and try to cut the hair in this position, you will not achieve a balanced shape. You need to move around the head as you work so that you are covering all angles of the haircut. This will help you to achieve an accurate cut, ensuring that you have even distribution of weight and balance throughout the style.

Cross-checking the haircut as you work will also help you to achieve even distribution and weight throughout the style. To cross-check a haircut you will need to take sections/meshes of hair in the opposite direction to the way in which you have carried out your haircut. You still hold them at the same angle as you did for the original haircut and continue to work in small methodical sections so that you are covering the whole of the haircut.

Your mirror is another good tool to use to check the shape, weight and balance of the haircut. If you stand directly behind your client and lift sections of hair, you will be able to use the mirror to confirm that they are of the same length, that you have

453

Unit

GB3

Cut hair using basic barbering techniques

Cross-check

To examine different sections of the hair to check the balance of the haircut.

Cut hair using basic barbering techniques

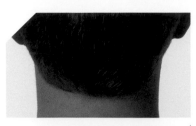

Rounded neckline

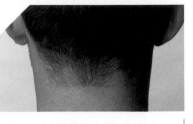

Tapered neckline

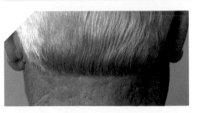

Square neckline

used the same angle on both sides and that you have achieved a balanced result. When you are more experienced, you will be able to carry out this process without using your mirror and check your sections through by feel, looking to see if the hair is 'sitting' in the style you have cut. You will be able to see if the weight left in the hair is working, giving you the effect both you and the client wanted to achieve.

By cross-checking and using your mirror to check the weight and angles of the cut, you are giving yourself and your client the opportunity to make any changes to the haircut before you get to the drying stage. It is important to check with your client that he is happy with what you have done and is ready for you to dry his hair into the finished result.

Neckline shapes

Cutting an accurate neckline shape in men's barbering is very important. Everyone's hairline grows differently and you will need to take this into account. It is always best to follow the natural growth pattern of the hairline. Any hair that is outside of the neckline shape will need to be removed by using clippers to give a clean, accurate finished result.

If the client doesn't have a preference, you could suggest one of the neckline shapes shown left. Clipper-over-comb/scissor-over-comb techniques can be used to achieve these effects.

Step-by-step rounded neckline

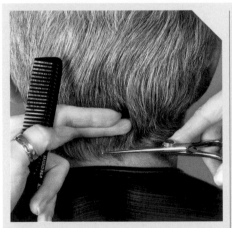

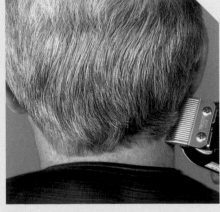

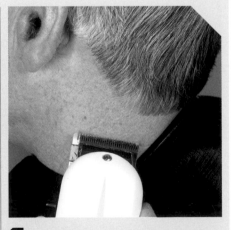

1 The hair is combed flat to the head and the extra length removed following the natural shape of the hair growth pattern.

2 Clippers are turned over so that a sharp edge can be given to the previously cut neckline shape.

3 Clippers are used to remove unwanted hair from outside the previously cut neckline shape.

Outline shapes

Sideburns

Facial hair growing in front of the ears.

The outline shape of the haircut is known as the perimeter. On many haircuts the perimeter shape is cut first, and the rest of the haircut will follow by taking small sub-sections from the perimeter. Because men's hair is generally worn shorter than in ladies' hairdressing, the outline shape can be a stronger feature of the haircut and needs to take into consideration the side hairlines, **sideburns** as well as front and back hairlines.

- *Natural* – if you are going to carry out a natural outline shape you will be working with the hair's natural growth patterns. This will produce a softer look that should be easier to maintain.
- *Created* – this is your chance to be creative. You may wish to use various texturising techniques, especially around the front hairline to achieve a certain look. The front area of the hair is usually the focal point and fringes act as a frame on the face so you need to work carefully, making sure that the methods and techniques you have chosen work for the client.
- *Tapered* – many short, layered cuts are tapered around the sides (ears) and back of the neck so the hair gradually disappears into almost nothing.

When cutting men's hair you will be required to shape and balance the client's sideburns. To do this you can use:

- scissor-over-comb techniques
- clipper-over-comb techniques
- freehand techniques
- club cutting techniques.

Scissor- and clipper-over-comb techniques will reduce the bulk from the sideburns, while club cutting and freehand cutting will remove length.

It is not always a good idea to judge the length of the hair by looking at where the hair sits in relation to the client's ears, as faces aren't always symmetrical and can be uneven. It is best to look at your client straight on in the mirror with a finger at the bottom of each sideburn to determine the correct balance and length.

Meeting client expectations and ensuring comfort

Client comfort is important throughout the service. If the client is not seated correctly, is wet from the shampoo or is covered in hair cuttings, he will not be comfortable. Throughout the service you should confirm with the client that he is happy with the way the service is progressing. These are the types of questions you could ask:

- Are you comfortable?
- Have I removed enough length? (Only cut one section of hair before asking this question!)
- Where would you like your fringe to sit? (Use eyebrows as a guideline.)
- How does the whole cut feel? (Let the client run his fingers through his hair.)

It is also important to use the back mirror to show the client the profile (side view) and back of his hair, again reaffirming that he is happy with the cut that you have completed. When using the back mirror:

- hold it at the height of the client's head
- spend time letting the client see all angles of the haircut
- do not stand too far back.

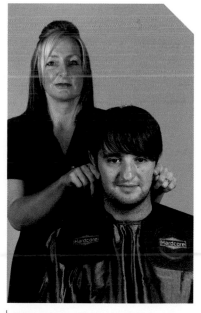

Balancing the client's sideburns

How to provide aftercare advice

Giving aftercare advice is an important part of the whole service. You would not expect to go to a hi-fi shop, purchase a stereo system and not receive information or instructions on how to use the equipment that you have bought. The same goes for giving information to your client following any service given in the salon.

The information on aftercare that you should give includes:

- How often he should come back into the salon for a trim to maintain the look.
- Which products are best suited to his hair type and will help him to recreate the look you have achieved.
- What the best tools (for example, correct size of brushes) and equipment are for achieving the look.

Basically, you are trying to give information that will help the client to maintain his hair and achieve the desired effect.

You can talk to him about the use of products and drying techniques during the service and give him information on how much the average head of hair grows each month, so that he will have a better understanding of why it is important to come into the salon for regular trims.

Check your knowledge

The following questions will help you to check your understanding of this unit.
The answers can be found on page 502.

1 Clippers should be used on:
- **a)** wet hair
- **b)** dry hair
- **c)** freshly washed hair
- **d)** either wet or dry – it doesn't matter.

2 One of the benefits of cutting the hair wet is that:
- **a)** your scissors will glide through the hair more easily
- **b)** it is quicker
- **c)** split ends are easier to see
- **d)** greater precision can be achieved.

3 The typical pattern of male baldness is:
- **a)** the client will lose all their hair by the age of 35 years
- **b)** total hair loss
- **c)** receding at the temples and crown
- **d)** round, circular, bald patches.

4 A uniform layer cut is where the hair is:
- **a)** held at 90 degrees all over the head
- **b)** held at 45 degrees all over the head
- **c)** held at 80 degrees all over the head
- **d)** held at 70 degrees all over the head.

5 How many different sizes of clipper grades are available?
- **a)** 4
- **b)** 6
- **c)** 8
- **d)** 5.

Getting ready for assessment

You will be assessed using a combination of assessment methods, as described below. Remember that within each of the services you carry out with a client, you will cover different units. For example, when cutting men's hair (GB3), you will also have to be aware of health and safety (G20) and advise and consult with clients (G7). You may also shampoo and condition hair (GH8). If you are not sure what you have covered in your service, always ask your assessor or supervisor for advice.

	NVQ	VRQ
Credit value	8	6
Guided Learning Hours	80	53

	NVQ	VRQ
Practical demonstrations, to be observed by assessor	You are required to complete ten cutting performances, two for each cutting look listed in the ranges (looks can be combined on one head). • Uniform layer • Graduation • With a fringe • Without a fringe • With a parting • Without a parting • Around the ear outline • With a fade You must complete all of the ranges listed. Simulation is not allowed for any evidence requirements within this unit.	You will need to complete eight competent performances and practically demonstrate that you have covered all ranges. Evidence must be gathered in a realistic working environment. At least 75 per cent of observation outcomes must be on real clients.
Service timings	Cut hair – 30 minutes Cut, blow-dry/dry and finish men's hair – 30 minutes	Cut, blow dry and finish men's hair – 30 minutes
Additional evidence	You will need to complete an independent written paper to show your understanding of the knowledge requirements.	There is one external paper that must be achieved.

Task mapping

When you have completed the tasks in this unit, check the table below to see which Performance Criteria (purple), Range (red), Knowledge (green) and Key Skills (blue) you have covered within GB3 to use as additional evidence within your portfolio. Information about which Functional Skills you have covered is available on the website.

Task and page reference	Mapping to Performance Criteria, Range, Knowledge and Key Skills
1 (page 437)	Performance Criteria: 1f, 1g, VRQ 2l Range: N/A Knowledge: 3, 8, 10, VRQ 1d, 2j, 2v Key Skills: C1.1, C1.2, C1.3, C2.1A, C2.2B, C2.3
2 (page 438)	Performance Criteria: 1g, 1h, 1i, VRQ 2l Range: 1a Knowledge: 3, 8, 11, 14, VRQ 1d, 1j, 2n, 2v Key Skills: C1.2, C1.3, C2.3
3 (page 440)	Performance Criteria: 1g, VRQ 2l Range: N/A Knowledge: 4, VRQ 1d, 2n, 2v Key Skills: C1.2, C1.3, C2.3

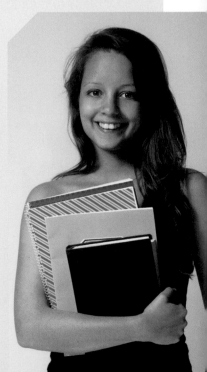

4 (page 440)	Performance Criteria: 1h, VRQ 1a, 2l Range: N/A Knowledge: 9, 12, 13, VRQ 1d, 1j Key Skills: C1.2, C1.3, C2.3
5 (page 441)	Performance Criteria: 1k, VRQ 2l Range: N/A Knowledge: 3, VRQ 1d, 2v Key Skills: C1.2, C1.3, C2.3
6 (page 443)	Performance Criteria: 2e, VRQ 1b, 1c, 2d Range: 2a–f, 6a–c, 7a–c Knowledge: 16, 24, VRQ 1i Key Skills: C1.2, C1.3, C2.3, N1.2, N2.2
7 (page 448)	Performance Criteria: 2d, VRQ 2d Range: 4a Knowledge: 17, 27, VRQ 2o, 2p, 2q Key Skills: C1.2, C1.3, C2.3
8 (page 453)	Performance Criteria: 2e, VRQ 1c, 2b, 2d Range: 2a–g Knowledge: 24, 26, VRQ 1e Key Skills: C1.1, C1.2, C1.3, C2.1A, C2.2B, C2.3

459

Unit

GB3

Cut hair using basic barbering techniques

Cut facial hair to shape
using basic techniques

What you will learn:

- **How to maintain effective and safe methods of working when cutting facial hair**
- **How to cut beards and moustaches to maintain their shape**
- **How to provide aftercare advice**

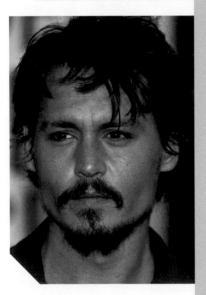

Introduction

In this unit you will learn how to cut beards and moustaches. Many unisex salons and barbers offer these services as part of a complete package to their clients. The cutting techniques you will be using are the same as those for cutting hair, but there are other factors that you will have to consider such as strong hair growth patterns, face shapes and the client's features. Your cutting techniques will need to be adapted to take these into account.

When you are learning to cut facial hair into a shape, it can be quite daunting as you are in close proximity to your client's face. Try not to feel intimidated by the closeness to your client as it is important to be extremely focused and concentrate fully on the area you are cutting. If you do not have full concentration while working on the facial area, you could cut the delicate skin of your client's ears, nose or lips. It is important to adhere to all health and safety rules and regulations due to the potential risks involved.

Some clients will automatically book for a beard and moustache trim, while others will expect it to be part of the haircutting service and will not necessarily book in separately for this service. It is therefore important to consider your clients' needs and ensure you ask the correct questions so that you understand their requirements. For example, some clients like to cut their top lip moustache hair themselves as this area grows particularly quickly and once it protrudes over the top lip it can be annoying and unsightly.

Cutting facial hair is an important component to being able to offer your client the 'full package' of grooming. If you can only offer a haircutting service and your client leaves the salon with an overgrown beard area, he will not look or feel fully groomed. You can practise beard and moustache cutting on a **male mannequin block** which is designed for this purpose and will build your confidence before working on living, breathing clients!

Fact or fiction?

Is this statement fact or fiction?

Pogonophobia is a fear of beards.

To check your answer see page 502.

Male mannequin block

A training head with hair, beard and moustache for practising cutting.

How to maintain effective and safe methods of working when cutting facial hair

When carrying out any hairdressing service, it is your responsibility to ensure the health and safety of your client and yourself while working. This section addresses all of the health and safety issues that you will need to consider when carrying out barbering services. You will look at the risk of infections and infestations that can be passed from one client to another. This element also covers the preventative actions you should take to avoid cross-infection (see page 144).

Preparing the client for a beard or moustache trim

Gowning

You should ensure that you correctly gown the client for this service, to prevent any hair from entering the client's clothing or falling down his neck and causing irritation.

When gowning for a beard or moustache trim:

- place a cutting cape/gown around the client and securely place a towel across the front of the client, tucking it slightly into the gown (not too tightly)
- over the top of the towel, use either a strip of cotton wool or neck tissue to prevent cuttings from falling inside the gown onto the client's skin. Cover the client's eyes with a protective strip or cotton wool pads to prevent cuttings falling into them.

It is also important to ensure that you remove any hair cuttings from your client's face and neck as you work, so make sure you have a neck brush and use it frequently to ensure client comfort.

Positioning

To enable you to work comfortably on the client during a beard or moustache trim, it is important that he is positioned correctly in the chair. Ensure that the client is sitting squarely with both feet flat on the floor or foot rest. This will prevent him from leaning to one side, making it awkward for you to work.

If your salon or training institution has a men's barbering chair, you need to recline the chair into the position that you require, then ask the client to sit down. Note: if you sit the client in the chair first and then recline the chair, the weight of the client may make the chair tip too far back, causing an injury to yourself or the client. Once your client is seated, you need to make adjustments to the chair. Ask him to sit forward before you recline the chair any further.

You also need to consider your own posture and position when you are working at your workstation. Some salons may have their workstations situated close together. If you work on a client without bending your knees, you may find that you will be bumping into the colleague working next to you. It will also put a strain on your back if you are not standing in the correct position, and this could cause back problems and fatigue.

Health, safety and hygiene

Health, safety and hygiene are the most important factors to be considered in the salon. You need to demonstrate good hygiene practice whenever you are working. Every client must be treated with care and attention from the beginning to the end of his barbering service and good health and safety practices must apply to all clients.

Potential hazards in the salon

These include:

- electric shock — remember, electricity and water do not mix!
- hair cuttings not swept up from the previous client
- trailing leads from electrical equipment
- client incorrectly gowned for a service
- bags or coats left on the floor
- spillages from previous services, for example a water spray used during a cut might have left the floor wet.

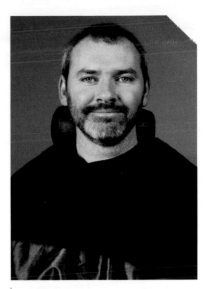

Correct gowning for a beard and moustache trim

463

Unit

GB4

Cut facial hair to shape using basic techniques

Using equipment safely to minimise damage to tools

- Do not use electrical equipment with wet hands.
- Check plugs and wires are not loose or damaged before use.
- Use the correct piece of equipment for the job you want to do.
- Replace equipment carefully after use, ensuring it is clean and in good working order.
- Switch off electrical items when not in use and unplug to avoid trailing wires.
- When putting away electrical equipment, avoid folding flexes too tightly as this will cause damage to the wires and will lead to faulty equipment.

In accordance with the Electricity at Work Regulations 1989, all electrical equipment should be checked annually (or every six months in a busy salon) by a qualified electrician, who should then place a sticker on the equipment to show that it is safe to use. A record of the visit should be kept by the salon for future reference. It is important for you to understand your responsibilities under the Electricity at Work Regulations 1989. Go to page 57 to get further information on this piece of legislation and how it affects you in the salon.

Cleaning and sterilisation of cutting tools

After each client, tools and equipment should be cleaned and sterilised to prevent cross-infection.

- Remove all hair cuttings.
- Wipe scissors and razors with spirit, alcohol wipe or sterilising spray.
- Dry metal tools thoroughly before putting them away.
- Change disposable blades after use and dispose of in the **sharps** bin.
- Spray clipper blades with sterilising spray after use.
- Wash all brushes and combs after use then sterilise them.
- Never use dirty or broken tools as this will increase the risk of damaging the skin and consequently cross-infection.

Sharps

The term used in hairdressing to describe any equipment that may cut or pierce the skin, for example scissors or razor blades.

Methods of sterilising tools and equipment

Tool/equipment		Method of sterilisation
Cutting comb		Wash in hot, soapy water to remove dirt and grease. Ultra-violet cabinet; Barbicide® solution.
Scissors		Ultra-violet cabinet; autoclave; alcohol/sterile wipes or sprays.
Clippers (and attachments)		Remove loose hair cuttings then spray blades with sterilising clipper spray.

Organising your working time

At the start of each day, you need to organise yourself so that you are ready to receive your first client. You should:

- check your appointments to see who your first client is
- get out the client's record (if appropriate)
- ensure you have all the correct tools and equipment for the service.

By making sure you are organised you will save time in the salon.

Using your time effectively

You should always be organised and ready for the client's arrival. Each salon has its own time allocation for services offered. As a trainee, you should be aware of the time it takes you to carry out a beard or moustache trim. If you took two hours for a basic trim, your salon would soon be out of business! However, it is expected that you will take longer than an experienced stylist while you are training. The maximum service times to be commercially viable are:

- tapered beardline = 15 minutes
- outlined beard = 15 minutes
- moustache shapes = 5 minutes

To make full use of your working time, you should always be prepared to receive your client. Tools and equipment should be clean and sterilised and within easy reach. If you are not prepared correctly, this will impact on the appointment time that you have with your client and could result in you running late for your subsequent appointments.

Protecting yourself and the client

You need to have a high standard of personal cleanliness. Nails should be well trimmed and jewellery should be minimal. Clean salon uniform or other appropriate clothing should be worn every day. Hands should be washed and dried thoroughly between each client. Any wounds or open sores on your hands should be covered with a suitable dressing, otherwise they may be a source of infection to the client or the client may infect you.

For your own health and safety, you need to be aware of potential hazards to yourself, for example the possibility of cross-infection from blood-borne diseases such as hepatitis and HIV. Prevention is better than cure. You can have a vaccination for hepatitis A and B if you are in a high-risk group, of which hairdressing could be considered one. You are at risk because of the potential for cuts from scissors and sharps which increase the risk of exposure to blood.

Before carrying out a beard or moustache trim, always cover the client's eyes – facial hair is coarser than normal hair and can fly up into the client's eyes. If you wish, as an extra safeguard, ask the client to close his eyes.

During the trim, you should be aware of the client's and your own position while you are working. Make sure that you stand in such a way that you don't strain your back. Remember to bend from your knees and not your back. Ensure that you have positioned the client correctly so that he is comfortable and you can work around him without difficulty.

Fact or fiction?

Is this statement fact or fiction?

Beards and moustaches are often used to hide facial features.

To check your answer see page 503.

465

Unit

GB4

Cut facial hair to shape using basic techniques

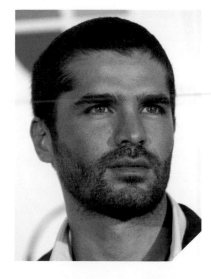

Some hygiene requirements that should be expected:

- Minimum amount of jewellery to be worn so that water and hair cuttings will not become trapped underneath, causing bacteria to grow.
- Flat shoes may need to be worn for health and safety and hygiene purposes.
- You will be required to sterilise all tools and equipment after each client.
- Make sure your personal presentation and hygiene are of a very high standard.
- Make sure you use a breath-freshening spray if you smoke or have had strong-flavoured food, such as curry, the night before.
- Wear cotton tops in the summer and use a good deodorant.
- Always wash your hands after a trip to the bathroom.
- Always keep cuts and open wounds covered with a plaster.

Most of these points are common sense and things that you will do on a daily basis without thinking about it. It is important to continue to follow good health and hygiene practices to maintain a professional appearance to clients and colleagues.

Tools and equipment

Electric and rechargeable clippers

Clippers work by the bottom blade remaining fixed while the top blade moves at a very high speed. You can add clipper attachments to vary/alter the length of the cut, depending on the size of the grade that you attach — the higher the number on the grade, the longer the hair will be left; the lower the number on the grade, the shorter the hair will be cut.

Rechargeable clippers are generally smaller than electric clippers and give a closer haircut. They can be used to trim behind the backs of the ears and other hard-to-reach areas.

You should oil both types of clippers after every use to maintain them and to make sure that they run smoothly This will help to prolong their life.

Clipper attachments

Clipper attachments, also known as grades, are added to your clippers to allow you to cut the hair to different lengths. They are available in different sizes ranging from a grade 1 (the smallest, leaving the hair 3 mm long) up to a grade 8 (the largest, which leaves the hair 25 mm long).

You should attach clipper attachments to the clipper head, making sure that they fit firmly and correctly. Once they are firmly in place you are ready to begin the beard trim. Clipper attachments should not be used if they have missing or broken teeth as this will result in an uneven cut.

You should confirm with the client the size of the clipper grade as you attach it to your clippers to double-check that you heard correctly and are using the correct grade. Most clients will know the number of the clipper grade they have, for example grade 2, but some clients will need guidance in this area.

You can sterilise the clipper attachments by brushing off the hair cuttings then either using a sterilising spray or by removing them from the clippers and immersing them in a solution of Barbicide® for the recommended time.

Use clipper oil after each use of the clippers

Fact or fiction?

Is this statement fact or fiction?

Traditionally, having a beard is a sign of masculinity.

To check your answer see page 503.

Top tips

Only use clippers on dry hair as water and electricity are not compatible and there is a potential risk of electric shock. Also, hair clumps together when wet and therefore your cut will not be as precise if you work on wet hair.

Identifying factors that may influence the service prior to cutting

Before beginning the consultation, you must always check the client for any skin conditions that may prevent you from carrying out the service (see page 468).

Your client's features will determine the size and shape of the beard or moustache.

- *Check the natural growth of the hair* – this may determine the shape of the moustache or how to finish off the neckline shape of a beard trim.
- *Check the density of the hair* – this may influence the cutting technique that you use. For example, if the beard is not very thick, you may want to use a scissor-over-comb technique so that you can leave the beard or moustache longer in places where the hair may be more sparse. However, if the beard is very dense, you may want to use clippers to give an even finish all over.

Safe disposal of used sharps

Salons should supply a yellow sharps bin for the disposal of blades and any equipment that may cut or pierce the skin. A sharps bin is a hard plastic bin that cannot be pierced, which is collected by the local health authority and incinerated. If you put a disposable blade from your razor/hair shaper in an ordinary black bin liner, the person emptying the bin may cut themselves and be at risk from cross-infection.

Task 1

Lewis had just completed a gents' haircut, moustache and beard trim on a client. He was new to the salon and did not know where the sharps bin was kept. He was in a hurry to get ready for his next client, so to save time Lewis threw the used sharps into the nearest bin.

1 What should Lewis have done?
2 What might be the consequences of his actions?

Task 2

Find out how long your salon allows for the following services:

- beard trim with clippers
- beard trim using scissor-over-comb technique
- moustache trim
- full beard and moustache trim.

Cut facial hair to shape using basic techniques

Top tips

- Check your clippers regularly to make sure that they have not been knocked out of alignment. (If the moveable top blade is above the bottom still blade, this will cut the client.)
- If your clippers are out of line, check the manufacturer's instructions to reset them.
- Special sterilising sprays should be used on your clippers after every use.
- Do not use clippers with broken teeth as they can pull, tear or cut the skin.

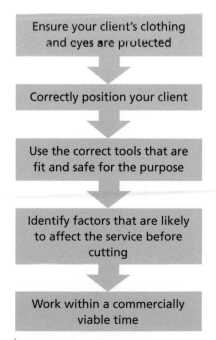

Ensure your client's clothing and eyes are protected

↓

Correctly position your client

↓

Use the correct tools that are fit and safe for the purpose

↓

Identify factors that are likely to affect the service before cutting

↓

Work within a commercially viable time

Facial hair cutting checklist

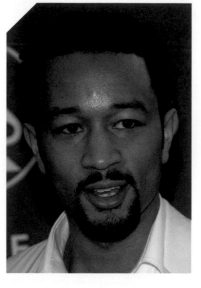

How to cut beards and moustaches to maintain their shape

This section looks at the cutting techniques required to complete a beard and moustache trim. As with other barbering services, you will need to take into account influencing factors.

Preparing the client

It is important that you follow the natural growth patterns of the hair.

- Comb the client's beard or moustache in the direction that it grows — this will also detangle the facial hair ready for cutting.
- Always complete a beard and moustache trim on dry hair.
- Check that the client is comfortable and that he is in a position that you can work around comfortably.
- Check that the client is correctly gowned and protected for the service.
- Check that your clippers are safe to use — make sure that the top moveable blade is not protruding above the bottom blade.

Consultation

During your consultation with the client, you are not only determining how much hair he wants removed or the shape of the beard or moustache he would like, you are also looking for any adverse skin conditions that may not allow you to carry out the service. If you suspect that the client has an infection or infestation, notify your salon manager or tutor. You will need to explain to the client as tactfully as possible why you are unable to carry out the service and refer him to his GP. Never diagnose a medical condition as you are not medically trained to do this.

Carrying out your consultation

Here are some guidelines to get you started.

- Refer to the client by name.
- Make eye contact, either face to face or through the mirror.
- Ask simple questions — do not use technical words that the client may not understand.
- Listen carefully to the answers to your questions and show an interest.

The consultation will involve finding out exactly what the client requires from the beard or moustache trim. You should ask the following questions:

- How short do you wish your beard or moustache to be? This will help you choose the clipper grade or scissor-over-comb technique you will use to remove length.
- What **beardline**/neckline shape would you like to see — tapered, round or square?
- When did you last have a beard or moustache trim? This will give you an indication of how often the client likes to have a beard or moustache trim and how quickly his facial hair may grow.

During your consultation with the client you should have established the length and shape of the beard or moustache that you will be trimming.

Beardline

The perimeter or outline shape of the beard.

Choosing your equipment and techniques

If the client had a very long, thick beard and wanted it cut very short, you would need to choose your equipment very carefully. You could use clippers with an attachment to shorten the beard, but you need to be aware that you might tug or pull the hair on a beard that is very long and thick. In this instance, you would be better off removing some of the length using a scissor-over-comb technique and then using the clippers for a closer finish.

In another instance, if the client had a very fine, soft beard that was not very long and was thin in places, you would choose to cut the beard using the scissor-over-comb technique. By using this technique you are able to leave the beard slightly longer in places to compensate for the thinner areas where the beard may not grow so thickly.

Normally scissors are used for moustaches because it is only a small area which is not suitable for clipper work, as in the first two pictures on page 471. You would also use scissors to cut and blend any **sideburns** into the beard area.

Scissors can be used to neaten off and shape the outside beardline before clippering to remove unwanted hair outside of the neckline shape. The edge of the clippers is used to give an even, blunt edge to the beard neckline shape.

Using the clippers with attachments will give an even look to the whole beard trim. Clippers are ideal for cutting thick, coarse hair.

There are special combs available for barbering which combine a rigid end and a thinner more flexible end. When cutting a beard you will need to use the rigid end of the cutting comb. When tapering in close to the neckline or carrying out a moustache trim, you should use the flexible end of the comb that will allow you to work in hard-to-reach areas. The fine teeth on a comb allow the hair to be controlled and closely cut; the coarser teeth allow for repeated combing and positioning of the hair.

Cutting techniques

When you are carrying out any cutting service, it is important that you work in a methodical manner; one that allows you to see where you are going next in a haircut and where you have already cut. When you are cutting beards and moustaches using either a scissor-over-comb technique or with clippers, you will find it easier if you work in channels. You could start in the middle or at either side, and by working in this way you will be able to see the areas of hair that you have cut and where you are working to next.

Scissor-over-comb

Refer to page 438 for cutting equipment.

This method of cutting is ideal for beard and moustache trimming as you can work closely to the head. The hair is lifted with the comb and the protruding hair is clipped off. Care must be taken when using this method to ensure that you do not leave a hard line or step in the hair. This is overcome by the correct use of the comb with the points of the teeth directed away from the skin and working in a flowing movement. If you feel the flow is lapsing, stop and move your scissors and comb away from the head then go back to it again. Cutting while the comb is stationary will create a hard line in the hair. The hair must be held at a 90-degree angle with the comb.

469

Unit

GB4

Cut facial hair to shape using basic techniques

Sideburns

Facial hair growing in front of the ears.

Top tips

- Sterilise all equipment after each client.
- Ensure the client is protected from hair cuttings entering the eyes or other uncomfortable areas.

470

Unit

GB4

Cut facial hair to shape using basic techniques

Step-by-step scissor-over-comb technique

1 Correctly gown, protect and position your client. Start in the centre section of the chin using a scissor-over-comb technique.

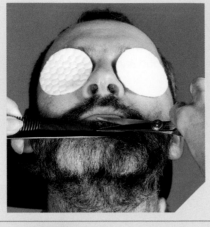

2 Using the central channel section as a guideline, cut the next channel by joining into the guideline.

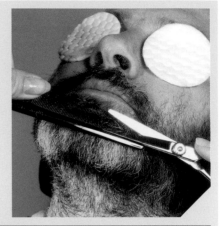

3 Remember to always close your scissors before using them to pick up the next section.

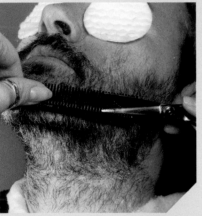

4 Work methodically in channel sections towards the ear. Remember to use your neck brush to remove hair cuttings during the service as they can become irritating.

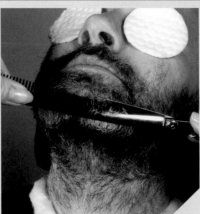

5 Use a flexible comb to follow the contours of the face to get an even scissor-over-comb result.

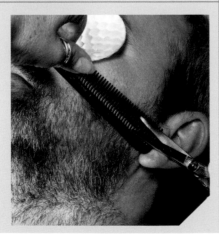

6 Blend the sideburns into the hair and repeat steps 1 to 5 on the other side of the beard.

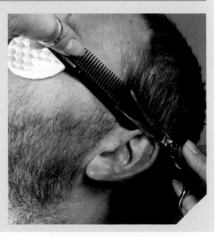

Eyebrow shaping/trimming

Scissor-over-comb is also useful when trimming eyebrows into shape. Some clients only have a few stray eyebrow hairs, which can be cut using the freehand cutting technique, but if the eyebrows are really overgrown and bushy you will need to use scissor-over-comb.

Top tips

When trimming your client's eyebrows, always ask your client to close his eyes so that the coarse eyebrow hairs do not fly off into the eyes.

Clippers with attachments

Refer to page 439 for more information on clipper attachments.

When using the clippers with an attachment, check that you have chosen the right grade to remove the length of hair required by the client. You will need to make sure that you fix the attachment firmly onto the clippers so that it does not fall off during the service.

When you put the clippers into the beard, they should be in contact with the skin. This will help you to maintain an even length throughout the beard trim.

Clipper-over-comb technique

This cutting technique is similar to the scissor-over-comb technique; the difference is that you will be using clippers rather than scissors to cut off the hair that is protruding from your comb. The same principles apply to clipper-over-comb as for scissor-over-comb – you need to cut the hair at a 90-degree angle to ensure you do not put any hard lines into the hair.

Freehand technique

This technique is mainly used for cutting the perimeter shape when trimming moustaches and when trimming eyebrows into shape. As the name of the technique suggests, you do not hold the hair with tension but comb the hair into place and cut freehand. The freehand technique gives you a truer indication of where the hair will sit because you will not have used tension by pulling the hair down.

Step-by-step moustache cutting

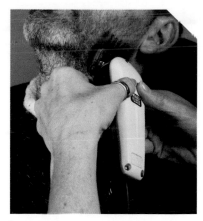

Clippers with attachment

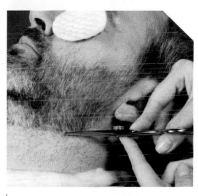

Freehand technique

471

Unit

GB4

Cut facial hair to shape using basic techniques

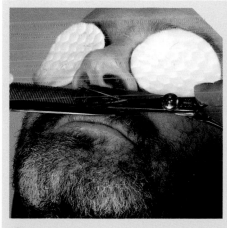

1 Gown and protect your client. Start scissor-over-comb technique in the centre section of the moustache. Use a barbering comb for flexibility.

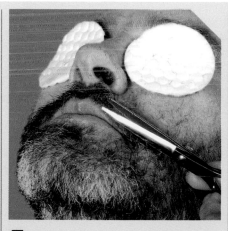

2 Use the centre section as a guideline for each subsequent section and join into the beard hair. Use a freehand cutting technique for neatening the edge of the top lip.

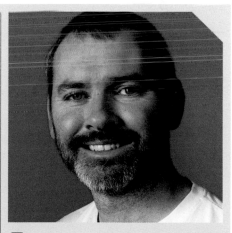

3 Remove hair cuttings with a neck brush. Check with your client that he is happy with the length of the moustache.

Top tips

Always double-check that the grade is properly attached before you begin to use the clippers. You will also need to take care not to push the clipper grade too firmly into the client's neck. Some clients have more sensitive skin than others, and you could cause the skin to turn pink or red and look sore.

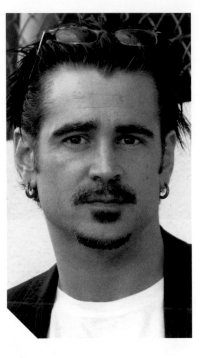

Factors influencing the cut

Head and face shapes

During the consultation with your client you will have looked at the client's head and face shape. If you have a client with a long face shape and you leave the neck outline long, you will emphasise the length of the face. Similarly, if the client has a very round face and you make the neckline very round, you will be emphasising the roundness of the face.

When cutting moustaches, the size of the moustache should correspond to the size of the facial features. Heavy facial features will require a large design, while small, fine, smooth features would suit a small design.

Critical influencing factors you should look out for are:

- length of the mouth
- size of the nose
- size of upper lip area.

Facial features and shape of moustache

Here are a few guidelines to get you started.

- *Large facial features* – heavy moustache.
- *Prominent nose* – large moustache.
- *Long, narrow nose* – narrow, thin moustache.
- *Extra-large mouth* – pyramid-shaped moustache.
- *Extra-small mouth* – narrow, short, thin moustache.
- *Smallish regular features* – small, triangular-shaped moustache.
- *Wide mouth with prominent upper lip* – heavy handlebar moustache or large divided moustache.
- *Round face with regular features* – semi-square moustache.
- *Square face with prominent features* – heavy linear moustache with ends curling slightly downwards.

Hair growth patterns

Not all hair grows in the same direction, and you will need to take this into account when you are trimming beards or moustaches. Some beards may have swirls in them; some moustaches may grow unevenly. When cutting facial hair, you may need to change the angle or the length of the cut to take these factors into account.

If the neck hair grows in a specific way, for example round or square, you will need to follow the natural growth patterns of the hair. If you try to alter the natural shape of the neckline, the client may have difficulty in maintaining the shape at home or the shape may grow out quickly and look untidy.

Hairstyles

The way in which the client is wearing his hair will need to be taken into account when deciding on the length, shape or thickness of the beard or moustache.

Task 3

If your client has a Grade 1 crew cut and you leave his beard thick and bushy, would that look right? In this instance, what do you think a better look for the client's beard would be?

Hair density

When you assess the hair's density, you are looking at the amount of hair that the client has on his face. An individual hair might be quite fine, but altogether there may be a lot of hairs. This is when you will refer to the density of the hair — that is, the amount of hair the client has per square centimetre. How would this influence your choice of method or cutting technique when carrying out a beard or moustache trim?

Task 4

Use the internet or style books to research a variety of men's haircuts. Look at the different hairstyles and discuss what shape and thickness of beard and moustache would best suit the different hairstyles you are looking at. If possible, draw in the type of beard or moustache that best suits the hairstyle in the picture.

Skin elasticity

The skin loses its elastic properties with age, and this can lead to a lack of tension in the skin. You need to assess the skin's elasticity before you start cutting. If there is a distinct lack of skin elasticity, you will need to pull the skin slightly to stretch it and improve the tension to limit the chance of cutting the skin.

Facial piercing

Facial piercing is a current fashion and therefore you will come across clients with these piercings. If they are in the beard or moustache area they will be very easy to catch with your scissors or comb, so you will need to either ask the client to remove the jewellery or try to avoid it when cutting.

Facial contours

The client's facial contours will need to be taken into account when cutting the beard and moustache area. You will need to ask your client to move his head at different angles to get into facial contours produced by the jaw and chin.

Task 5

Sally was booked to complete a beard trim on a client she had never met before. She was very busy that day and felt pushed for time when she carried out the consultation. The client wanted a very short beard so Sally decided to use a Grade 1. When she had finished she realised that the client had some scars underneath his beard — it looked as if the client had bald patches in his beard.

What should Sally have done?

Adjusting your position to ensure an even, accurate, balanced cut

As you are progressing through your trim, you will need to adjust the position in which you work so that you cover the whole area in a methodical manner. You should ensure that you have not missed any area and that you have achieved an even, balanced result.

If you stand 'square' on to the client and try to cut the hair in one position, you will not achieve a balanced shape since people tend not to have a symmetrical head and face. You will need to move around your client as you work so that you are covering all angles of the face. This will help you to achieve an accurate cut, ensuring that you have an even distribution of weight and balance throughout the beard and moustache trim.

A mirror is a good tool to use to check the shape, weight and balance of your cut. If you sit your client up in the chair and stand directly behind him, you will be able to use the mirror to confirm that you have achieved the same length and have attained a balanced result.

By using your mirror to check the beard or moustache trim, you are giving yourself and your client the opportunity to make any changes to the cut that may be required. It is important to check with your client that he is happy with what you have done and feels that you have achieved the desired result.

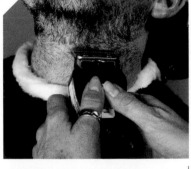

Turn the clippers upside down and use the edge of the blade to create a definite line

Task 6

In groups, discuss the types of questions that you can use to confirm with the client that he is happy with the desired look. Remember to think about using open questions rather than closed questions, which will help you to gain more of a response from your client.

- Closed questions usually only need one-word answers. For example, 'Do you normally have your beard cut with clippers?' This type of question confirms or eliminates information: 'Yes, I do' or 'No, I don't'. Sometimes you will need to ask a closed question if you just require facts, but try to keep this type of questioning to a minimum.
- Open questions help to make the conversation flow as they require a fuller response. For example, 'How are you today?' Since open questions encourage more detailed answers, they are good to break the ice with, as the client cannot respond with a simple 'yes' or 'no'.

Removing unwanted hair outside the desired outline

As part of the complete look, you need to make sure that you 'clean up' any hair that is outside of the outline shape of the cut.

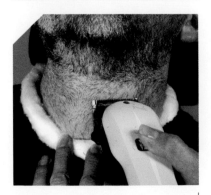

Turn the clippers so the flat side is against the client's neck

You will need to confirm with the client the neck shape that you are going to cut, and do that first. You can do this by turning your clippers upside down and using the edge of the blade to gently make a definite line. Once you have put the shape in that you require, you then turn your clippers so that the flat side of the clippers is sitting against the client's neck, and can continue to remove the unwanted excess hair.

Meeting client expectations and ensuring comfort

When you are showing the client the end result you should:

- ensure he is sitting upright
- remove the towel, tissue and cotton wool from his neck so he can see the result
- give him a hand mirror so he can look closely at what you have done
- show him all angles using a hand mirror (if appropriate).

If any hair is sticking to the client, you can use a small amount of talcum powder to absorb the moisture and help to remove the hair cuttings. You should also be able to give your client the correct aftercare advice on home maintenance and discuss a suitable time for him to come back for a trim.

How to provide aftercare advice

Giving accurate advice and recommendations on the maintenance of the beard and moustache trim is essential to complete the service. You need to use good communication techniques so that the advice you are giving is clear and constructive. It is useful to advise your client on the best way to carry out any maintenance he may need to do at home before his next appointment with you, and the most appropriate tools to use for this.

Examples of information to give your client:

- how often he will require regular trims to maintain the cut
- how fast hair grows on average
- how you have cut the neck shape, and explain to him how to carry out the same process at home
- suitable equipment to use at home.

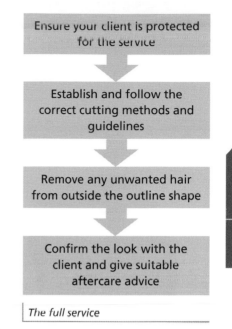

Ensure your client is protected for the service

↓

Establish and follow the correct cutting methods and guidelines

↓

Remove any unwanted hair from outside the outline shape

↓

Confirm the look with the client and give suitable aftercare advice

The full service

475

Unit
GB4

Cut facial hair to shape using basic techniques

Salon life

Eye eye!

Scott's story

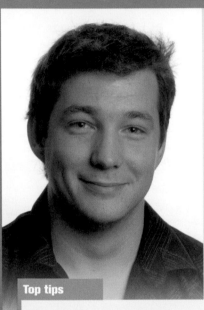

When I was an apprentice I was asked to cut a male client's hair, which I did with guidance from my tutor. When I had finished and showed the client the back in the mirror, he said it was fine and I thought I had finished. Then he asked me to trim his eyebrows! I was shocked, as I had never had to do this before. I went over and said very quietly to my tutor, 'Help, he wants me to cut his eyebrows!' She told me not to worry and said that she would show me how to trim the eyebrows. Once I had seen how to do one eyebrow I had a go at the other one, and it was quite easy really – just a bit of scissor-over-comb and freehand. I think it was just fear of the unknown that freaked me out when asked to do it for the first time. Now I see trimming my clients' eyebrows as a part of the service.

Top tips

Don't be afraid to remove excess hair from your clients' ears and eyebrows. Many elderly clients grow excess hair in these places and find it hard to remove themselves. Think of it as part of your complete service.

Ask the expert

Q *What do I do if a client asks me to do something I have not been trained in?*

A Ask a more senior member of staff for their guidance and they will be able to use their expertise and experience to help you.

Q *Why is it necessary to cut a client's eyebrows?*

A Some clients' eyebrows grow very bushy and sometimes they get stray hairs that grow really long (commonly known as 'cat brows'). If they are not trimmed they can make the client look and feel quite unkempt. Some clients are unable to trim their own eyebrows and will ask you to do this for them as part of their haircutting service.

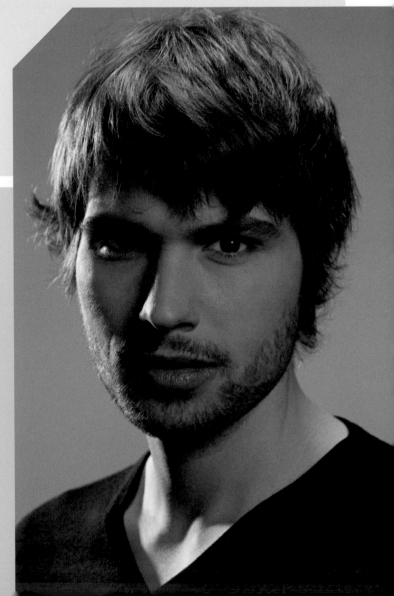

Check your knowledge

The following questions will help you to check your understanding of this unit.
The answers can be found on page 502.

1 What is the correct gowning procedure for a beard and moustache trim?
 a) Gown, and a towel in case you cut the client by accident
 b) Gown, towel and either a strip of cotton wool or neck tissue to prevent cuttings dropping down onto clothes
 c) Gown only, as blokes don't like too much fuss
 d) Gown and either a strip of cotton wool or neck tissue to prevent cuttings dropping down onto clothes

2 What are the legal requirements for the disposal of sharps?

_____

3 What are your responsibilities under the current Electricity at Work Regulations?
 a) All electrical equipment you use should have been tested once or twice a year for safety.
 b) All electrical equipment you use should have been tested every two years.
 c) All electrical equipment you use should have been tested every three years.
 d) Only really old equipment needs testing to see if it is still working properly.

4 Why is it important to avoid cross-infection and infestation in the salon?

_____

_____

_____

5 Why is it important to cut to the natural facial hairline?

_____

_____

_____

6 What is the average rate of hair growth?
 a) 1 inch per month
 b) 1 cm per month
 c) 1.25 inches per month
 d) 1.25 cm per month

7 List the methods of sterilisation used in barber shops.

_____

_____

_____

477

Unit

GB4

Cut facial hair to shape using basic techniques

8 What is meant by the term 'factor'?

_____

_____

_____

9 List the four cutting techniques you have learned about in this unit which can be used when cutting facial hair.

_____

_____

_____

10 What sort of aftercare advice should you give to your client?

_____

_____

_____

Getting ready for assessment

Remember that within each of the services you carry out with a client, you will cover different units. For example, when cutting facial hair to shape (GB4), you will also have to be aware of health and safety (G20) and advise and consult with clients (G7). If you are not sure what you have covered in your service, always ask your assessor or supervisor for advice.

	NVQ	VRQ
Credit value	4	4
Guided Learning Hours	37	37

	NVQ	VRQ
Practical demonstrations, to be observed by assessor	Your assessor will observe you on at least four different occasions, covering: • one tapered beardline • one outlined beard • two different moustache shapes. Simulation is not allowed for any performance evidence within this unit.	Your assessor will observe you on at least four different occasions, covering: • one tapered beardline • one outlined beard • two different moustache shapes. Simulation is not allowed for any performance evidence within this unit.
Service timings	Tapered beardline – 15 minutes Full beard outline – 15 minutes Moustache only – 5 minutes	Tapered beardline – 15 minutes Full beard outline – 15 minutes Moustache only – 5 minutes
Additional evidence	Most evidence of your performance will be acquired from the observations made by your assessor. If your assessor has not been present, you may be required to produce other forms of evidence to support your performance. There is no external paper requirement for this unit.	Most evidence of your performance will be acquired from the observations made by your assessor. If your assessor has not been present, you may be required to produce other forms of evidence to support your performance. There is no external paper requirement for this unit.

Task mapping

When you have completed the tasks in this unit, check the table below to see which Performance Criteria (purple), Range (red), Knowledge (green) and Key Skills (blue) you have covered within GB4 to use as additional evidence within your portfolio. Information about which Functional Skills you have covered is available on the website.

Task and page reference	Mapping to Performance Criteria, Range, Knowledge and Key Skills
1 (page 467)	Performance Criteria: –, VRQ 2i Range: –, VRQ N/A Knowledge: 3, 13, VRQ 2R Key Skills: C1.2, C1.3, C2.3
2 (page 467)	Performance Criteria: Practising 1g, VRQ N/A Range: –, VRQ R3a–c Knowledge: 2, VRQ N/A Key Skills: C1.2, C1.3, N1.1, N1.2, N1.3, N2.1, N2.2, N2.3
3 (page 473)	Performance Criteria: Practising 2b, 2d, VRQ 1c, 2h Range: 2c, 2e, VRQ R3a–c Knowledge: 19, 20, 24, VRQ 1d, 2o Key Skills: C1.2, C1.3, C2.3

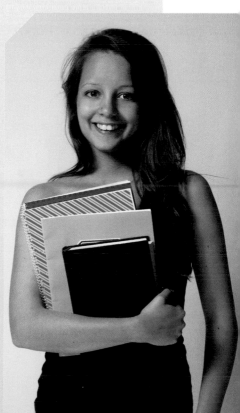

Cut facial hair to shape using basic techniques

4 (page 473)	Performance Criteria: Practising 2b, VRQ 1c Range: 2c, 4a–c, VRQ R2c, R2e, R3a–c Knowledge: 22, VRQ 1d, 1e, 1f, 2m, 2o Key Skills: C1.2, C1.3, C2.3
5 (page 473)	Performance Criteria: Practising 2b, 2d, 1j, VRQ 1b, 1c, 2a, 2d Range: 1a–d, VRQ R2b Knowledge: 20, VRQ 1e–g,, 1j, 1l, 1s Key Skills: C1.2, C1.3, C2.3
6 (page 474)	Performance Criteria: Practising 2b, 2k, VRQ 1b, 1c, 2a Range: 4a–g Knowledge: 23, VRQ 1J, 2s Key Skills: C1.1, C1.2, C1.3, C2.1a, C2.2B, C2.3

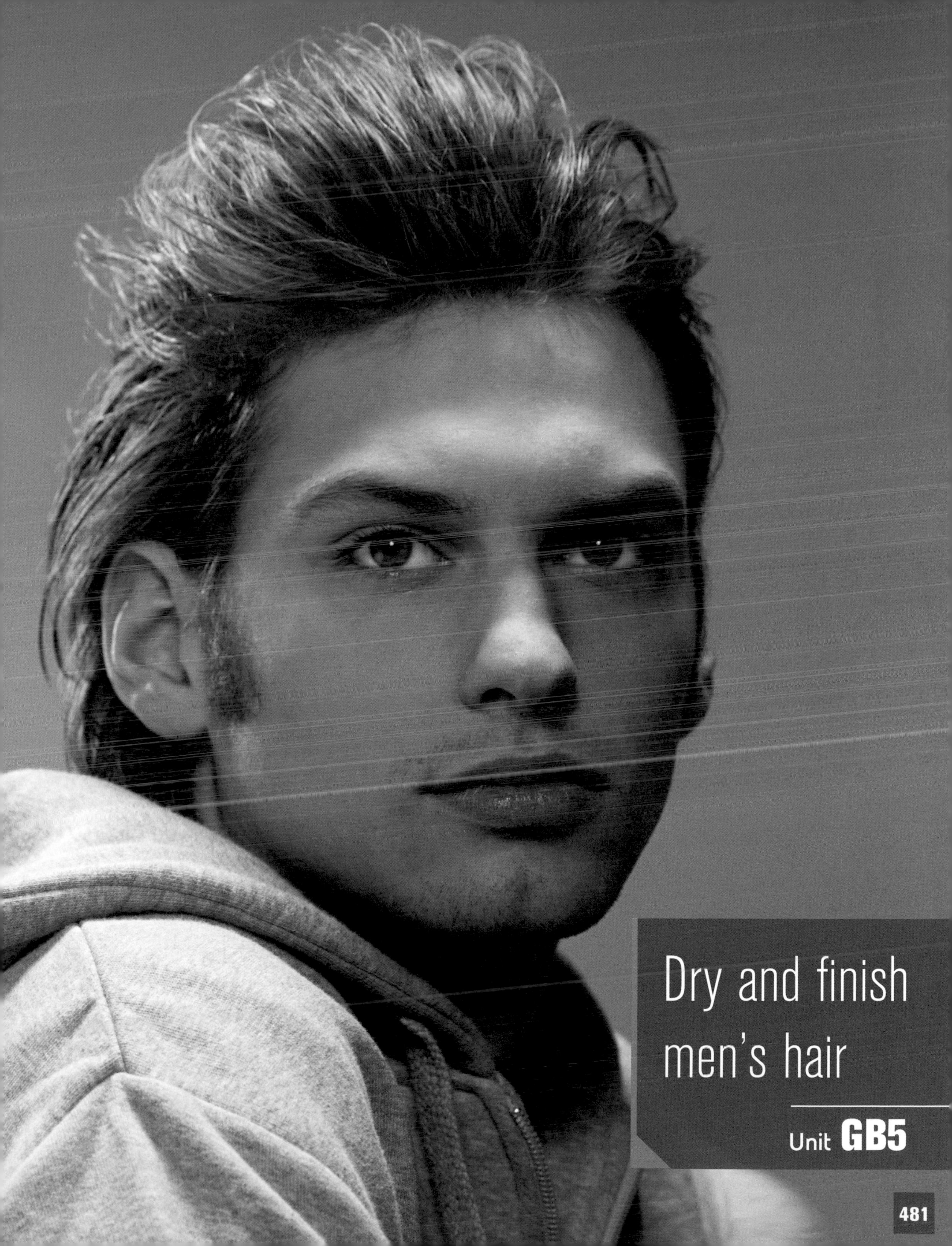

Dry and finish
men's hair

Unit **GB5**

What you will learn:

- **How to maintain effective and safe methods of working when drying and finishing hair**
- **How to dry and finish hair**
- **How to provide aftercare advice**

Introduction

In many unisex salons, you will be required to carry out blow-drying services on men's hair. These services are offered to produce an end result from a cutting or colouring service and should complement the style in which the hair is cut or coloured.

In this unit you will be looking at using different styling techniques to create a wide range of finished looks, taking into account any critical influencing factors and working with a range of styling and finishing products. Many of the products, tools and techniques that you will use are very similar to those in ladies' hairdressing (see GH10, GH11 and GH12).

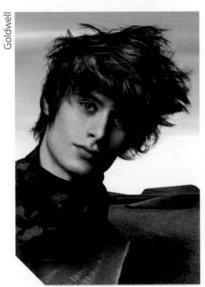

Goldwell

How to maintain effective and safe methods of working when drying and finishing hair

The essential underpinning knowledge and skills you will need are covered in GH10, pages 243–70. They are:

- Preparing your client (page 244)
- Your position while working (page 245)
- Personal hygiene (page 251)
- Safe working area (page 245)
- Safe use of tools (pages 261–62)
- Organisation of working area (page 245)
- Consultation (pages 251–52).

Variations for men's services

However, there are one or two variations for men's services that you need to be aware of.

Products

As a stylist, you need to know the effects of different products on different hair types to help you ensure the services you carry out are successful. There is a wide range of products available, from those that make the hair more pliable to those that protect the hair from added heat and the effects of **atmospheric moisture**.

Atmospheric moisture

Water in the air as water vapour, in the form of raindrops, steam, fog, etc.

Product	Application	Suitability	Comments
Gel (wet or dry)	Usually applied to wet hair. If you require the hair to stand up then apply at the root area. Can also be spread evenly through the hair for a firm hold throughout. Note: gels can also be used as a finishing product and come in a spray form, to be used similarly to hairsprays.	Suitable for most hair types, but avoid very fine or thinning hair as this will accentuate (emphasise) the fineness of the hair. Good for short spiky styles. Note: a gel spray is a heavier product than hairspray so should be avoided on very fine hair.	If left to dry naturally it will produce a 'wet' look. If a hairdryer is used, the use of gel will not be so apparent. Note: if you want to still work with the hair while applying a finishing product, a gel spray allows you to do this; you can work the hair into spikes and create more texture.
Dressing cream	Apply small amounts evenly throughout the hair.	Light hold – large amounts will produce a slicked-back look.	Leaves the hair sticky to touch.
Blow-drying lotion/heat protector	Applied evenly to towel-dried hair by spraying into the hair. Note: if the product is a heat protector spray only, it should be applied to dry hair before any electrical heated equipment is used.	Good for most hair types and will produce a soft, natural look. Ideal for fine hair that requires extra body. Note: heat protector sprays are suitable for hair that is in poor condition, and to prevent healthy hair from becoming dry.	Some products contain chemicals that protect the hair from heat. Standalone heat protector sprays will put a slight barrier on the hair to protect from the effects of electrical heated styling equipment.
Hairspray	Apply sparingly (not too much) onto styled hair from a distance of 20 cm.	Suitable for most hair types and will hold the finished style in place.	This product can have a drying effect on the hair. If sprayed too close or overused will leave white flakes in the hair.
Wax	Applied to dry hair. Can either be applied evenly throughout the hair or used on the ends of the hair to create texture.	No real hold, but will clump the hair together, creating texture.	Too much on very fine hair will weigh the hair down. Ideal for coarse, thick hair and styles where you want to define the cut.

Styling and finishing products

Tools

Choosing the right tools

As well as understanding how styling products affect the way hair behaves, you also need to know the effects different types of equipment can help you to achieve.

When blow-drying, the length of hair dictates the size of the brush that you would choose. This is why most stylists have a wide and varied range of brushes. To start with, you will only need a basic range of brushes. As you gain experience and master different techniques, you should add to your equipment.

Fact or fiction?

Is this statement fact or fiction?

Only sprays will coat the hair with a protective barrier to prevent the effects of atmospheric moisture.

To check your answer see page 503.

Top tips

By having *all* of your equipment clean and sterilised, you will always be ready to receive a client.

Styling tools and techniques

Tool		Effect	Suitability
Denman brush		Used to create a smooth finish and can 'pull' out waves in the hair.	Hair only requiring a slight curve or straight finish; curl cannot be created.
Vent brush		Produces a soft, broken-up effect.	Good for producing a quick casual effect. Not suitable for curling the hair.
Circular brush		Produces a curled effect. The smaller the brush, the tighter the curl.	Large round brushes are ideal for long hair, while shorter hair will require a smaller brush.

Timing

Organising your time effectively

Organising yourself and your time at work is an important part of your role as a stylist. Every salon allows a set amount of time for every process that is carried out, from shampooing to colouring.

A good trolley layout with all the necessary equipment will allow you to spend more time with the client on the service.

Task 1

Most salons allocate a set amount of time for each service that is offered. Find out your training establishment's times for the following services:

- shampoo and conditioning
- conditioning treatment
- blow-drying
- finger-drying.

How to dry and finish hair

In this section you will learn how to carry out a consultation, use equipment safely and effectively, apply the correct styling and finishing products and take into account critical influencing factors.

Consultation

The consultation is the first communication that you have with the client. It is important to spend time questioning him on his requirements and expectations of the service. It is also the time when you need to complete a blow-drying analysis. It may be useful to prepare a checklist to help you. During the consultation, check:

- for anything that may not let you carry out the service such as infections and infestations – this is a contraindication to the service
- the type of hair you are working on — look at the texture and density of hair as this will influence the choice of styling product (these are classed as 'factors')
- any critical influencing factors that may influence the blow-dry, such as head and face shape
- how the client is currently wearing his hair — if he wants the same style, you have an advantage by seeing the hair before it is shampooed
- how much natural movement there is in the hair — this will affect your product choice and the choice of equipment
- whether there are any natural partings — it is always better to allow the hair to fall into its natural partings as the style will last longer and look more natural.

Examples of questions to ask during the consultation:

- Would you like a styling product on your hair?
- How would you like your hair blow-dried? (Use style books to help.)
- Do you get any problems with particular parts of the hair? (Let the client identify what he considers to be awkward areas.)

Blow-drying

For tools, see GH10 pages 247–48.

You need to be able to control the hair as you blow dry it. The way in which you manage the hair is very important, as this will affect the finished result and determine whether the style is manageable for the client.

Task 2

Some questions are provided on the website to use to recap your knowledge. You can refer back to GH10 once you have attempted to answer them!

A worksheet for this task is provided on the website for you to complete and add to your portfolio.

Step-by-step finger-dry to create volume and movement

1 Apply the desired amount of product and distribute evenly through the hair.

2 Dry the hair into the desired style, using your fingers as the tools, making sure that the hairdryer is at the correct angle so that the airflow is moving from root to points and produces the correct amount of root lift.

3 Confirm the finished result with the client. Apply a finishing product if required and provide the correct aftercare advice.

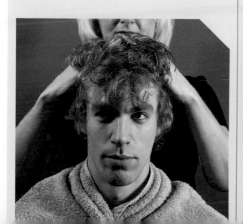
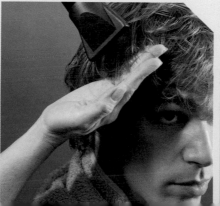
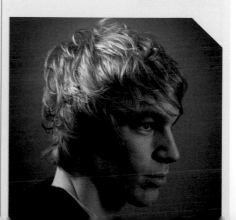

Top tips

Men do not always have such elaborate blow-dries as women. You will need to be more aware of where double crowns and natural partings sit, so that you are working with the hair's growth patterns.

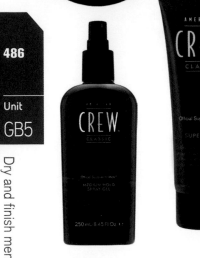

Styling and finishing products

Hygroscopic

Able to absorb water. In hairdressing, this refers to the hair's ability to absorb moisture from the atmosphere, i.e. via rain, steam, etc.

Hydrogen bonds

Weaker bonds in the cortex that are broken down with water and re-formed by using added heat.

Alpha keratin

Hair in its natural state.

Beta keratin

Hair in its stretched state.

Plasticiser

An ingredient in products that coats the hair with a protective barrier.

Styling and finishing products

It is important that you understand the drying techniques, products and equipment available to help you to achieve a wide variety of styles (see pages 482–83).

Task 3

Gather together some styling products that you have in your salon or college/training institution. Using the chart provided on the website, decide which products are suitable for the hair types listed.

A worksheet for this task is provided on the website for you to complete and add to your portfolio.

Basic science

Hair is **hygroscopic**; this means it has the ability to absorb water (allowing you to shampoo the hair). Atmospheric moisture is also water and is around us every day in the form of rain and steam from baths and showers. When water penetrates into the cortex through the cuticle, it breaks down the weaker bonds in the hair known as the **hydrogen bonds**. This allows you to change the shape of the hair many times by simply shampooing the hair and drying it around a brush or using your fingers to help it take on a new shape.

By shampooing the hair and then blow-drying it into a new shape, you are changing the hair from its natural state, known as **alpha keratin**, into its new stretched shape, **beta keratin**. By using styling and finishing products you are putting a protective barrier (plastic film) on the hair that helps to prevent atmospheric moisture from entering into the cortex and breaking down the hydrogen bonds.

Modern products are made of **plasticisers**, for example polyvinyl pyrolidone, a clear film which dissolves in hot water and shampoo. It is therefore easily removed from the hair. They soften the hair shaft, allowing shapes to be formed readily, preventing the hair from becoming 'fly-away', which makes it more manageable for styling. They also protect the hair from added heat.

Incorrect use of heat

When you carry out drying techniques on the hair, it is important to ensure the heat of the hairdryer flows over the cuticle layer the correct way. Failure to do so could result in burns to the scalp and over-drying of the hair. The flow of air from the hairdryer should go from root to point (tip). This will help to keep the cuticle layer flat, which in turn gives the hair a more shiny appearance.

You should also keep the hairdryer moving so that the heat from the dryer is not focused on one area. This requires a wrist action and not a full arm action (you will get tired very quickly by using your whole arm when drying the hair).

If you continue to use the hairdryer when there isn't any moisture left in the hair, you will be over-drying the hair. If the hair dries before you have styled it in the required way, you must re-dampen the hair using a water spray.

Allowing the hair to cool

By allowing the hair to cool before you dress or 'play' with the end result, you help the hair to 'fix' into its new shape, which will help your finished result to last longer.

If you are working with a brush, dry the section of hair around the brush then remove the heat for a few seconds, keeping the brush in place. The hair will cool into this position and the bonds will be fixed more firmly into place.

Critical influencing factors

When choosing products, equipment and blow-drying techniques, you should take into account the following factors:

- *Hair texture* – very fine hair will need a product that stops it becoming fly-away. Some products also have a 'thickening' effect on the hair, for example mousse.
- *Haircut* – the length of the layers and style will determine what brush size to use. They will also influence the type of product you choose.
- *Head and face shape* – this will influence your drying technique and how you style the hair. You may need to dress the hair to take the emphasis away from a prominent feature that the client is not happy with.
- *Hair growth patterns* – a firm-hold product may be needed to help you disguise a double crown or a fringe with a cowlick.

Communicating with the client throughout the blow-dry

Throughout the blow-dry service you should check the following:

- Are you working towards the style desired by the client? Is his parting in the right place?
- Are you achieving the amount of texture or spikiness that the client requires?
- Is the heat of the hairdryer comfortable for the client?
- Would the client like you to apply any finishing products?
- Is the client happy with the finished result?

How to provide aftercare advice

You should always end every service with suitable aftercare advice. This does not necessarily mean that you are trying to get the client to purchase every product that you have used on them. However, if you have used a product that you think has particularly suited their hair and given a good result, this would be a prime opportunity to discuss the features and benefits of that product.

You should be advising the client on the best way to maintain the 'look' you have achieved, whether they will need to apply any more product, and when they should next shampoo their hair.

Salon life

Faith in your products

Amy's story

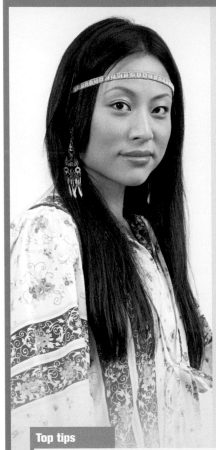

I am halfway through my training and I have just managed to find a work placement in a salon at the weekend. It's really great – everyone is so friendly and I am learning masses! We have a regular team meeting every Friday morning, mainly to tell us about the offers and promotions that the salon is offering that week. We can earn commission on the retail sales that we make and some of the stylists seem to be doing really well. I was finding it really hard so I decided to speak to the senior stylist, to ask her for any hints or tips that might help.

She explained that I need to build trust with clients so they are confident with the advice I am giving them. She said that the only way to give the correct advice is by getting to know the products and believing in them and what they can do. She then sent me off to list all the styling and finishing products that we have in the salon and even set me homework! I had to research each product on the internet and write up the information to take in the following week. I was also encouraged to try out as many products as I could each week, so I could see the benefits of each and decide what I liked.

Her advice worked wonders! Once I learned about the products I found I could use them with confidence and was happy to talk about what they could do for my clients. I now never recommend anything unless I am convinced it will do exactly what it says it will! I also earn regular commission from retail sales, but more importantly I feel really confident about the information I am giving to my clients.

Top tips

Many styling products can be used on both ladies' and men's hair. If you can't find a specific men's hair product to suit your client, don't be afraid to use a product that you know works well on your female clients.

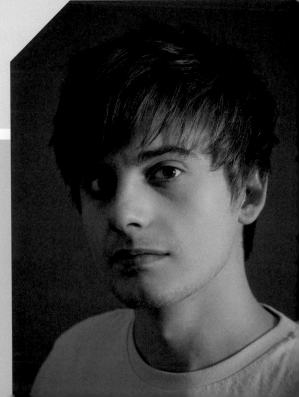

Ask the expert

Q *My salon doesn't give us commission on our product retail sales. How do I go about taking this further? Who should I speak to?*

A There is no law that requires salon owners to pay commission. Most salons do this as an incentive to staff and as a way for them to boost their staff wages. My suggestion would be to keep a record of how much you are selling and then approach the salon owner with a proposition that suits both parties.

Check your knowledge

The following questions will help you to check your understanding of this unit.
The answers can be found on page 503.

1 What is the best way to minimise cross-infection when working in the salon?
   a) Only allow clients in that have clean hair.
   b) Sterilise tools and equipment after every client.
   c) Wear gloves for every service.
   d) Ensure the correct gowns are used for every service.

2 A heat protector product is designed to:
   a) stop the client from getting sunburnt
   b) put a curl into the hair as it is blow-dried
   c) coat the hair with a slight film to prevent the hair from becoming over-dry
   d) stop the hydrogen bonds from re-forming into the wrong position.

3 An infestation is caused by:
   a) parasites
   b) an infection
   c) a disease
   d) unclean hair.

4 By allowing the hair to cool you will:
   a) prevent atmospheric moisture entering the cuticle
   b) put a barrier on the hair
   c) break down the hydrogen bonds
   d) fix the hair in its new shape.

5 Styling and finishing products coat the hair with:
   a) atmospheric moisture
   b) plasticisers
   c) water
   d) oil.

Getting ready for assessment

You will be assessed using a combination of assessment methods, as described below. Remember that within each of the services you carry out with a client, you will cover different units. For example, when styling men's hair (GB5), you will also have to be aware of health and safety (G20) and advise and consult with clients (G7). If you are not sure what you have covered in your service, always ask your assessor or supervisor for advice.

	NVQ	VRQ
Credit value	4	3
Guided Learning Hours	29	30

	NVQ	VRQ
Practical demonstrations, to be observed by assessor	You must practically demonstrate in your everyday work that you have met the standard for drying and finishing men's hair. Your assessor will observe these aspects of your performance on at least three occasions, which must include the use of three different styling and finishing products. From the range, you must show that you have: • used three out of the five styling and finishing products • dried and finished all hair types • considered all the factors • used all the styling techniques • achieved all the finished looks • given all the advice. Simulation is not allowed for any performance evidence within this unit.	You are required to complete three competent performances, and practically demonstrate that you have used all the: • techniques • products • factors and equipment. You must also prove that you have met all of the behavioural expectations. Evidence for this unit must be gathered in a real or realistic working environment; simulation is not allowed for any performance evidence within this unit.
Service timings	There are no maximum service times that apply to this unit.	Blow-drying hair, above shoulder – 30 minutes Blow-drying hair, below shoulder – 45 minutes
Additional evidence	There is one external paper that must be achieved.	There is no external paper for this VRQ unit.

Task mapping

When you have completed the tasks in this unit, check the table below to see which Performance Criteria (purple), Range (red), Knowledge (green) and Key Skills (blue) you have covered within GB5 to use as additional evidence within your portfolio. Information about which Functional Skills you have covered is available on the website.

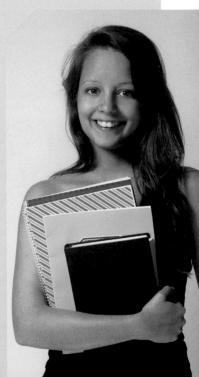

Task and page reference	Mapping to Performance Criteria, Range, Knowledge and Key Skills
1 (page 484)	Performance Criteria: 1i Range: N/A Knowledge: 1, 2 Key Skills: C1.2, C1.3, C2.3, N1.1, N1.2, N1.3, N2.1, N2.2, N2.3
2 (page 485)	Performance Criteria: N/A Range: N/A Knowledge: 9, 11, 20, 21, 23, 31, 32, 33 Key Skills: C1.2, C1.3, C2.3
3 (page 486)	Performance Criteria: 2c, 3a, VRQ 2a, Range: 1a–e, 6a, VRQ R2a–h Knowledge: 25, 26, 27, VRQ 2d Key Skills: C1.2, C1.3, C2.3

Working in the hair industry

Fact or fiction?

Page 21: Self-development is important for you only, not your employer. – *FICTION. Self-development is important to both you and your employer. If you improve your skills, this will benefit both yourself and your salon.*

Page 21: Your employer can decide the minimum amount they pay you per hour. – *FICTION. All employers are bound by the National Minimum Wage Regulations, which stipulate the minimum amount that employees can be paid, according to their age group. Apprenticeship wages are slightly different, but there is still a minimum amount that employers can pay apprentices*

Check your knowledge

1   At a hairdressing exhibition, you would see a display of hairdressing products and tools, and demonstrations of hairdressing techniques.
2   Wella, L'Oréal, Schwarzkopf, Goldwell and Tigi are hairdressing product manufacturers.
3   The hairdressing industry allows for a range of flexible working patterns, including full time, part-time and seasonal work.
4   CPD stands for Continuing Professional Development.
5   COSHH stands for Control of Substances Hazardous to Health.
6   It is important for you to understand what is required of you in your job role and what your work responsibilities are, in order to ensure that you will fulfil what your boss expects of you, work safely and responsibly, and contribute to the success of the salon.
7   Your job responsibilities are recorded in your contract of employment and job description.
8   Your strengths and weaknesses should be reviewed when setting regular targets, and during the appraisal process.
9   The Working Time Regulations state how long you can work before you must have a break.
10 The National Minimum Wage states the least amount employers can pay their staff.

Employment awareness in the hair and beauty sector

Fact or fiction?

Page 32: To be successful working in the hairdressing industry you need to enjoy working with others. – *FACT. A career in the hairdressing industry is based on working with lots of different people.*

Page 32: The *Hairdressers Journal International* is a trade magazine containing a huge amount of industry information. – *FACT.*

Page 33: HABIA is the hairdressing industry's awarding organisation. – *FICTION. HABIA is the industry's government-appointed sector skills body, not awarding organisation.*

Page 38: RIDDOR stands for Reporting of Injuries, Diseases and Dangerous Occurrences Regulations. – *FACT. RIDDOR requires employers, the self-employed and people in control of work premises (the responsible person) to report serious workplace accidents, occupational diseases and specified dangerous occurrences (near misses).*

Page 39: COSHH stands for Control of Substances Hazardous to Hands. – *FICTION. COSHH stands for Control of Substances Hazardous to Health (not Hands).*

Page 40: Employers must pay their staff at or above the levels of the National Minimum Wage. – *FACT. The National Minimum Wage is a minimum amount per hour that most workers in the UK are entitled to be paid. Check out this website to see those not entitled to NMW:* http://www.direct.gov.uk/en/Employment/Employees/TheNationalMinimumWage/DG_175114

Check your knowledge

1   HABIA stands for Hair and Beauty Industry Authority.
2   HABIA's function is to determine the standards for hairdressing, beauty, barbering, African-type hair, nails and spa qualifications.
3   Personal qualities could include: reliable, friendly, approachable, enthusiastic, motivated, creative, well-presented, good personal hygiene, good communication skills.

4   If you decide to become a freelance stylist you must ensure you have public liability insurance in order to protect yourself and your clients.

5   The National Minimum Wage is a minimum amount per hour that most workers in the UK are entitled to be paid.

6   Your answer can include any five of the following:
   • your name and your employer's name
   • your job title or a brief job description
   • the date when your employment began
   • your pay rate and when you will be paid
   • your hours of work
   • your holiday entitlement
   • where you will be working (if you are based in more than one place it should say this along with your employer's address)
   • sick pay arrangements
   • notice periods
   • information about disciplinary and grievance procedures
   • any collective agreements that affect your employment terms or conditions
   • details of pensions and pension schemes
   • how long your employment is expected to continue (if you are not a permanent employee), or (if you are a fixed-term worker) the date your employment will end.

7   Five things you should find in your job description are:
   • your duties
   • your responsibilities
   • the most important contributions and outcomes needed from the job role
   • required qualifications of candidates
   • lines of reporting, e.g. specified line manager.

Unit G20 Ensure your own actions reduce risks to health and safety

Fact or fiction?

Page 57: Around 1,000 electric shock accidents at work are reported to the HSE each year. — *FACT.*

Page 59: All employees must take responsibility for their deeds and actions, and are liable if they do not. Insurance cover will be null and void if it is proven that legislation or establishment rules have been broken and an accident or damage has occurred. — *FACT.*

Page 63: Barbicide® is approved by the United States Environmental Protection Agency for use as a hospital disinfectant. — *FACT.*

Check your knowledge

1   HASAWA stands for Health and Safety at Work Act.

2   A hazard is:
   b) something with the potential to cause harm.

3   A salon policy is:
   a) having rules and regulations for staff to follow to ensure safe practice.

4   What is the purpose of the Manual Handlings Operations Regulations 1992?
   c) To make sure that the correct lifting, pulling, pushing, etc. postures are used

5   Under the Health and Safety at Work Act employees have responsibilities to take reasonable care of themselves and other people affected by their work and to cooperate with their employers to follow the law.

6   What does RIDDOR stand for?
   c) Reporting of Injuries, Diseases and Dangerous Occurrences

7   Under the Electricity at Work Regulations 1989 all equipment should be checked
   a) at regular intervals — every 6 moths to 1 year.

8   The purpose of sterilising tools and equipment is to:
   c) kill all organisms including bacteria, fungi and parasites.

9   How many people have to be employed at a workplace before a fire risk assessment has to be in writing?
   b) 5

10 What type of fire extinguisher can be used on electrical fires?
   c) Dry powder, vaporising liquid and carbon dioxide

11 What is meant by the term 'workplace policies'?
   b) A set of rules that the salon expects staff to follow to ensure safe working practices

12 What is meant by the term 'code of practice'?
   a) A document stating the behaviour, professional appearance etc. that is expected in the salon

13 What are the responsibilities of the employer under the Health and Safety at Work Act?
   b) Plan safety and security, provide information, update systems and ensure the safety of individuals and visitors

14 Which of these is the responsibility of the employee under the Health and Safety at Work Act?

d) To report flaws or gaps within the system or procedure when in use

15 What is the main purpose of health and safety legislation?

d) To ensure employers provide safe systems of work

16 What is a PAT test?

c) A portable appliance test

17 Which colour fire extinguishers could be used on an electrical fire?

c) Black, green or blue

Unit G4 Fulfil salon reception duties

Fact or fiction?

Page 83: You have to be a qualified hair stylist to work as a receptionist in a salon. — *FICTION.*

Page 90: You do not need to keep your client records secure. — *FICTION. If you do not keep your clients' personal details private, you are breaking important laws of confidentiality. If you keep clients' details on paper or computer, you must follow the requirements of the Data Protection Act 1998.*

Check your knowledge

1 A salon's procedure for maintaining client confidentiality will vary depending on individual salon rules, but generally you must not give out clients' contact details or private information to anyone else. You must not discuss any personal information your clients disclose to you.

2 What are the consequences of breaking client confidentiality?

d) The client could sue the salon

3 Methods of ensuring that cash and other payment types are kept safe and secure will vary according to individual salon procedures; however, generally cash and other payment types should be kept in a locked till/drawer which can only be accessed by designated salon staff. Large amounts of cash should not be kept on the premises as this can attract thieves.

4 Who you refer a payment discrepancy to if you cannot resolve the problem will vary according to individual salon procedures; however, generally either your salon owner/manager or the senior person in charge of reception should be informed.

5 How you check for invalid cash payments will vary according to individual salon procedures; however, generally cash can be checked for validity by ensuring you look for the watermark — every note has a watermark, which can be seen when the note is held up to the light. Look for the metallic strip which is woven into the paper — it should be unbroken. Test the feel of banknote paper — often a forged note is not printed on the same quality of paper and may have a thin, papery feel.

6 If a cheque payment is acceptable, certain checks and precautions need to be carried out. Always check that:

- the date is correct — day, month and year (this is especially important just after New Year!)
- the name of the salon is spelled correctly — the client could be offered a stamp with the full name pre-printed on it
- the amount is correct and that the amount in words and figures are the same
- the signature is included and that it matches the signature on the cheque guarantee card.

7 Effective communication is vital to the salon's business as every aspect of salon life revolves around communication. From client first impressions at reception to effective relationships between staff and owners/managers, to ensuring staff communicate regarding stock reordering — everything hinges on good, effective communication.

8 State how you would deal with a client who is angry.

a) Keep calm and do all you can to help

9 How do you ensure you give clients the correct change when they pay cash with a note?

a) Make sure you remember what note you were given by leaving it out of the till drawer until you have given the change to the client

10 Why it is important for the reception area to be clean and tidy at all times?

c) To ensure the first impression the client has is of a well-maintained, clean and tidy business

Unit G17 Give clients a positive impression of yourself and your organisation

Fact or fiction?

Page 109: Behaviour breeds behaviour so it is acceptable to get angry if a client gets angry with you. – *FICTION. You need to stay calm in order to deal with an angry client situation.*

Page 110: If a client didn't tell you her scalp was burning during a chemical process, you are not responsible for the scarring resulting from this problem. – *FICTION. You have a duty of care to the client and therefore you must take every step necessary to ensure she is kept safe. Ask your client if everything is all right throughout the service, so that if any problems occur your client will not be too afraid to say.*

Check your knowledge

1 Why is it important to follow your salon's rules for appearance and behaviour?
b) To ensure you maintain your salon's set standards

2 As a stylist, you should be:
a) pleasant, patient and helpful to everyone coming into the salon.

3 What is needed to help build a rapport with clients?
d) Trust and effective communication

4 If the salon is busy, who should greet a client arriving at reception?
d) Whoever is free greets the client first

5 To ensure a positive impression of the salon and yourself, the client should be made to feel:
a) valued and respected.

6 You must make sure you identify your clients' needs and also confirm their expectations so that:
a) you are positive you know their requirements.

7 If you find yourself in a situation you feel you cannot deal with yourself, you should:
b) ask the client to take a seat and find someone who can help you.

8 What are the three types of communication within the salon?
d) Verbal, non-verbal and written

9 There are many different ways to give clients the information they need about products or services offered in your salon. The methods can be:
d) talking to your client, printing information on the back of appointment cards, sending out information flyers or emails/text messages stating promotional offers, or posters in salon windows.

10 Sometimes it is not possible to carry out your client's wishes. This may be because:
c) either a) the client's hair is too fine, b) the client's hair is too damaged, or d) a contraindication is present.

Unit G18 Promote additional products or services to clients

Fact or fiction?

Page 121: It is only necessary to check with manufacturers once a year for updates. – *FICTION. Offers and promotions will change from week to week. You don't want to miss out so you need to make sure you are constantly checking what offers are happening with all the different wholesalers.*

Check your knowledge

1 The five Acts/legislation that need to be taken into account when selling additional products or services are:
• Consumer Protection Act 1987
• Cosmetic Products (Safety) Regulations 1996
• Trade Descriptions Act 1968 (and 1987)
• Sale of Goods Act 1979
• The Supply of Goods and Services Act 1982

2 Positive body language includes:
• smiling
• good eye contact
• good posture (no slouching)
• positive tone of voice
• nodding in agreement
• arms and legs unfolded/not crossed.

3 The benefits of promoting additional services and products in your salon are:
• increased salon profits
• good client relations
• ensuring the client has the correct tools and products to maintain the service at home.

4 If you were absent when a new product was introduced at work, you could find out about the product by discussing the product launch with other staff members, speaking with your salon manager to arrange formal training, and reading all the information on the product.

5 For this answer, you should choose one product or service that your salon provides and list five positive points about it that you could discuss with a client. For example: A deep conditioning treatment — helps to restore lost moisture, nourishes both the hair and scalp, is relaxing, stimulates the blood flow, helps to close the cuticle and even out porosity.

Unit G7 Advise and consult with clients

Fact or fiction?

Page 144: A head louse (pediculosis capitis) can live off the scalp for up to 72 hours. This means that once it has crawled off a client it can live in your brush or comb, or on your workstation, for three days. — *FACT*.

Check your knowledge

1 Salon rules for maintaining client confidentiality include:
- never give out a client's personal information
- treat anything you are told confidentially.

2 It is important to carry out a thorough hair and scalp analysis during your client consultation to:
b) assess the client's requirements and to check for any contraindications.

3 The seven skills required for a professional consultation are:
- technical knowledge about services
- observation skills
- clarification techniques
- advice
- product knowledge
- questioning techniques
- effective communication, including listening skills.

4 The questioning technique more commonly used to make conversation with a client:
b) Open questions

5 State how and when you carry out the following tests:
a) *Porosity* – how to carry out a porosity test is explained on page 141. It should be carried out before chemical processes.
b) *Elasticity* – how to carry out an elasticity test is explained on page 141. It should be carried out before chemical processes. Hair that is in good condition will stretch and then return to its original length due to its good internal strength (found in the cortex).

c) *Skin* – how to carry out a skin test is explained on page 141. It should be carried out 24–48 hours before a colouring process.
d) *Test cutting* – how to carry out a test cutting is explained on pages 142–43. It should be carried out before colouring.
e) *Incompatibility test* – how to carry out an incompatibility test is explained on page 142. It should be carried out if the colouring history of the hair is doubtful before colour or perming.
f) *Pre-perm test curl* – how to carry out a pre-perm test curl is explained on page 143. It should be carried out before perming.
g) *Strand test* – how to carry out a strand test is explained on page 142. It should be carried out during the colouring process.
h) *Development test curl* – how to carry out a development test curl is explained on page 143. It should be carried out during the perming process.

6 A contraindication is any reason that prevents a service from taking place, such as the presence of a disease, hair disorder or infestation of the scalp or infection of the skin.

7 Psoriasis is not contagious.

8 The cause of impetigo is bacteria.

9 Pediculosis capitis is an infestation of head lice.

10 The cause of folliculitis is bacteria entering the follicle.

Unit G8 Develop and maintain your effectiveness at work

Fact or fiction?

Page 158: As a stylist you have to carry out 30 hours' CPD every year. — *FICTION. If you are an assessor or verifier, CPD is compulsory. If you are a stylist, it is highly beneficial to keep up to date with new products, techniques and styles and is great for inspiration and confidence-building.*

Page 166: You should never attempt to do a job that you have not been trained to do. — *FACT. This could result in serious consequences and your salon's insurance will be null and void.*

Check your knowledge

1   You can get information about your job, responsibilities and the standards expected of you from your job description, contract of employment and your boss/salon manager.

2   Who would you ask for information on your salon's appeal and grievance procedures?
    a) Salon owner

3   You identify your own strengths and weaknesses through performance appraisals, reviews and reports.

4   What does CPD mean?
    c) Continuing Professional Development

5   Who is responsible for developing the National Occupational Standards for Hairdressing?
    a) A government-approved organisation called HABIA

6   You need to be aware of current and new trends and developments in hairdressing to enable you to offer the best and most current services to your clients.

7   If you had a difficulty with a colleague in the salon, who would you report it to?
    c) Your salon owner/manager

8   The eleven qualities of a good team are:
    • clear objectives and a sense of direction
    • good balance of planning and action
    • the right number of people
    • good communication
    • flexibility and tolerance
    • clear job roles
    • a sense of humour
    • the right mix of skills
    • good listening skills and exchange of ideas
    • enthusiastic, committed team members
    • a fair but decisive leader.

9   The five skills needed for effective communication are:
    • listening skills
    • positive body language
    • clear written skills
    • good eye contact
    • verbal skills.

10 It is important to be a good team member in the salon because everybody within the salon has a job to do, and if everyone does their job well the salon will function effectively and harmoniously.

Unit GH8 Shampoo, condition and treat the hair and scalp

Fact or fiction?

Page 179: Expensive conditioners can permanently repair split ends and damaged hair. — *FICTION. Once hair is damaged, you can only temporarily repair it with conditioners. The only way you can permanently repair it is to cut the damaged hair off!*

Check your knowledge

1   Why are we recommended to wear gloves during shampooing?
    b) To avoid the risk of dermatitis.

2   The health and safety legislation which covers the use of electrical equipment is the Electricity at Work Regulations 1989.

3   It is important to carry out a thorough consultation before shampooing in order to analyse the hair and scalp, choose the correct shampooing, conditioning and scalp service products, and to check for any contraindications.

4   The health and safety legislation that deals with the handling, storage and disposal of hairdressing products is the Control of Substances Hazardous to Health (COSHH) Regulations 2003.

5   It is important to have a good knowledge of the shampooing and conditioning products used in the salon in order to ensure that you are fully aware of the product range available to use for specific hair and scalp conditions.

6   The shampoo to use before a perm is a soapless-based shampoo with no additives, since these may cause a barrier between the perm lotion and the hair and stop the perm working properly.

7   A surface conditioner smooths and coats the cuticle scales.

8   A penetrating conditioner smooths and coats the cuticle scales and helps to temporarily rebuild bonds within the cortex, thereby helping to improve the hair's strength and elasticity.

9   Which do you apply first to remove a hot oil service from the hair?
    b) Neat shampoo — use neat shampoo first to help emulsify the oil before adding water

10 What types of heat are ideally used during conditioning treatments?
   a) Moist heat from hot towels or a steamer

Unit GH9 Change hair colour

Fact or fiction?

Page 201: PPE (personal protective equipment) only refers to towels and gowns used on the client. – *FICTION. PPE takes into account all protective equipment used to protect both the client and the stylist.*

Page 206: You cannot carry out a highlighting/lowlighting service on hair that is below shoulder length. – *FICTION. The cap method would be unsuitable, but mesh or foils could be used.*

Page 222: High lift tint can lighten other tints of a base 8 and below. – *FICTION. Tint will not lift tint.*

Check your knowledge

1 The purpose of a skin test is to determine:
   b) whether the client is allergic to a colouring product.
2 Barrier cream is used to:
   c) prevent the tint from coming into contact with the skin and staining.
3 Quantities of colour and developer/peroxide should be mixed accurately:
   b) to ensure the target colour is achieved.
4 The highest strength of peroxide that is used in hairdressing is:
   a) 40 volume.
5 A colour that sits on the cuticle and can slightly diffuse into the cortex is known as:
   d) semi-permanent colour.
6 What two colours are mixed on the colour wheel to obtain violet?
   c) Blue and red
7 Using the ICC system, the second number of a colour after the point or slash is:
   d) the secondary tone.
8 Opposites on the colour wheel will:
   b) neutralise one another.
9 Quasi-permanent colours have the ability to:
   c) add depth and tone.
10 The best type of added heat to use during a bleaching service is:
   a) a steamer.

11 An incompatibility test is to determine whether:
   d) there are any metallic salts present in the hair.
12 A skin test should be carried out:
   b) 24–48 hours prior to the service.
13 Application of tint to virgin hair should begin at:
   c) the mid-lengths, ends then roots.
14 What action should you take if the hair is too yellow?
   a) Reapply the bleach or use a violet toner
15 How many levels of lift can be achieved with bleach?
   d) 7
16 Products need to be mixed in a well-ventilated room because:
   c) this will prevent breathing problems.
17 What are the three primary colours on the colour wheel?
   c) Red, yellow, blue
18 What colour should be used to neutralise unwanted yellow tones in the hair?
   a) violet
19 What is meant by the 'depth' of a colour?
   b) How light or dark the colour is
20 It is important to use an anti-oxy conditioner after a colouring service in order to:
   a) prevent creeping oxidation and return the hair to its natural pH balance.

Unit GH10 Style and finish hair

Fact or fiction?

Page 245: If a client sits with her legs crossed for the hairdressing service, you could end up with a lopsided result. – *FACT. The client's posture will mean that she has one shoulder higher than the other. You may compensate for this which would result in an uneven result.*

Page 251: If you do not identify infestations before you shampoo, then you are obliged to complete the service. – *FACT.*

Check your knowledge

1 What is the best way to gown your client for a blow drying process?
   d) Gown, towel and disposable plastic cape
2 The styling product gel is suitable for which hair type?
   c) Short textured styles

3   A Denman brush is used to:
    b) give a smooth finish, for example to a 'bob' style.

4   The purpose of glosses and serums on the hair is to:
    a) reduce frizz and add shine.

5   A manufacturer's data sheet is:
    b) information on the ingredients, handling and storage
    of a product.

6   If you discover an infestation when halfway through a
    service, you should:
    c) continue with the service and give the client advice
    on whether she should visit her GP.

7   When blow-drying the hair the airflow of the hairdryer
    should go:
    a) from root to point.

8   When blow-drying in the nape area you should position
    the client:
    c) with head tilted forward so you can work freely in
    this area.

9   When blow-dried hair comes into contact with
    atmospheric moisture it will:
    c) start to drop and return to its natural state.

10 Styling products coat the hair with:
    b) plasticisers.

11 Hair in its natural state is called:
    d) alpha keratin.

12 Hair is hygroscopic. This means that it has the ability to:
    c) absorb moisture.

13 Styling products will protect the hair against:
    a) heat and moisture.

14 Heated styling equipment should be checked by a
    qualified electrician every:
    c) 6 months.

15 The bonds that are broken down during a blow-drying
    process are:
    d) the hydrogen bonds.

16 What effect will humidity have on the hair structure?
    c) It will break down the hydrogen bonds, causing the
    style to collapse

17 How will overuse of heat affect the hair and scalp?
    b) Hair condition will deteriorate; severe damage may
    include yellowing of the hair, split ends or breakage,
    and burns to the scalp

Unit GH11 Set and dress hair

Fact or fiction?

Page 272: If your client sits with crossed legs, this may
affect the dressing-out process and produce an unbalanced
end result. – *FACT. If your client sits with crossed legs,
one shoulder could be 'thrown up' slightly higher than the
other, and this could cause an uneven, unbalanced result.*

Page 274: All hairdressing equipment can be sterilised
using Barbicide®. – *FICTION. There is a wide range of
sterilising methods that should be used for different tools
and equipment. For example, electrical equipment should
not be immersed in a liquid; a sterilising wipe or spray
should be used.*

Page 279: It is up to the client to inform you of any critical
influencing factors. – *FICTION. These should be identified
during the consultation and discussed throughout the
hairdressing service.*

Page 279: Hair should only be dry set when it is clean. –
*FICTION. If hair is freshly washed, it can sometimes be too
soft and fly-away to work with and will not hold as well.
However, you can't work with very dirty, oily hair, so ask the
client to shampoo her hair one to two days before coming
into the salon.*

Page 285: You can rough-dry the hair and then use heated
styling equipment to add curl, volume and movement. –
*FICTION. This shouldn't be done and won't demonstrate
good practice. The set will not last very long if the hair's
hydrogen bonds aren't broken (during shampooing) then re-
formed around the new shape when the hair is dry.*

Check your knowledge

1   Coloured mousses and setting lotions should be
    applied to:
    c) towel-dried hair.

2   The purpose of a hair net used in setting the hair is to:
    a) prevent any small hairs escaping from the rollers.

3   What effect does a 'dry' setting process have on the
    hair's structure?
    d) It will 'bake' the hair into its new shape

4   When you carry out a directional set, you will place the
    rollers:
    b) in the direction you want the hair to be dressed.

5   A flat barrel pin curl will produce:
    a) an open middle, with a curl that is even from roots
    to points.

6   Pin curling techniques are used in setting:
    d) for shorter hair that may not wind around a roller easily.

7   The purpose of hot brushes is to:
    b) produce a soft, casual look.

8   The angle at which the hair is held during setting will determine:
    c) the amount of root lift created.

9   'Baggy' ends are created by:
    b) the section of hair taken being too large.

10 Good, even tension will:
    d) distribute the hair evenly around the roller, ensuring a uniform curl result.

11 Why is it important to give aftercare to the client after the service?
    b) To ensure the client understands how to maintain the look at home

12 Why is it important to allow the hair to cool before removing rollers?
    c) To allow the curl to set

Unit GH12 Cut hair using basic techniques

Fact or fiction?

Page 304: Washing tools and equipment will ensure you won't pass on any infections. – *FICTION. Equipment needs to be properly sterilised in order to kill the micro-organisms responsible for infection.*

Page 309: Clippers can be used on wet and dry hair. – *FICTION. Clippers are an electrical piece of equipment and should not be used on wet hair. Furthermore, you will not achieve an accurate cutting line on wet hair.*

Check your knowledge

1   Thinning scissors are also known as:
    b) serrated scissors.

2   It is important to sterilise equipment after every client to:
    c) minimise the risk of cross-infection and infestation.

3   'Sharps' is the term given to:
    d) the blades in safety razors.

4   When the hair's 'texture' is referred to, this means:
    d) whether a single strand of hair is fine, medium or thick in diameter.

5   Critical influencing factor means:
    a) any factor that you have to take into account when adapting your haircut.

6   A freehand cutting technique involves:
    b) not using tension on the hair.

7   The purpose of club cutting the hair is to:
    b) make the ends of the hair blunt and level.

8   The scissor-over-comb technique is used when:
    c) you need to get in close to the head, where the hair is too short to pick up.

9   Clippers are sterilised using:
    d) sterilising wipes and sprays.

10 During a one-length cut the head is tilted forward to prevent:
    a) unwanted graduation.

11 It is important to cross-check your haircut because:
    b) you can check you have achieved a balanced shape.

12 Tension is important when cutting hair because:
    c) it ensures you achieve a balanced result.

13 Using a scissor-over-comb technique will allow you to:
    d) cut the hair shorter in the nape of the neck.

14 If you cut the hair using a 90-degree angle all over the head you will achieve a:
    b) uniform layer.

15 A hair growth pattern is:
    c) the movement of the hair at the root area.

16 A short graduated haircut is cut at a:
    a) 45-degree angle

Unit GH13 Plait and twist hair

Fact or fiction?

Page 326: Cornrow plaiting originated in India. – *FICTION. Cornrow plaiting originated in Africa and has been passed down through generations of families, thereby creating intricate plaiting designs.*

Page 331: Cornrow plaiting is also known as cane row. – *FACT. Cornrow is sometimes referred to as cane row.*

Check your knowledge

1   Traction alopecia is hair thinning or hair loss due to excessive tension on the hair follicle. This can be the result of wearing the hair in tight plaits or twists.

2   Why is it important to minimise the risk of cross-infection and cross-infestation when plaiting and twisting hair?
    b) To ensure that you do not pass on any infections or infestations to clients and colleagues

499

3 What are the potential consequences of excessive tension on the hair when plaiting and twisting?

   a) The client may lose hair through a condition called traction alopecia

4 Section hair accurately when plaiting and twisting hair to ensure you work neatly and accurately and produce precise plaits and twists.

5 Students can choose any three of the following methods of securing plaits and twists:

   • covered bands
   • silicone bands
   • grips
   • tiny jaw clips
   • pipe cleaners.

6 It is important to use products economically when plaiting and twisting hair:

   • so that you do not overload the hair and make it look greasy
   • so that you are being cost-effective with your products.

7 It is important to recommend homecare advice to your client after plaiting or twisting services because if your client goes home without knowing how to care for her plaits or twists they are unlikely to last for the time generally expected.

8 It is important to give good advice to your client regarding removing the plaits or twists. If your client is unaware of the correct procedure and rips out the bands securing the plaits and tries to pull the plait out from the root, it will not only cause knotting but will also be painful and damage the hair.

9 A client's lifestyle can influence the choice of style when plaiting and twisting hair. If the client is an active sportswoman, a style which keeps the hair away from the face and which needs little maintenance (cornrows) may suit her more than twists, which may come loose/out as she is competing in a sports event. However, some plaiting or twisting styles which result in the hair being tightly secured to the scalp may not be considered suitable by certain employers.

10 Everyone loses between 80 and 100 hairs a day, and if these hairs are not able to fall out because they are stuck in a plait or twist, then you will see them all fall out once the plait or twist is removed.

Unit GH14 Perm and neutralise hair

Fact or fiction?

Page 343: You can temporarily perm hair. — *FICTION. Once the disulphide bonds are chemically changed, this is a permanent process.*

Page 350: It is important to ask your client questions during the consultation before perming and to record the client's responses to these questions. — *FACT. If, in the unfortunate event you are sued by a client and you have evidence of your client's responses to the questions asked, this can be seen as a significant benefit during legal proceedings.*

Check your knowledge

1 The personal protective equipment you should wear during the perming and neutralising processes are gloves and an apron.

2 The perming information that should be recorded on your client's record is:

   • perm lotion used
   • winding technique
   • whether pre-perm lotion was used
   • how long it took to process
   • end curl result
   • price charged.

3 Why is it important to keep your work area tidy during the perming and neutralising processes?

   c) For health and safety reasons and to avoid accidents

4 Why is it important to minimise wastage of perming and neutralising products?

   a) To be cost-effective and keep salon profits up

5 Name two perming tests that should be carried out before perming.

   b) Pre-perm test curl and elasticity test

6 Development test curl is a perming test carried out during the perming process.

7 Five influencing factors for perming are:

   • hair condition
   • hair texture
   • hair length
   • hair density
   • direction and degree of movement/curl required.

8 The three different types of perm lotion are acid, alkaline and exothermic.

9   Barrier cream and cotton wool are used to protect the client's hairline during perming.

10 Nine-section, directional and brickwork are the three perm winds you need to perfect for this qualification.

11 You should always check water temperature and flow during rinsing of perm lotion and neutraliser to ensure the temperature is appropriate for your client and the flow of water is not too fierce.

12 Types of heat used to help the perm process are body heat and heat from processors/climazones.

13 It is important to use personal protective equipment in order to prevent dermatitis and avoid clothes being ruined.

14 Accurate timing is important during the perming and neutralising procedures to avoid under- or over-processing the perm.

15 In order to know how long the perm lotion should be processed for, check the manufacturer's instructions.

16 It is important to section accurately when winding a perm in order to ensure accurate placing of rods and that no hair is missed, which will ruin the finished result.

17 Perm rod rubbers positioned too tightly will put too much pressure on the root area, which will fracture the hair and eventually cause hair breakage.

18 To resolve the problem of a frizzy perm result, carry out restructurant conditioning treatment and cut if possible.

19 The three stages of the perming process are softening, moulding and fixing. A description of each stage is given on page 343.

20 To be commercially competent, you are allowed 45 minutes for winding a perm on assessment.

Unit GH15 Attach hair to enhance a style

Fact or fiction?

Page 372: You are required by law to take a non-refundable deposit from the client for a hair extension service. — FICTION. *This is a salon policy, not a requirement of law. It makes good business sense to ask for a deposit (which most clients are happy to pay and will expect to pay), as the hair needs to be matched to the client's specific hair colour and may not be able to be used again.*

Page 373: The client is required to pay for the full service on the initial consultation. — FICTION. *The client need only pay for the hair that is ordered for her service.*

Check your knowledge

1   By maintaining the correct posture when applying extensions, you:
    b) prevent backache and incorrect positioning of the extensions.

2   To prevent the hair from becoming tangled, you must brush or comb the hair from:
    c) point to root.

3   The hair is sometimes pre-cut before added hair is applied:
    d) to remove any hard blunt, lines from the hair.

4   To avoid incorrect application of added hair:
    a) ensure the correct positioning and tension when applying the added hair.

5   A contraindication to a service for applying added hair would be:
    b) breakage at the root area.

6   'Pre-consultation' is a consultation carried out before the actual service, usually when the client comes in to book the appointment.

7   When positioning your client for the service, she should have feet flat on the floor with the base of the back touching the back of the chair.

8   Regular swimming would dry hair extensions out and cause them to knot and tangle.

9   Traction alopecia is hair loss due to excessive tension at the root area.

10 To carry out a pull test, the hair is gently pulled at the root (follicle) to see whether it is strong enough to take the weight of the hair extensions.

Create an image based on a theme within the hair and beauty sector

Check your knowledge

1   What is the purpose of a mood board?
    a) To record the development of your initial idea through to your final concept

2   What is meant by the term 'media images'?
    a) Images from the internet, books, cinema, magazines etc.

3   What is the recommended length of time for your presentation?
    b) Ten minutes

4 What should you use to protect your client from coloured hairsprays?
a) A chemical gown, a towel and a face shield

5 Why is feedback important?
b) To identify strengths and weaknesses

Unit GB2 Change men's hair colour

Fact or fiction?

Page 413: A skin test should be carried out before every colouring service. — *FACT. This is a legal requirement to ensure that your client is not allergic to any colouring products. The only exception is coloured mousse.*

Page 415: A client who has had a root retouch in the past and experienced a reaction to the barrier cream should be advised not to have any further colouring services. — *FICTION. You can use petroleum jelly (Vaseline) as this doesn't contain any added colours or perfumes.*

Page 418: A porosity test is only carried out if the hair looks in bad condition. — *FICTION. A porosity test should be carried out before every colouring service to determine if the cuticle is in good or bad condition as this will affect the product choice, application and development of the colouring product.*

Page 419: A client may have 'hot' and 'cold' spots on his head that will affect the development of the colour. — *FACT. Heat will speed up the development of the colour.*

Check your knowledge

1 White hair is taken into account during a consultation because it affects:
a) product choice and the application techniques used.

2 When a tint is mixed up it will begin to:
d) oxidise.

3 Block colouring is a technique where the hair is:
b) sectioned into two or more sections and coloured.

4 The Electricity at Work Regulations are designed to ensure:
c) that equipment is fit and safe for use and all staff are trained in using the equipment.

5 What is a 'hypersensitivity' test also known as?
d) Patch test

6 Why should powder lighteners be mixed in a well-ventilated room?
b) To prevent breathing problems

7 What tests are carried out before a colouring process?
c) Elasticity test, porosity test, skin test

8 What are the natural colour pigments contained in the hair called?
c) Eumelanin and pheomelanin

9 What part of the hair is affected by permanent colouring products?
c) Cortex

10 How many levels of lift can be achieved when using 20 volume (6 per cent) peroxide?
a) 0–1

Unit GB3 Cut hair using basic barbering techniques

Fact or fiction?

Page 437: Good posture is essential to portray a professional appearance and reduce the risk of injury or unnecessary fatigue. — *FACT. If you do not have good posture, you will strain muscles and may cause yourself injury.*

Page 440: A neck brush and water spray cannot be sterilised, only washed in warm soapy water. — *FICTION. Both of these pieces of equipment can be sterilised using Barbicide® solution.*

Check your knowledge

1 Clippers should be used on:
b) dry hair.

2 One of the benefits of cutting the hair wet is that:
d) greater precision can be achieved.

3 The typical pattern of male baldness is:
c) receding at the temples and crown.

4 A uniform layer cut is where the hair is:
a) held at 90 degrees all over the head.

5 How many different sizes of clipper grades are available?
c) 8

Unit GB4 Cut facial hair to shape using basic techniques

Fact or fiction?

Page 462: Pogonophobia is a fear of beards. — *FACT. 'Phobia' means 'fear of', and 'pogono' is the Greek for 'beard'!*

Page 465: Beards and moustaches are often used to hide facial features. — *FACT. Sometimes clients use beards and moustaches to distract from facial features.*

Page 466: Traditionally having a beard is a sign of masculinity. — *FACT. Through the ages, many males have believed growing and maintaining a beard shows masculinity.*

Check your knowledge

1 What is the correct gowning procedure for a beard and moustache trim?
   b) Gown, towel and either a strip of cotton wool or neck tissue to prevent cuttings dropping down onto clothes

2 Sharps should be disposed of in a sharps bin which is collected by the local council.

3 What are your responsibilities under the current Electricity at Work Regulations?
   a) All electrical equipment you use should have been tested at least once or twice a year for safety.

4 It is important to protect everyone working and visiting the salon from the risk of infections and infestations because these could cause harm to you, colleagues or clients

5 It is important to cut to the natural facial hairline so that the client can maintain the shape at home; if this is not done, the shape may grow out quickly and look untidy.

6 What is the average rate of hair growth?
   d) 1.25 cm per month

7 Methods of sterilisation used in barber shops are:
   • Barbicide® solutions
   • sterilising clipper spray
   • UV cabinet
   • sterilising wipes.

8 The term 'factor' means anything that influences the service. These must be assessed before the start of the beard or moustache trim.

9 The four cutting techniques which can be used when cutting facial hair are:
   • scissor-over-comb
   • clippers with attachment (grade)
   • clipper-over-comb
   • freehand.

10 Aftercare advice to give to your client: it is useful to advise your client on any maintenance he may need to do at home before his next appointment with you, the best way to carry this out and the most appropriate tools to use.

Unit GB5 Dry and finish men's hair

Fact or fiction?

Page 483: Only sprays will coat the hair with a protective barrier to prevent the effects of atmospheric moisture. — *FICTION. All styling and finishing products will coat the hair with a protective barrier to help against the effects of atmospheric moisture; refer to GH11 to refresh your memory.*

Check your knowledge

1 What is the best way to minimise cross-infection when working in the salon?
   b) Sterilise tools and equipment after every client.

2 A heat protector product is designed to:
   c) coat the hair with a slight film to prevent the hair from becoming over-dry.

3 An infestation is caused by:
   a) parasites.

4 By allowing the hair to cool you will:
   d) fix the hair in its new shape.

5 Styling and finishing products coat the hair with:
   b) Plasticisers

Index

Index

Index

H

Index